MANAGERIAL EPIDEMIOLOGY
Practice, Methods, and Concepts

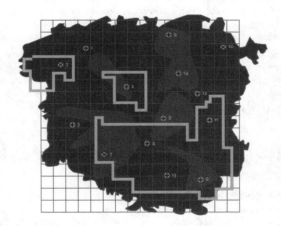

G.E. Alan Dever, PhD, MT, MD (Hon.)

Associate Vice President, Health Policy
Director, Center for Organ Donation, Education, and Health Policy
Grassmann Chair of Rural Medicine
Professor, Department of Community Medicine
Mercer University School of Medicine

JONES AND BARTLETT PUBLISHERS
Sudbury, Massachusetts
BOSTON   TORONTO   LONDON   SINGAPORE

World Headquarters
Jones and Bartlett Publishers
40 Tall Pine Drive
Sudbury, MA 01776
978-443-5000
info@jbpub.com
www.jbpub.com

Jones and Bartlett Publishers Canada
2406 Nikanna Road
Mississauga, ON L5C 2W6
CANADA

Jones and Bartlett Publishers International
Barb House, Barb Mews
London W6 7PA
UK

Jones and Bartlett's books and products are available through most bookstores and online booksellers. To contact Jones and Bartlett Publishers directly, call 800-832-0034, fax 978-443-8000, or visit our website www.jbpub.com.

Substantial discounts on bulk quantities of Jones and Bartlett's publications are available to corporations, professional associations, and other qualified organizations. For details and specific discount information, contact the special sales department at Jones and Bartlett via the above contact information or send an email to *specialsales@jbpub.com*.

Copyright © 2006 by Jones and Bartlett Publishers, Inc.

Library of Congress Cataloging-in-Publication Data
Dever, G. E. Alan.
  Managerial epidemiology : practice, methods, and concepts / G.E. Alan Dever.
     p. ; cm.
  Includes index.
  ISBN 0-7637-3165-X (hardcover)
  1. Health services administration. 2. Epidemiology.
  [DNLM: 1. Delivery of Health Care--organization & administration. 2. Epidemiology--organization & administration. WA 105 D285m 2005] I. Title.
  RA971.D48 2005
  362.1'068--dc22

                              2004022321

Production Credits
Acquisitions Editor: Michael Brown
Production Director: Amy Rose
Editorial Assistant: Kylah Goodfellow McNeill
Production Assistant: Kate Hennessy
Associate Marketing Manager: Marissa Hederson
V.P of Manufacturing and Inventory Coordinator: Therese Connell
Composition: Northeast Compositors, Inc.
Cover Design: Kristin E. Ohlin
Printing and Binding: Malloy Incorporated
Cover Printing: Malloy Incorporated

Printed in the United States of America
09 08 07 06 05   10 9 8 7 6 5 4 3 2 1

Contents

Preface

Managerial Epidemiology: Practice, Methods, and Concepts is a book that emphasizes the basic principles of epidemiology applied to the management and utilization of health services. In the most basic sense, the book brings a perspective to the field of epidemiology that provides the standard and traditional applications to public health and managerial problems. However, to set the book apart from the traditional approach to epidemiological analysis, *Managerial Epidemiology* incorporates a philosophy which encompasses methods necessary to perform managerial and public health analysis from a broad-based holistic point of view. Specifically, Chapter 1 emphasizes the role of preventive medicine as a major contributor to understanding the management and utilization of health services from a public health perspective. Chapter 2 presents a review of health policy issues and how such policy must be utilized to drive the management of services focusing on the very basic tenets of a broad-based holistic epidemiological model. The classic difference between clinical-based medicine and population-based health (medicine) is highlighted in Chapter 3 with an emphasis on how population-based health must be considered as a practical approach to understanding the effective and efficient delivery of services from a population—not clinical—perspective.

Chapter 4 outlines the basic measurement tools utilized in epidemiological investigation and analysis. Managers and public health investigators must enhance their basic measurement skills for monitoring and evaluating progress in the management of programs. In Chapter 5, *Identifying Problems, Determining Priorities*, decision-makers are presented with some basic methods to quickly and simply identify problems and determine priorities. Measures such as the standardized mortality ratio (SMR), proportionate mortality ratio (PMR), years of life lost (YLL), and risk factor methods are summarized. To effectively describe the epidemiology of disease and health services utilization, Chapters 6 and 7 outline the methods for portraying characteristics by person, place, and time. These descriptive epidemiological parameters are essential and basic to the study of epidemiology. No general analysis and no analysis of management issues can be complete without having a strong knowledge and basic understanding of demographic trends and the specific tools by which to analyze such trends. Thus, Chapter 8, *Demographics: Epidemiological Tools*, provides the necessary components for analyzing population components, distribution, trends, and forecasts.

Managerial Epidemiology offers four unique chapters to the study of epidemiology, generally, and to the management of health services, specifically. Notably, chapters on evidence-based health services management, small area analysis, marketing, and geographical information systems (GIS) are topics usually not seen in epidemiological textbooks. The intent of *Managerial Epidemiology* is to offer these concepts with the understanding that the management of health services cannot be comprehensive without being cognizant of the importance of such topics to health planning, evaluation, and policy components of managerial epidemiology. The chapters outline very specific and practical steps with concrete examples to follow for applying to managerial problems. These four chapters form a basic and comprehensive cornerstone to the expansion of epidemiological principles to nontraditional problems as conceived by epidemiologists. Of particular significance is Chapter 13, the marketing chapter. Finally, a chapter on health services utilization outlines the factors and variables that contribute to the variation in use of such services.

As students of epidemiology progress through this text, they will become skilled and trained in a new epidemiology that enhances tradition. Furthermore, this new epidemiology recognizes that epidemiologists must expand their horizons and apply their methods in a most practical and skillful manner so as to meet the needs of managers, researchers, planners, evaluators, and policymakers in this new century. The intent in writing *Managerial Epidemiology* was to expand and improve upon the existing books of epidemiology. However, the major driving focus was the need to outline basic, practical, understandable methods for application in the applied world of business, marketing, and epidemiology.

Acknowledgments

This book has years of relationships contained between its covers. As an author I would have been unable to write without the benefit of many creative and long-standing friends who provided both insight and wisdom to the many concepts and ideas that are presented in this, my most recent book, *Managerial Epidemiology: Practice, Methods, and Concepts.* I thank all of these individuals who have touched my life and have given me the energy and excitement to consider my voyage in the "book world." Their ideas, comments, and constructive evaluations have been of great value to produce a more thorough and comprehensive view of epidemiology from a managerial perspective.

I wish to thank my colleagues and professional acquaintances for all their support in this endeavor. In particular, I thank Douglas Skelton, MD, Director of Public Health, Central Savannah Region, for always supporting my ideas and giving me the opportunity to participate. A never endless thank you to Ms. Bunnie Stamps, my research clerk, who reviewed chapters, tracked down graphics, sought permissions and reviews, and proofread chapters with a well-trained eye. If one ever needs assistance with accuracy, focus on detail, and completion of any given task—ask Ms. Bunnie. Thank you Diana Wilson, Colette Caldwell, and Leah Smith for performing various activities related to tracking down research articles, typing some critical chapters, and producing graphics. Thank you for your support. Thanks to Mercer University School of Medicine. Thank you, Dr. Sanjay Reddy, for his major contribution to the GIS chapter.

As most authors know, when you agree to pursue the challenge of writing a book, many of your friends and relatives realize that you become part of the lost generation for a significant period of time. My wife Georgie, my friend, has always understood and her understanding has given me the support and encouragement I needed to complete this endeavor. I am, without question, one of the most fortunate men to have such a true companion for life. Her humor, compassion, and zest for life enable me to do this. Thank you, Georgie. I am so fortunate to have such a wonderful family who always understands what Dad is working on. To my daughter Tammy and my son Jamie and his wife Micky, thank you. I am blessed with six wonderful grandchildren—Andrew, Anna, Jennie, Sophie, Natalie, and Cealie—all of whom I am sure don't understand why they do not see me at every event, but curiously I know they wonder. A half dozen beautiful treasures wrapped by my love for all of them—who could ever imagine such a gift. Thank you, all of my family.

Thanks to Mike Brown who saw the future by prompting me to create a new and fresh book on the management aspects of epidemiology. The staff at Jones and Bartlett are absolutely delightful people who are masters in the business of customer and author satisfaction. It was their myriad skills and expectations wrapped in laughter and persuasiveness that kept the project on schedule. They exuded magic and miracles. Thank you Kate Hennessy and Kylah McNeill, two wonderful and talented individuals.

1

Epidemiological Preventive Care: Health Services Management

Introduction

As stated by David Satcher in January 2000, "We have witnessed a great deal of progress in public health and medicine [and health services management] since"[1] the 1979 publication of *Healthy People: The Surgeon General's Report on Health Promotion and Disease Prevention*.[2] This report was followed by the 1990 *Healthy People 2000* and subsequent to 1990 the report we are now offered *Healthy People 2010*, which represents the third effort to document ten-year health objectives for the nation by the U.S. Department of Health and Human Services.[3]

The basic recurring theme over the decades has been health promotion and disease prevention. Public health officials and communities fostering healthy environments have embraced this with zeal but have met with frustration as a result of government funding priorities and industry reluctance to adapt prevention strategies due to reimbursement issues and unclear messages that convey contradictory approaches to adopting a healthy lifestyle. Clearly, as the level of evidence mounts for the practice of prevention and as the science of behavioral change is more understood, we will see some rocketing changes in the adoption of prevention principles and practices.[4]

Certainly, if the United States is to improve the health of its citizens, it must press these priorities in health care and continue to put greater emphasis on the prevention of disease and the promotion of health. All providers have to join in this effort by broadening their comprehension of their patients' health problems and by extending their activities into communities or target populations.

Healthy People 2010

Healthy People 2010 reflects the evidence-based advances that have evolved since the initial 1979 report in areas such as preventive medicine, disease surveillance, vaccine and therapy development, and information technology. All these are critical to the improvement of health in communities, but they are certainly of major importance to the management of health care services. The current 2010 report also is cognizant of the changing demographics in the United States, the shifts in the management of our health care system, and the impact of "thinking globally" on the health status of our nation and our communities. It is these characteristics concerning the improvement of health status that will be reviewed in the context of managing health services, utilizing some basic epidemiological principles and methods applied to the management of health care services.

The concepts of disease prevention and health promotion not only encompass the tenets expressed in *Healthy People 2010*, but also are of critical importance to the application of health services management.

The mere statement of goals and objectives in the 2010 report cannot by itself improve the health status of any given geographical area or population group. Generally, the improvement process must embrace a systematic process of four elements:

- Goals
- Objectives
- Determinants of health
- Health status[5]

Whether this systematic approach is used to improve health on a national level, as outlined in *Healthy People 2010*, or to organize community action on a particular health issue, such as promoting smoking cessation, the components remain the same. The **goals** provide a general focus and direction. The goals, in turn, serve as a guide to develop a set of **objectives** that will actually measure progress within a specified amount of time. The objectives focus on the **determinants of health**, which encompass the combined effects of individual and community lifestyle; history (biology); environments as they relate to the policies; and interventions used to promote health, prevent disease, and ensure access to quality health care. The ultimate measure of success in any health improvement effort is the **health status** of the target population.

Healthy People 2010 is built on this systematic approach to health improvement.[6]

The disease prevention and health promotion framework adopted in this book suggests a need for a broader consideration of a patient who presents with health problems. Rogers and colleagues[7] in their recent monograph on *Living and Dying in the USA* provide evidence-based support for continuing to embrace a broader policy on the determinants of health and, as a consequence, recognize that the management of health services must in fact concern itself with a broader health policy.

Furthermore, health care providers need to extend their services into the community in an effort to reach not only the patients who initiate contact but also all others who might be at risk from their environment, lifestyle, or heredity (biology). Providers should be committed to the health of the community as a whole and of its individual members and to involve them in programs before they become sick.[8]

The objectives for the nation 2000 and 2010 reports were established to provide a road map for health and benchmarks to measure and monitor performance. There has been criticism of this approach, stating that the program is unwieldy, lacks balance in number of objectives by the identified focus areas, is inconsistent in the issues being addressed by each objective, and, because the document identifies all sectors of the nation, the role of the federal government is naturally absent.[9] In response to these concerns, the objectives for 2010 orient our thoughts toward a broad health policy that can be utilized by communities and health service workers who establish programs to monitor progress toward the national objectives and goals. Several criteria were used to develop the objectives for the nation in 2000 and 2010. Table 1-1 shows the basic comparison of the criteria used for each decade's health objectives for the nation. There are several similarities, notably the objectives must be measurable, have continuity, be understood by the public, and be compatible with or comparable to previous measures established. However, there are important differences. The two most significant are those objectives that must be supported by sound *scientific evidence* (the cornerstone of epidemiology and its application to health service management) and the objectives must be *prevention oriented* and should address health improvements that can be achieved through population-based health programs and health services management interventions.

The logical extension of these two significant additions to the criteria is that the determinants of health must be driven by sound epidemiological principles that embrace the broad concepts of health policy, and that the health services managers must focus beyond the individuals in clinics and hospitals and expand their efforts to include population-based programs or focus on specific populations in communities.

TABLE 1-1 Comparison of Criteria for Developing *Healthy People* Objectives 2000 and 2010

Healthy People 2000 *Criteria*	Healthy People 2010 *Criteria*
1. **Credibility:** Objectives should be realistic and address the issues of greatest priority.	1. The result to be achieved should be **important and understandable** to a broad audience and relate to the two overarching *Healthy People 2010* goals.
2. **Public comprehension:** Objectives should be understandable and relevant to a broad audience, including those who plan, manage, deliver, use, and pay for health services.	
3. **Balance:** Objectives should be a mixture of outcome and process measures, recommending methods for achieving changes, and setting standards for evaluating progress.	2. Objectives should be **prevention oriented** and should address health improvements that can be achieved through population-based and health-service interventions.
4. **Measurability:** Objectives should be quantified.	3. Objectives should **drive action** and suggest a set of interim steps that will achieve the proposed targets within the specified timeframe.
5. **Continuity:** Current objectives should be linked to previous objectives, where possible, but reflect the lessons learned in implementing them.	4. Objectives should be **useful and relevant**. States, localities, and the private sector should be able to use the objectives to target efforts in schools, communities, worksites, health practices, and other settings.
6. **Compatibility:** Objectives should be compatible, where possible, with goals already adopted by the community as a whole and by major groups within the community, such as the public health department and/or major health care providers.	5. Objectives should be **measurable** and include a range of measures—health outcomes, behavioral and health-service interventions, and community capacity—directed toward improving health outcomes and quality of life. They should count assets and achievements and look to the positive.
7. **Freedom from data constraints:** The availability or form of data should not be the principal determinant of the nature of the objectives. Alternate and proxy data should be used when necessary.	6. **Continuity** and **comparability** are important. Whenever possible, objectives should build upon *Healthy People 2000* and those goals and performance measures already established.
8. **Responsibility:** The objectives should reflect the concerns and engage the participation of professionals, advocates, and consumers, as well as state and local health departments.	7. Objectives must be supported by sound **scientific evidence**.

Sources: U.S. Department of Health and Human Services, *Healthy People 2000: National Health Promotion and Disease Prevention Objectives* (Washington, D.C.: U.S. Government Printing office, 1991), p. 90; U.S. Department of Health and Human Services, *Healthy People 2010, Conference Edition* CD (2000).

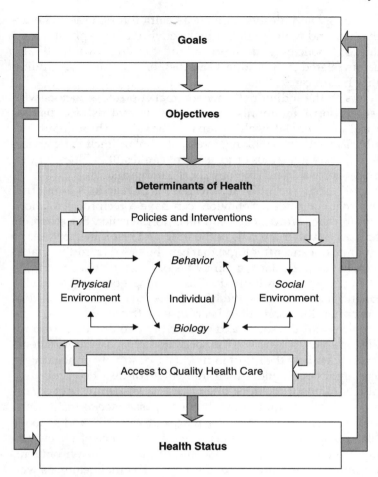

FIGURE 1-1 Healthy People in Healthy Communities. *Source:* U.S. Department of Health and Human Services, *Healthy People 2010, Conference Edition* CD (2000).

Healthy People 2010 outlines the array of influences that determine the health of individuals (clinic-based programs) and the health of communities (population-based programs). Figure 1-1 outlines a policy process for creating programs to ensure healthy people in healthy communities.

For example, individual behaviors and environmental factors are responsible for about 70 percent of all premature deaths in the United States.[10] Developing and implementing policies and preventive interventions that effectively address these health detriments can reduce the burden of illness, enhance quality of life, and increase longevity.[11]

Individual biology and lifestyle influence health through their interaction with each other and with the individual's environment—physical and social. In addition, policies and interventions can improve health by addressing factors related to individuals and their environments, including access to quality health care.

Biology refers to the individual's genetic makeup (those factors with which he or she is born), family history that can suggest risk for disease, and the physical and mental health problems acquired throughout life. Aging, diet, physical activity, smoking, stress, alcohol or illicit drug abuse, injury or violence, or an infectious or toxic agent can result in illness or disability and can produce a "new" biology for the individual.

Behaviors or lifestyle are individual responses or reactions to internal stimuli and external conditions. Behaviors can have a reciprocal relationship to biology; in other words, each can react to the other. For example, smoking (behavior) can alter the cells in the lung and result in shortness of breath, emphysema, or cancer (biology) that can then lead an individual to stop smoking (behavior). Similarly, a family history that includes heart disease (biology) can motivate an individual to develop good eating habits, avoid tobacco, and maintain an active lifestyle (behaviors), which in turn can prevent his or her development of heart disease (biology).

Personal choices and the social and physical environments surrounding individuals can shape behaviors. The social and physical environments include all factors that affect the life of individuals, positively or negatively, many of which might not be under their immediate or direct control.

The social environment includes interactions with family, friends, coworkers, and others in the community. It encompasses social institutions such as law enforcement, the workplace, places of worship, and schools. Housing, public transportation, and the presence or absence of violence in the community are among other components of the social environment. The social environment has a profound effect on individual health, as well as on the health of the larger community, and is important because of cultural customs; language; and personal, religious, or spiritual beliefs. Conversely, individuals and their behaviors contribute to the quality of the social environment.

The physical environment can be thought of as that which can be seen, touched, heard, smelled, and tasted. However, the physical environment also contains nontangible elements, such as radiation and ozone. The physical environment can harm individual and community health, especially when individuals and communities are exposed to toxic substances; irritants; infectious agents; and physical hazards in homes, schools, and work sites. At the same time, the physical environment can promote good health, for example, by the provision of clean and safe places for people to work, exercise, and play.[12]

Policies and interventions can have a powerful and positive effect on the health of individuals and the community. Examples include promotional campaigns to prevent smoking; policies mandating child restraints in cars and the use of seat belts; disease prevention services, such as immunization of children, adolescents, and adults; and clinical services, for example, enhancing mental health care. Policies and interventions that promote individual and community health can be implemented by a variety of agencies such as transportation, education, energy, housing, labor, justice, and other venues, including places of worship, community-based organizations, civic groups, and local businesses. The health of individuals and communities also depends greatly on easy access to quality health care. Access includes enhancing the proximity of clinics and health facilities by means of public transportation and reducing costs of services rendered. Thus, expanding access is important to eliminate health disparities and to increase the quality and years of healthy life for all people living in the United States. Health care in the broadest sense not only includes services received through health care providers but also health information and services received through other venues in the community.

The determinants of health—individual biology and behavior, physical and social environments, policies and interventions, and access to quality health care—have a profound effect on the health of individuals and communities. An evaluation of these determinants is an important part of developing any strategy to improve health and must become a part of a health services manager's approach to identify the provision of services to communities.

Understanding these determinants and how they relate to one another, coupled with knowledge of how individual and community health determines the health of the nation, is perhaps the most important key to achieving the *Healthy People 2010* goals to increase the quality and years of life and eliminate the nation's health disparities.

Expansion of Services

Prevention and health promotion also represent a way to deal with changes in the field and to expand services. Many changes are affecting the industry. Health care costs have risen steadily, while hospital occupancy rates and average length of stay have decreased. At the same time, survival rates for many chronic diseases have increased and the population of those 65 and older has grown. Obviously, these last two trends point to the increasing need for secondary and tertiary prevention. Primary prevention represents an opportunity for providers to cope with these and other changes.

The entire burden to improve the practice of disease prevention and health promotion cannot be carried entirely by the institution or the medical professional. The health promotion market must be widened, however, so that people slowly but surely become motivated to take more responsibility for their own health.

In spite of this, changes are occurring and although health care providers might not have control over them, they can anticipate and plan for them. For example, they can manage their services creatively and effectively to gear them to the needs of their target communities. That is what this book is all about.

A Framework for Health Concepts

To look at associations between risk factors and states of health and disease, an overall framework or conceptualization of health and its determinants is needed. This framework and its attendant policies must be broad, comprehensive, and manageable. It also must accommodate two epidemiological models—those involved with multiple cause/multiple effect factors and those associated with risk factors, as opposed to the more traditional limited emphasis on strict causality as purported in a single cause/single effect model.

The Traditional Model

The traditional epidemiologic model of disease has three components: agent, host, and environment (Figure 1-2). As noted by Friis and Sellers, this is a venerable model that has been used for many decades and is embraced by epidemiologists today.[13] Agents of disease include infectious organisms, physical agents, allergens, chemical agents, and dietary excesses and deficiencies.[14] Host factors are intrinsic elements influencing the individual's susceptibility to the agent. Environmental factors are extrinsic entities that influence exposure to the agent. Factors in each of these categories interact

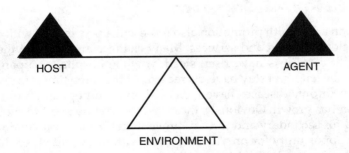

FIGURE 1-2 The Traditional (Ecological) Model. *Source:* Reprinted from *Community Health Analysis* by G. E. Alan Dever with permission of Aspen Systems, Inc., ©1980, 11.

to produce disease. A change in any of the three will alter an existing equilibrium to increase or decrease the frequency of disease.

The model in Figure 1-2 was developed when infectious disease was the main, if not sole, preoccupation of epidemiologists who studied diseases in an effort to explain the etiology. Today the model (ecological) is less appropriate; however, with the resurgence of infectious diseases, a more complex multivariate model is being embraced.[15] Infectious organisms were accorded a status separate from other factors and were identified as agents. With the shift in disease patterns and in the focus of epidemiological studies, new models were developed by stretching the traditional one—de-emphasizing agent, and broadening host and environmental factors.

This expansion does not alter the fact, however, that the traditional framework was developed with the assumption of a single cause/single effect model. Host and environmental factors simply influence the exposure and susceptibility of the individual but do not correspond adequately to present comprehension of most noninfectious diseases.

Some experts talk about the "human host as a causative factor" and "environmental causative factors."[16] However, the author believes it is much simpler and more appropriate to adopt a framework that is broader, more comprehensive, and more fitting to a multiple cause/multiple effect and risk view of health and disease. This multidimensional framework allows health care executives to approach the management of services from a broader epidemiological population-based perspective.

Models for 2005 through 2010

In the 80s and 90s, several specific epidemiological models for health policy development were used in the management of health service. Table 1-2 examines the history of some of these models and illustrates those conceptual components as they have evolved during recent years. In addition, the epidemiological models proposed for health policy development and health services management in 2005 and 2010 are presented in this table.

The models of the 90s are clearly still viable and applicable where they concern the etiology of disease, specifically lifestyle, environment, biology, and the health care delivery system. However, for 2005 through 2010, the expansion to partnerships, networks, and community development becomes significant as hospitals, communities, and health professionals forge collaborative partnerships to have an impact on the health status of the population in the communities served. The progression of these epidemiological models for use in health service management clearly delineates this evolution of health policy models for advancing the health of populations, eliminating disparities, adding years of quality life, and assessing accountability.

TABLE 1-2 Conceptual Epidemiological Models for Health Determinants in the Management of Health Services: A Selected Review

Epidemiological Model	Conceptual Components	Author/Source
1. Health Field Concept	Environment, Lifestyle, Biology, Health Care Delivery System	Lalonde (1974)[17]
2. Epidemiological Model for Health Policy Analysis	Environment	Dever (1976)[18]
	▪ Social	
	▪ Psychological	
	▪ Physical	
	Lifestyle	
	▪ Employment Participation and Occupational Risks	
	▪ Consumption Patterns	
	▪ Leisure Activity Risks	
	Biology	
	▪ Maturation and Aging	
	▪ Complex Internal Systems	
	▪ Genetic Inheritance	
	Health Care Delivery System	
	▪ Restorative	
	▪ Curative	
	▪ Preventive	
3. Expanded Behavioral Model of Health Services Utilization	Health Policy	Aday et al. (1980)[19]
	Characteristics of Population at Risk	
	Characteristics of Health Delivery System	
	Utilization of Health Services	
	Consumer Satisfaction	

TABLE 1-2 Conceptual Epidemiological Models for Health Determinants in the Management of Health Services: A Selected Review *(continued)*

Epidemiological Model	Conceptual Components	Author/Source
4. Achieving Health for All	Aim	Epp (1986)[20]
	Health Challenges	
	■ Reducing Inequities	
	■ Increasing Prevention	
	■ Enhancing Coping	
	Health Promotion Mechanisms	
	■ Self-care	
	■ Mutual Aid	
	■ Healthy Environments	
	Implementation Strategies	
	■ Fostering Public Participation	
	■ Strengthening Community Health Services	
	■ Coordinating Healthy Public Policy	
5. Determinants of Health Model	Individual Response	Evans and Stoddart (1990)[21]
	■ Behavior	
	■ Biology	
	Social Environment	
	Physical Environment	
	Genetic Endowment	
	Prosperity	
	Well-being	
	■ Health and Function	
	■ Disease	
	■ Health Care	

TABLE 1-2 Conceptual Epidemiological Models for Health Determinants in the Management of Health Services: A Selected Review *(continued)*

Epidemiological Model	Conceptual Components	Author/Source
6. Community-Oriented Health Systems Model	Needs Assessment System Design System Performance Assessment Organizational Performance Assessment	Rohrer (1999)[22]
7. Seven Patterns of a Healthy Community	Healthy Environment Vital Economy Personal Well-being ■ Mind ■ Body ■ Spirit Participation in Civic Life ■ Practices Ongoing Dialogue ■ Embraces Diversity ■ Shapes Its Future ■ Cultivates Leadership Everywhere ■ Creates a Sense of Community ■ Connects People and Resources ■ Knows Itself	Norris and Pittman (2000)[23]

TABLE 1-2 Conceptual Epidemiological Models for Health Determinants in the Management of Health Services: A Selected Review *(continued)*

Epidemiological Model	Conceptual Components	Author/Source
8. Healthy People in Healthy Communities Model	Determinants of Health Policies and Interventions ■ Social Environment ■ Biology ■ Behavior ■ Physical Environment Access to Quality Care Health Status	*Healthy People 2010 (2000)*[24]
9. A Framework for Health Care System Development	Health Care Policy Stable Local Health Care Systems ■ Regional/Rural Partnerships ■ Community Participation Access to Primary Care ■ Health Insurance ■ Support Service Improved Health Status ■ Monitor/Surveillance of Epidemiological Data	Georgia Rural Development Council (2001)[25]

Source: G. E. A. Dever, © 2005.

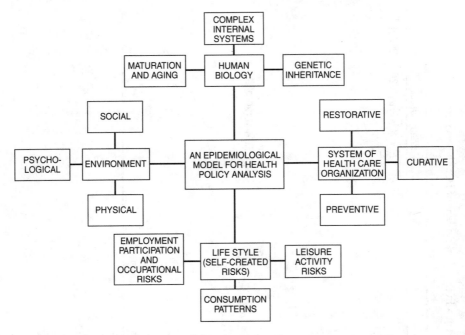

FIGURE 1-3   An Epidemiological Model for Health Policy Analysis. *Source:* Reprinted from "An Epidemiological Model for Health Policy Analysis" by G. E. Alan Dever, *Social Indicators Research* 2, ©1976, 455.

One plan that came into play in the 80s and 90s was developed by Laframboise, who proposed a conceptual framework for analysis of the health field.[26] This framework, later described as the "health field concept" in a Canadian governmental working paper[27] that became the basis for that country's policy, holds that health is determined by a variety of factors that fall into four primary divisions: lifestyle, environment, health care organization, and human biology.

In 1974, Blum proposed an environment of health model, later titled the "Force Field and Well-being Paradigms of Health." In 1976 Dever, building on the Laframboise and Lalonde model, labeled it "An Epidemiological Model for Health Policy Analysis" (Figure 1-3).

Blum suggests that the width of the four inputs [in his model which contribute] to health indicate assumptions about their relative importance. The four inputs relate to and affect one another by means of an encompassing wheel containing population, cultural systems, mental health, ecological balance, and natural resources. On the other hand, the assumptions of Lalonde and Dever are that the four inputs are weighted equally and must be in balance for health to occur. The important question to answer is, How do these four inputs operate when analyzed for specific diseases; or, alternatively, how do these four inputs operate when no disease exists (that is, a state of wellness)? The analysis of risk factors for disease categories within the framework of Dever's epidemiological model for policy analysis provides results similar to those hypothesized by Blum.[28]

To validate the numbers Dever produced in 1976, CDC in 1978 and 1993 analyzed the causes and determinants of death as applied to the epidemiological model for health policy. Further, McGinnis and Foege (1993)[29] and Fielding and Halfon (1994)[30] provide a similar analysis. The results are displayed in Table 1-3. All the studies document lifestyle and environment as major risk factors contributing to mortality and morbidity. As previously stated, an overall framework or conceptualization of health is needed for examining and studying the relationship between risk factors and states of health and disease. An underlying framework forces the epidemiologist, health services manager, or other investigator to consider all factors coming into play in the preservation and restoration of health. As Kerr puts it:

> I would agree that the mechanistic or reductionistic view of health and disease should be supplemented by this broader psychobiological view, . . . starting with his aliquot of genes, enters a life of complex internal and external transactions that are as yet only vaguely understood. . . . The need for a theoretical framework that does not require all noxious agents to be physical, chemical, or biological and that leaves room for such complex deleterious influences on health as noise pollution, jet fatigue, occupational stress, domestic violence, inadequate parenting, and sexual strife is readily apparent.[31]

The health field concept is this type of framework, allowing the broad psychosociobiological analysis of any state of health or disease. It is a comprehensive structure that forces the equal examination of lifestyle, environmental, and biological elements as well as health care organization factors. The model also is ideally suited to collaboration among partnerships, networks, and cooperatives that are objectively focused in the main issues of improving the health status of the population. In fact, Table 1-2 highlights the evolution of health policy models from the basic agent, host, and environment concepts to the more advanced Framework for Health Care System Development focusing on these within the context of collaboration, partnerships, networks, and cooperatives. The U.S. government embraced this model in *Healthy People 2010* (Figure 1-1).[32]

Epidemiological Futures

No one has a crystal ball to see the future, but a long view is critical to plan for strategic challenges to understand the changing role of epidemiology in the management of health services.[33,34,35] Several groups have developed

TABLE 1-3 Determinants of Health: An Epidemiological Model for Health Policy

Factors Influencing Health	Allocation of Mortality to Factors Influencing Health							
	Dever Model (1976)[36]		CDC Model (1978)[37]		CDC Model (1993)[38]		McGinnis/Foege Fielding/Halfon Model[39,40]*	
	%	Cumulative	%	Cumulative	%	Cumulative	%	Cumulative
Lifestyle	43	43	53	53	51	51	34	34
Environment	19	62	21	74	19	70	21	55
Biology	27	89	16	90	20	90	28	83
Health Care Delivery System	11	100	10	100	10	100	17	100

Source: G. E. A. Dever, © 2005.

*Funding allocation based on their "plus" system analysis

scenarios in an attempt to understand current facts and provide perceptions as to what might become reality in the future of health care management. In a 1992 report by Dubnicki, three scenarios suggest ways to guide the management of health services to the year 2001.

Specifically, Dubnicki designates these future scenarios as Constant Crunch/High Tech, Hard Times/Government Leadership, and New Civilization. Although none of these scenarios can be predicted with certainty, they do provide a portrait by which health care leadership can consider the issues of access, health status, and health services in a changing environment. Specifically, advances in understanding of the aging process (including the demographics of aging), disease, and genetics will allow us to predict and evaluate changes in illness trends and improvements in the health care arena.

Elements framed against these scenarios are advanced therapies and disease prevention (primary, secondary, and tertiary) that will provide direction in the management of health services and forecast the impact of these trends on morbidity and mortality levels. A thumbnail sketch of these scenarios is provided in Table 1-4.

When health care leaders and health services managers were asked about these strategies they suggested that new transformational competencies and values would be needed for the twenty-first century.[41,42] Specifically, they indicated that mastering change, system thinking, shared vision, continuous quality improvement, redefining health care, and serving the individuals and the community were essential to meet the new challenges forecasted for the twenty-first century. The importance of putting a greater emphasis on prevention (primary, secondary, and tertiary) and healing, along with appropriate health care coverage that was directed toward the community and that was population-based, was the expected outcome of the new millennium. More recently, Coile outlined three scenarios for the twenty-first century that expounded on the ones developed by the health care leaders noted here.[43] However, these new scenarios were not considerably different from the ones proposed in 1992 for the year 2001; although of major interest is the document by the Institute for the Future that forecasted health care trends for the year 2010.[44] Specifically, they suggest three trends with novel names: Sunny Side of the Street, Long and Winding Road, and Stormy Weather (Table 1-5).

The major distinctions among these trends are the nation's economic outlook, health care reform, and the impact of technology. Each of these trends will have significant consequences for the health services manager, directly affecting the provision of population-based services and, subsequently, the prevention programs that will be developed to understand and thus combat disease patterns of the new millennium. According to Coile, a new era of growth in the health industry is signaled based on advancing age demographics, technology, and consumers who seek prevention programs

TABLE 1-4 Health Care Management Scenarios, 1992 Projections for the Year 2001

Scenarios	Basic Predictions
Constant Crunch/High Tech	1. U.S. health care system expands—represents 17 percent of GNP by 2001
	2. High tech proliferates, providing cures and life extension at a high cost
	3. No national health care reform
	4. Managed care grows—patchwork health care coverage persists
	5. Poverty and unequal access to health care are still problems
Hard Times/Government Leadership	1. Economic recession leads to political revolt in mid-1990s over health care costs
	2. A frugal Canadian-like national health insurance system with rationing of services (especially high tech) will develop
	3. Heroic life-saving measures decline and a more frugal approach to innovation is adopted
	4. U.S. health care systems represent 11 percent of GNP by 2001
New Civilization	1. Dramatic change in service, technology, society, and government hastens health care change
	2. Health care broadens its focus from the individual in clinics to populations in the community and home environment
	3. Health care reform favors managed care through a government/business partnership with discretion at the community level
	4. Basic coverage for all is provided with emphasis on continuum of care: primary, secondary, tertiary prevention
	5. Alternative medicine therapies are common along with high tech
	6. Health care represents 12 percent of GNP by 2001

Source: Adapted from C. Dubnicki, "Bridging Your Own Leadership Gap," *Healthcare Forum Journal* 35, no. 3(1992):43–65.

TABLE 1-5 Epidemiology and the Management of Health Care Services in 2010: Three Scenarios

Health Care Management Scenarios	Potential Trends	Potential Outcomes
Sunny Side of the Street	▪ Spending growth 1% above GDP ▪ Competition among providers drives prices down ▪ Efficient health care organizations emerge from wave of consolidation ▪ Cost pressure closes hospital beds ▪ Public/private partnerships ▪ Effective risk adjustment for Medicare risk ▪ Prospective payment works for ambulatory care ▪ Clinical information technology improves care processes and outcomes	▪ NHE 15% of GDP $8,100 per capita ▪ 30 million uninsured; 10% of Americans ▪ System well equipped to absorb Baby Boomers after 2010 ▪ Population and alternative preventive services prevail ▪ Best practices minimize practice variation ▪ Tiers of care by amenities, access, quality ▪ Medicare and private plans reward population management
Long and Winding Road	▪ Spending growth 1% above GDP ▪ Benefit cuts drive out-of-pocket costs up; utilization down ▪ Employees keep pressure on plans ▪ Continued "hassling" and rate pressure by plans ▪ Limited adoption of organizational innovation ▪ Government limits Medicare and Medicaid expenditures ▪ Turbulent unorganized change ▪ Open competition	▪ NHE 16% of GDP $8,600 per capita ▪ 47 million uninsured; 16% of Americans ▪ Continued 3 tiers of health care ▪ Safety net muddles through as usual ▪ Fragmented delivery of individual care ▪ No major policy reform in health care

TABLE 1-5 Epidemiology and the Management of Health Care Services in 2010: Three Scenarios (*continued*)

Health Care Management Scenarios	Potential Trends	Potential Outcomes
Stormy Weather	▪ Spending growth 2.5% above GDP ▪ Managed care fails to contain costs or improve quality ▪ MD/consumer backlash ▪ Hospital oligopolies ▪ Large employers pay up; small ones drop insurance benefits ▪ New medical technologies are costly and in high demand ▪ IT systems costly and ineffective ▪ No social consensus on limiting end-of-life spending ▪ Safety net in tatters	▪ NHE 19% of GDP $10,200 per capita ▪ 65 million uninsured; 22% of Americans ▪ 60% of Americans worried about security of benefits ▪ Radical tiering of access and care ▪ Several major public hospitals go under ▪ Spending on Medicaid overwhelms state budget ▪ Baby Boomers hit Medicare unprepared—meltdown

Source: Adapted from the Institute for the Future, *Health and Health Care 2010: The Forecast, the Challenge* (San Francisco: Jossey-Bass Publishers, 2000).

or, as he notes, want "the best medicine."[45] He listed ten health care trends that will fuel a technology-driven future. The trends that are most critical to health services management leadership are health politics (budget surplus and coverage for the poor); HMOs are out and PPOs are in (attempts to bring costs under control); competing for excellence (ratings and rankings are important: top 100 lists—hospitals, providers, wellness programs, etc.); and clinical care improvement (deciding on the most important cost-management strategies, especially considering the approach to the levels of prevention).[46]

Prevention and Health Services Management

Epidemiology is the cornerstone to understand disease patterns and therefore the development of prevention programs (primary, secondary, and tertiary). Leavell and Clark[47] outlined five strategies and Davis[48] showed the relationship of a population's disease status to these three levels of prevention and the subsequent effect on the incidence, prevalence, and disability of disease. Figure 1-4 illustrates these preventive medicine strategies as they relate to a population's disease status and the effects on the burden of illness in a society. More recently, Ratzan and others[49] outlined a twenty-first-century field model that incorporates the determinants of health as they relate to the primary, secondary, and tertiary levels of prevention. These two approaches evoke the basic principles of descriptive epidemiology that are the person, place, and time characteristics of a disease measured by incidence and prevalence. The health services manager will need these tools and methods to analyze the health care market from the community (population-based) and the institutional (patient-based) perspectives.

As noted in both approaches, the three basic levels of prevention are significant to the attainment of a more holistic health. The three levels of prevention are:

1. **Primary:** The inhibition of the development of a disease before it occurs, or "How do we keep ourselves well?"
2. **Secondary:** The early detection and treatment of disease, or "If we are getting sick, how can we detect these conditions early?"
3. **Tertiary:** The rehabilitation or restoration of effective function, or "If we are sick, how do we get the best care?"

Primary Prevention

In the prepathogenesis period, prevention consists of measures designed to promote optimum general health and of specific protective elements (Figure 1-4). The latter includes immunization, environmental sanitation,

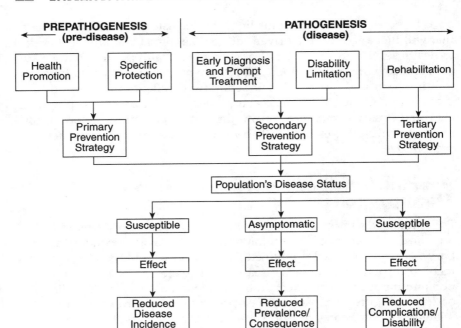

FIGURE 1-4 Preventive Medicine Strategies, Population Disease Status, and Effects. *Source:* Adapted from *Preventive Medicine for the Doctor in His Community* by H. R. Leavell and E. G. Clark with permission of McGraw-Hill Book Company, ©1965, 20. Also, adapted from *Chronic Disease Epidemiology and Control* by R. C. Brownson et al. with permission of APHA, © 1993, 7.

and protection against accidents and occupational hazards. This is prevention in its conventional sense. These measures prove very effective in reducing mortality and morbidity from infectious diseases. General health promotion measures incorporate lifestyle, environmental, and biological factors. This area can contribute the most to the reduction of mortality and morbidity. "Health can be delivered only in a small part; it must largely be lived."[50]

Secondary Prevention

Secondary prevention consists mostly of the early diagnosis and treatment of diseases through measures such as screening and periodic health examinations. The early detection of cancer, hypertension, sexually transmitted diseases, and other treatable illnesses is the aim of secondary prevention. For certain diseases, such as arthritis or other morbid conditions associated with the aging process, secondary prevention consists mostly in limitation of the disability—prevention of complications or sequelae.

Tertiary Prevention

Where disease has already occurred and left residual damage, tertiary prevention is the avoidance of complete disability after anatomical and physiological changes are more or less stabilized. The aim is to restore an affected individual to a satisfying and self-sufficient life.

Figure 1-5 delineates some diseases as a "continuum for preventability." The shading represents the possibility of preventing diseases or disabilities by applying known intervention methods. The darkest area, at the left end of the shaded bar, indicates conditions that can be prevented unequivocally. In the center are some conditions where drastic, sizable, or at least some reductions in risk can be achieved. The lightest area, at the right, illustrates conditions where no progress in reducing risks can be expected until breakthroughs in medical science are made.

The Surgeon General stated quite succinctly the sum context of prevention as it must be conceptualized in the twenty-first century:

> As we begin a new century with a rapidly aging population, vast disparities in health status among various segments of our society, and increasing numbers of people burdened with chronic conditions, we are more aware

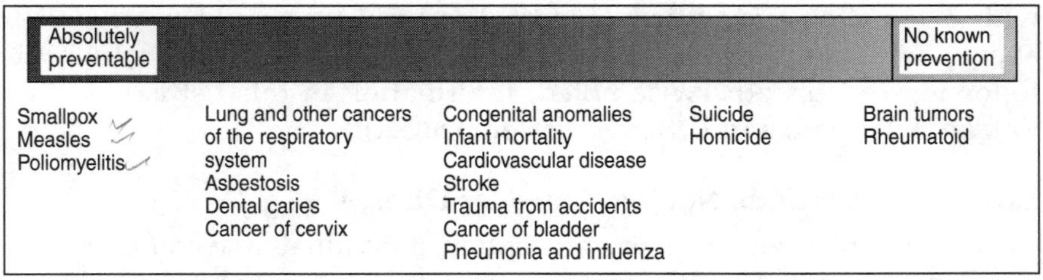

Absolutely preventable				No known prevention
Smallpox Measles Poliomyelitis	Lung and other cancers of the respiratory system Asbestosis Dental caries Cancer of cervix	Congenital anomalies Infant mortality Cardiovascular disease Stroke Trauma from accidents Cancer of bladder Pneumonia and influenza	Suicide Homicide	Brain tumors Rheumatoid

FIGURE 1-5 A Continuum for Preventability. *Source:* U.S. Department of Health and Human Services, *Health, United States, 1980* (Washington, D.C.: U.S. Government Printing Office, 1980). *Note:* The order and placement of the diseases and conditions listed are intended only to be illustrative.

than ever of the need for greater attention to health promotion and disease prevention. . . . Without minimizing the importance of curative efforts, it is now clear that we need a health system that balances cure with health promotion, disease prevention, and early detection, that provides universal access to care, that is community-based, and that includes a balance between individual medical care and public health.[51]

The application of these levels of prevention to health services management problems can achieve the following purposes:

1. Professionals involved in patient care can determine quickly where their resources should be concentrated to prevent (and intervene) in the disease process.
2. Health services managers should be able to realize the vast potential for using prevention strategies in managing the health care institution.

Shifting Disease Patterns: 1900–2010

Agricultural and industrial changes in society resulted in a shift in disease patterns. The transition currently underway from an industrial and even postindustrial society to a service and information-transfer society (knowledge/information revolution) brings new patterns of disease. The leading causes of illness and death have changed significantly over the past one hundred years and will undergo a dramatic shift in the next ten years (2010). See Table 1-6.

Holistic global/local health will not be attained unless it is guided by certain tenets. Health services managers must begin to guide health systems with more than technology, with more than bottom lines, but with a focus on prevention outcomes, which eventually protect their above-mentioned beliefs. The tenets that will guide them include the following (unless otherwise noted, information in this list is based on Ratzan, Filerman, and LeSar. See reference 52.):

1. **Pursue Health, Not Just Cures for Disease**

   By emphasizing primary prevention, individuals and communities can avoid health conditions that would require treatment or cause loss of productivity.

   An ideal health system includes primary prevention by incorporating better communication, education, and vaccination.

   Another way to focus on attaining health rather than treating disease is to develop new ways to measure health. International

TABLE 1-6 The Ten Leading Causes of Illness and Death in the United States, Ranked by Age-Adjusted Death Rates

	1900[53]	1950[54]	1998[55]	2010[56]
1.	Tuberculosis	Diseases of the heart	Diseases of the heart	Diseases of the heart
2.	Pneumonia	Cancer	Malignant neoplasms	Cancer
3.	Diarrhea and enteritis	Cerebrovascular disease	Unintentional injuries	Aging/mental illness
4.	Diseases of the heart	Accidents	Cerebrovascular diseases	Coping/adaptability
5.	Nephritis	Pneumonia/influenza	Chronic obstructive pulmonary diseases	Obesity/nutritional disorders
6.	Accidents/violence	Tuberculosis	Diabetes mellitus	Violence
7.	Cerebrovascular disease	Arteriosclerosis	Pneumonia and influenza	Cerebrovascular disease
8.	Cancer	Nephritis	Suicide	Accidents
9.	Bronchitis	Diabetes mellitus	Homicide and legal intervention	Suicide/Drugs/Alcoholism
10.	Diphtheria	Suicide	HIV	AIDS

Source: G. E. A. Dever, © 2005.

surveillance systems could focus on health indicators rather than just tracking the path of diseases.

2. **Strive for Ideal Health, Not "Best" Health**

The definition of health needs to be broadened.

Health is measured by the quality of individuals' lives rather than simply the absence of disease.

The health of an individual or population is best assessed within the relevant socioeconomic and environmental setting.

Ideal health requires a basic set of values and services; it is not equivalent to "free" health for all or "longest life" for all.

The surest way to attain ideal health is to focus on actions that will have the greatest impact: Increase economic development; reduce poverty; educate the public; deter poor individual health habits (such as smoking and unprotected sex); provide basic housing and clean water; and build an effective health sector.

3. **Reduce Economic and Social Disparities**

Reducing poverty is one of the toughest challenges of the new century, but it would bring the largest rewards.

Rapid population growth often hinders poverty reduction in low-income countries. High fertility creates a large dependent-child population that requires costly educational, social, and health services.

Population pressure and poverty can lead rural populations to waste and destroy resources, which can contribute to environmental, economic, and eventually, health problems.

Slowing population growth in the low-income countries can help reduce poverty.

4. **Acknowledge That Behavior, as Well as Microbes, Spreads Disease**

Human behavior, including the allocation of resources within populations and among institutions, determines the health status of a population.

At least in the short term, the way to stem the AIDS epidemic lies with changing human behavior, not medical research.

Health policies need to look beyond the causes of specific diseases and strengthen the health sector by mobilizing resources from international, private, national, or other sources.

These resources can enhance the delivery and management of health services and can thwart the spread of disease by focusing on primary prevention.

5. **Seek Health Knowledge from Individuals and from Traditional Cultures, Not Just from Medical Research**

Knowledge about what keeps people healthy can be gleaned from the experiences of people in their villages, towns, cities, and within their families.

Traditional and non-Western healing practices can also reveal important links between disease and behavior and introduce effective treatments not found in Western familiar medicine.

6. **Empower Individuals Through Health Literacy**

Health literacy embodies the ideals of education and health.

Health literacy is the capacity of individuals to obtain, interpret, and understand basic health information and services necessary for appropriate health decision making.

Health literacy involves developing the skills to care for others or teaching healthy behavior to other family members.

As parents become better informed about healthy behaviors, their children will develop a greater health literacy.

Health literacy not only prepares individuals to enhance their own health and the health of family members, it also empowers them to advocate for a health-friendly environment with appropriate services and preventive care.

7. **Make Health a Global and Multisectoral Issue**

British scientist Sir Geoffrey Vickers suggested a need to stimulate the "world of the well" to mobilize private and public organizations to create living and working conditions and public organizations to inform public attitudes that support heath and well-being.[57] World Health Organization (WHO), the World Bank, UNICEF, and a number of nongovernmental organizations (NGOs), as well as the for-profit multinational pharmaceutical industry, are the principal actors involved in the delivery of health services.

Multinational groups and NGOs promote health on many fronts: education, immunization campaigns, research and analysis, and policy formation. WHO, for example, supports a treaty that would standardize the marketing, production, and promotion of tobacco to limit the health hazards related to tobacco use.

Health issues can be integrated into the activities and agreements among the growing number of organizations that govern trade. The World Trade Organization and the World Intellectual Property Organization can promote the development of health delivery, provision of medicine and foodstuffs, advancement of health literacy in communications and management, and sanctions against the marketing of illegal drugs and other health hazards. The North American Free Trade Agreement (NAFTA), Mercosur (Southern Cone Common Market in Latin America), Asian Pacific Economic Cooperation (APEC), Association of Southeast Asian Nations (ASEAN), and the Andean Community could also put health on their agendas.

Nongovernmental organizations are also becoming important components in the efforts to attain global health. They include relief and welfare agencies, technical innovation organizations, public service contractors, development agencies (such as Oxfam), grassroots development organizations, and advocacy groups and networks. In addition to administering their own programs, NGOs can influence the policy agenda at international conferences and in national legislatures.

Public and private organizations and national governments need to work together to advance global health. The most obvious areas that would benefit from cooperative effort are health service delivery and policies concerning treatment of diseases. As previously stated, worldwide surveillance systems are another prime opportunity for international cooperation.

Another potential for cooperation includes integration of activities that affect social, economic, and environmental factors important for health. Many international organizations support actions crucial to these other factors that determine health.

8. **Implement and Enforce Policies That Strengthen Health Systems and Encourage Health Literacy**

The creation and implementation of effective policies could include the following:

- Promoting public–private partnerships. Resolutions by soap manufacturers to join governmental handwashing campaigns, for example, can decrease the spread of disease, and pesticide manufacturers can work with health workers on malaria eradication.

- Adopting best-practice guidelines and incentives to adopt and evaluate health policies.

- Encouraging policy change at the local level to create healthier environments.

- Supporting global conventions that address health threats, for example, the global convention on tobacco.

- Rewarding agencies that report disease and health issues.
- Linking economic policy and development with the goal of improving health.
- Developing ethical standards and moral leadership for media conglomerates.

9. **Harness the Information Revolution to Improve Health Systems**

   New technologies make health information available faster than it can be absorbed by health systems. Health care systems need help to capitalize on the wealth of information and new means of communicating.

   Passive public health delivery systems include primary prevention interventions such as smart airbags in automobiles, food fortified with micronutrients, new vaccines for endemic regions, and fluoridated water.

   Active interventions are being developed for cancer: chemotherapy to prevent the spread of cancer, earlier detection and treatment, cancer vaccines, and cancer-fighting viruses and antibodies.

   New indexes and measurements can be developed to capitalize on new technologies and allow individuals to take a more active role in their health. Data on an individual's blood pressure, body mass index, cholesterol, and other indexes can be used as interventions.

   The development of comprehensive global health awareness could also help focus society on prevention. Credible international organizations (such as WHO) could receive publicity in the news media and could be adapted locally so that every citizen could compare his or her individual and community's health.

The leading causes of death are frequently used to describe the health status of a nation as a whole. However, the leading causes of death in the United States generally result from a mixture of injury, violence, and other behaviors within a community; environmental factors; and the unavailability or inaccessibility of quality health services. Understanding and monitoring these health detriments is more useful for health services managers than focusing on the death rates that reflect the cumulative impact of these factors. This approach can serve as the basis for using epidemiology in the management of health services.

The turning point for deaths from infectious and chronic diseases in the United States occurred circa 1925 (Figure 1-6). Collectively, deaths due to

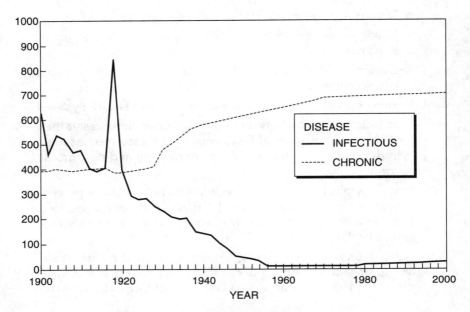

FIGURE 1-6 Adapted from Infectious and Chronic Disease Death Rates in the United States, 1900–2000. *Source:* Reprinted from *Dynamics of Health and Disease* by C. L. Marshall and D. Pearson, p. 131, with permission of Appleton & Lange, ©1972.

infectious diseases declined from approximately 650 deaths per capita 100,000 in 1900 to approximately 20 deaths per capita 100,000 in 1970, a decline of 96 percent. Because of the epidemic of influenza in 1918, the death rate from infectious diseases mounted to 850 deaths per 100,000 population at that time.

Chronic diseases, on the other hand, collectively accounted for approximately 350 deaths per capita 100,000 in 1900 and increased to approximately 690 deaths per capita 100,000 in 1970, an increase of 97 percent. Since 1980, deaths from infectious diseases (namely, AIDS) have increased, whereas deaths from chronic diseases remain relatively stable. This disease transition—not unlike a demographic transition—was caused by the societal shift from an agrarian to an industrial society. An excellent example of this shift in disparities is shown in Figure 1-7 for New York City. In the late 1800s, deaths were five to six times as high as in 1990 and 2000. In 2000, the majority of diseases were chronic, whereas in the 1800s they were infectious.

SUMMARY OF VITAL STATISTICS
THE CITY OF NEW YORK

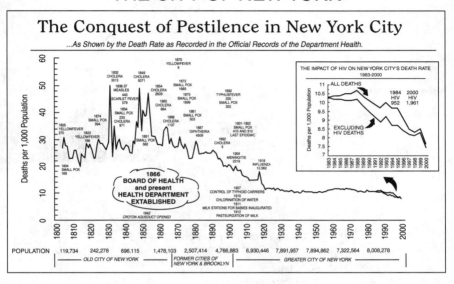

FIGURE 1-7   The Conquest of Pestilence in New York City. *Source: Summary of Vital Statistics 2000: The City of New York* (New York: Office of Vital Statistics, New York Department of Health, 2002), cover.

Infectious Disease Cycle

The agrarian society generated a cycle of events that is portrayed in the infectious disease model (Figure 1-8). The fertility rate was high in the agricultural era, as large families were needed to farm the land. Thus, in 1900, 52 percent of the population was under 21 years of age, and only 3 percent was over 65. This population pyramid is typical of today's inner cities, rural counties, and developing countries where the infectious disease model is still applicable. With no specific medical treatment available, however, parasitic diseases, infectious diseases, and malnutrition contributed to high infant and preschool mortality. In fact, 34 percent of all deaths occurred between birth and 5 years of age.

Chronic Disease Cycle

The cycle of disease during the industrial era is demonstrated by the chronic disease model (Figure 1-9). Deleterious social, physical, emotional, and environmental ways of life resulted from affluence, changing values, and

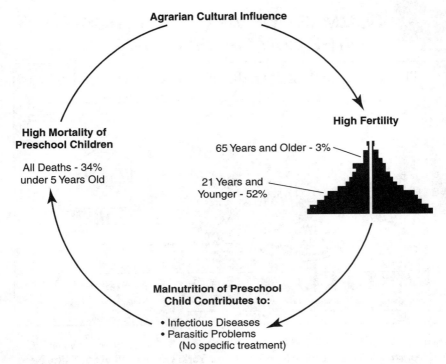

FIGURE 1-8 Cycle of Disease Patterns, Infectious Disease Model. *Source:* Reprinted from *Social Indicators Research*, vol. 4, with permission of Kluwer Academic Publishers, ©1977, 485.

increased leisure time. With this overall societal change, the fertility rate dropped; the population under 21 years decreased to 40 percent; and the population over 65 years increased from 8 percent in 1970 to 12.6 percent in 1990. Consequently, the diseases of an older age group became more prevalent, and 51 percent of all deaths occurred among those 65 and older. The big three—heart disease, cancer, and stroke—accounted for a little more that 60 percent of all deaths in 1970, and in 1998 the big three still accounted for only 61 percent of all deaths.[58] Presently, society is in a knowledge/information, e-world, dot.com revolution in which intellectual capital is becoming the key to strength, prosperity, and social well-being. This is in stark contrast to the material- and labor-intensive products and processes that characterized the industrial revolution.[59] As a result of these changes, a new cycle is emerging—the social transformation disease model—that has several parallels to the infectious and chronic disease models.

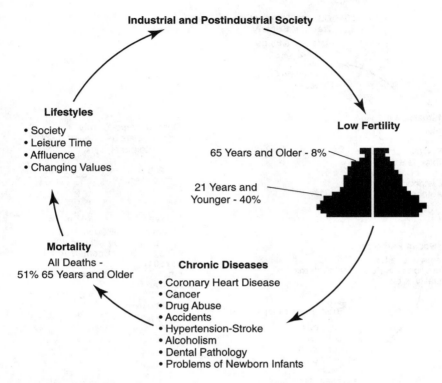

FIGURE 1-9 Cycle of Disease Patterns, Chronic Disease Model. *Source:* Reprinted from *Social Indicators Research*, vol. 4, with permission of Kluwer Academic Publishers, ©1977, 486.

Social Transformation Disease Cycle

Analysts now need a conceptual framework that goes beyond the infectious and chronic disease models. The social transformation model was developed to reflect the new disease patterns (Figure 1-10).[60] It outlines societal and demographic patterns that produce "dys-ease" and social pathology. It assumes that society will face an increasing number of social dysfunctions, environmental dislocations and disasters, and major demographic challenges. Completing the cycle of the social transformation model are societal values and ethical dilemmas.

A Service and Information Transfer Society—e-world dot.coms   The move from an industrial manufacturing economy to a service, information transfer society (knowledge/information revolution/e-world) is reflected in

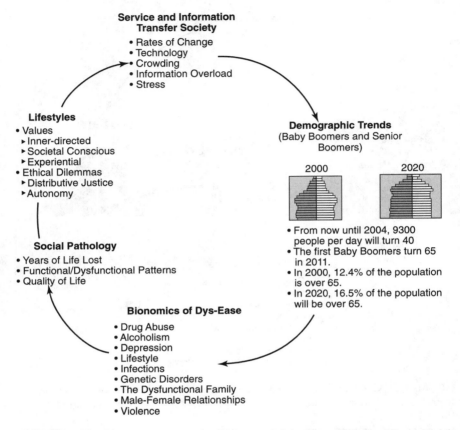

FIGURE 1-10 Social Transformation Disease Model. *Source:* Adapted from *Social Transformation Model: Human Development and Disease Patterns*, Datalog File 87-1153 by J. W. Alley, G. E. A. Dever, and T. E. Wade, with permission of SRI International, ©1986, 9.

changing employment patterns. In 1978, 21 million people held manufacturing jobs, and 16.5 million performed jobs in the service industry; however, by 1983, 19.2 million worked in service jobs, and 18 million worked in manufacturing.[61] In the new millennium and beyond, this continuing shift to service occupations and e-world technology players will assume a major role in formulating disease patterns. The interaction of the increasing rate of change, technology shifts, population density, information overload, and stress—all characteristics of the service and information transfer society—plays a role in creating new disease patterns (Figure 1-11).[62]

Population crowding accompanies increased urbanization. In the United States, the population density is 80 people per square mile, yet in

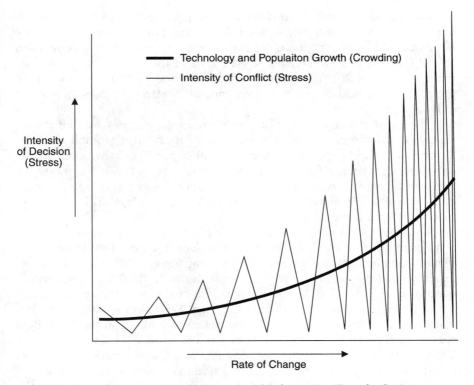

FIGURE 1-11 Characteristics of a Service and Information Transfer Society. *Source:* Modified from G. E. A. Dever, "Future Shock and You" (unpublished paper, 1974).

2000, 74 percent of the population lived in urban areas.[63] In Manhattan, the density exceeds 60,000 people per square mile, leading to numerous problems. Lesse suggested that overcrowding will create a conflict between the individual's need for privacy and desire for group security.[64] No one knows, however, at what level of population density societal breakdown is likely to occur, if at all.

Associated with density and urbanization is information overload, a problem in many U.S. cities. This overload of information forces people to make endless choices among options, which causes stress and eventually social shock. Nonetheless, restricting the opportunity for choice transforms the desire to choose into the "need" to choose.

Demographic Trends: The Baby Boom/Senior Boom   Between 1946 and 1964, 76.4 million babies were born in the United States; these individuals now make up one-third of the current population. The post–World War II increase in the fertility rate also occurred in many other countries, including Canada, New Zealand, Australia, and the Soviet Union. This Baby Boom created birth cohorts considerably larger than the Great Depression cohort (i.e., those between ages 45 and 49) and the Baby Bust cohort (i.e., those under age 20). The population distribution of people over age 50 resembles a typical population pyramid, as deaths decrease the size of older age groups.

The great upsurge in fertility between 1946 and 1964 still affects all aspects of contemporary society. Because of its relatively small size, the Depression cohort experienced relative abundance. The Baby Boom cohort can expect continued frustrations as it passes through life. For example, this group encountered overcrowded classrooms and a shortage of teachers during the 1960s and 1970s and faced school closings and unemployment problems throughout the 1980s.

The recent increase in the number of births and in the crude birth rate is an echo effect of the Baby Boom that reflects the arrival of the cohort's female members at the prime childbearing ages of 20 to 29. Analysts expected this rise in the number of annual births in the 1980s, even with a continued fertility rate of approximately 1.8 births per woman. The number of births remained high during the early 1990s, but should then have decreased (fertility rates remaining constant) as females in the Baby Bust cohort reached childbearing age between 1995 and 2005. From the early 1990s on, the number of births should remain constant because the age-sex profile will change from a pyramid to a stationary rectangular profile.

As the Baby Boom generation ages and as fertility remains low, the median age of the population will increase. In fact, as a result of declining birth rates and a progressively aging population, people 65 and over (particularly those 85 and over) are the fastest growing group in the United States. Because the Depression cohort is small, this growth will slow in the 1990s and in the first decade of the new century. Thereafter, however, the Baby Boom of the 1950s will become a Senior Boom, and the proportion of the population over 65 will grow rapidly to 16.5 percent in 2020 and 18 percent in 2030. After 2030, that group's relative size will probably decrease sharply again as the Baby Bust cohorts of the 1960s and 1970s become 65 and older.

The Bionomics of "Dys-ease"   Disease in a society usually results from the convergence of preconditions, or bionomics. For example, the preconditions set by demographics and the service and information transfer society are partially responsible for the current cycle of disease. The "dys-eases" typical of this cycle can be grouped as psychological, lifestyle, genetic, and social problems.

Psychological Problems.   Drugs, alcohol, and depression will be the major causes of psychological problems in the future. These problems have already increased dramatically and could easily reach epidemic proportions.

Increased use of marijuana and cocaine is particularly notable. Marijuana use increased from 1974 to 1982 in all groups, except for the current users aged 12 to 17. The greatest increase is in the adult group (26 and older)—a 4.6 percent increase in the current user group, and a 13.1 percent increase in the ever used group. Young adults (18 to 25) show the greatest percentage of current users (25.2 percent) and people who have used drugs in the past (64.1 percent). Substantial increases occur in all age groups for both categories of cocaine use.

Depression and associated psychological disturbances often occur with the advent of middle age. In 1986, approximately 9,300 persons per day reached the age of 40, and this rate continued up until 2004. For the 15 to 44 age group, 1983 hospital discharge records listed neurosis as the most common problem for males and the second most common problem for females. For the 45 to 64 age group, neurosis dropped to third and fourth positions, respectively, for males and females.[65]

From 1974 to 1982, all age groups increased their use of stimulants, sedatives, and tranquilizers—the prescribed drugs of choice—to combat neurosis and depression. Selby suggests the following reason for this enormous consumption of psychotropic drugs:

> [They are] taken more as a means of defense than for a therapeutic effect; they provide momentary escape or support rather than cure, relief from fatigue, monotony, anguish, frustration, or even minor anxieties arising in everyday life. Curiously, as the stresses of modern life increase, so is the threshold of tolerance to [those stresses] becoming progressively lower, so that substances which at one time were taken only for some pressing cause, such as severe insomnia or profound anxiety, are now ingested almost routinely in anticipation of such minor stresses as starting school or occasional insomnia. These drugs are too often looked on as panacea, as a chemical screen behind which to escape from the stress of everyday life, as the ultimate recourse in the face of conflict situations.[66]

Alcohol use in the United States has contributed to many diseases and will continue to do so in the future. Violence—including motor vehicle accidents, homicide, and suicide—is often a result of alcohol use. Research shows that 65.2 percent of youths and 94.6 percent of young adults have used alcohol at least once. The corresponding figure for adults is 88.2 percent.

Psychological patterns of disease (depression, drug use, and alcohol) are fueled by the stresses of the service and information transfer society, as well as by demographic pressures. Of grave concern, the age groups that use mind-altering drugs will grow rapidly over the next 15 to 20 years, creating a potentially volatile situation.

Lifestyle Problems.   Both infectious and chronic diseases can stem from destructive lifestyles. The social transformation disease cycle, however, suggests that two of the major diseases plaguing U.S. society—AIDS and violence—are bionomically unique. AIDS has reached epidemic proportions among homosexuals and intravenous drug users, and it is now spreading to the general population. Social conditions and time/space clustering contributed to the evolution and spread of AIDS in the United States. Furthermore, homophobia and ignorance still frighten some groups, causing regression to medieval values of control and prevention. AIDS could become even more devastating in the next 15 years, as the number of AIDS cases increased approximately 150 percent per year since 1981.[67]

Violence, the other major lifestyle disease pattern, threatens the social fabric of the United States; it is the fourth leading cause of death in this country. In many instances, suicide, homicide, and motor vehicle accidents can be traced to depression, alcohol abuse, and drug use. Again, societal and demographic preconditions led to these disease patterns. For the most part, the rates of violence show a downward trend, but they still remain persistently high. Violence, however, will have more impact in the next 5 to 10 years.

Genetic Problems.   Scientific change has occurred most dramatically in the field of genetics. In 1970, scientists identified only a few genes on any chromosome; by 1975, more than 100 genes were mapped on human chromosomes.[68] It is estimated, however, that there can be as many as 100,000 genes in a single human chromosome, which indicates the magnitude of the work still to be done in this area.

Genetic research has important consequences for biological medicine. Clearly, genetic mapping or engineering introduces enormous risks and ethical dilemmas. Because it could lead to disasters comparable to the thalidomide crisis, some degree of control is essential. On the one hand, too much change at too rapid a pace could produce dysfunctional products with overwhelming destructive consequences. On the other hand, genetic engineering promotes greater understanding of human development, facilitates the diagnosis of birth defects, and can make it possible to predict inherent susceptibility to disease.[69] Interferon, which helps to arm the body against viral infections, is one positive outcome of genetic engineering. Furthermore, the ability to combine segments of deoxyribonucleic acid (DNA) to produce hybrid molecules could contribute to scientists' understanding of cancer and other diseases. Lesse underscores the ethical dilemmas that are some of the many "stop/go" decisions that society must make.

> The potentialities of genetic manipulations are theoretically endless. . . .
> The prevention of or effective treatment of a variety of diseases that have
> hereditary propensities (diabetes mellitus, hemophilia, hematologic ailments, renal and cardiac problems) are valid possibilities.[70]

Lesse also notes the potential for minor or even cataclysmic problems if recombinant DNA research proceeds without controls.[71]

The dilemma is to control genetic engineering so that it produces positive outcomes while preventing negative effects of re-engineered bacteria or genetically changed human, animal, or plant life. Society has a responsibility to temper its desire for scientific research with careful exploration, and control, of possible negative outcomes.

Social Problems.   In the social pathology of dysfunctional families and male-female relations, the most telling statistic is the divorce rate. In 1970, the rate was 41 per 1,000 people; by 1984, it increased to 89 per 1,000 people.[72] In 1996, one of every two marriages ended in divorce.[73] The health of a community depends in part on the quality of family life, and divorce jeopardizes the family's ability to act as a force for stability.

Prison population is another indicator of family breakdown. The number of adults under correctional supervision (jail, prison, parole, or probation) increased dramatically from 1979 to 1983—from 113 per 10,000 adults over age 18 in 1979 to 143 per 10,000 in 1983.[74] The number of prisoners in all institutions has jumped drastically since 1950, with the greatest increase between 1980 and 1984.[75] In 1950, the rate was 110 prisoners per 100,000 people. In 1980, the rate climbed to 139 per 100,000, and by 1984, it reached 188 per 100,000.

In the future, relationships between men and women will be in a state of flux and will be a major source of stress. During the industrialization era, men increasingly participated in hierarchical organizations, whereas women, as a group, did not. One result is that men are more likely to speak as "we," as a reflection of their group orientation and their power. Women, on the other hand, traditionally have the status of the "other," while men in power made decisions affecting women.[76] Between 1948 and 1985, however, the percentage of women in the labor force rose from 29 to 55 percent, and it reached 59.5 percent in 2000.[77] Conflict is likely to grow as women show greater psychological similarity to men, becoming "we"-oriented. Friction will result from role shifts[78] and women's refusal to accept "other" or "object" status.

Epidemiology: Aims, Types, and Methods

Aims

Epidemiology has three main aims:

1. To study the occurrence, distribution, and progression of disease problems and, more generally, to describe the health status of human populations so as to provide a basis for the planning, evaluation, and management of health promotion and rebuilt systems.
2. To provide data that will contribute to comprehension of the etiology of health and disease.
3. To promote the use of epidemiological concepts for the management of health services.

Table 1-7 illustrates the three main aims of epidemiology in relation to their associated type of strategies and methods. Traditionally, Aims 1 and 2 foster the general principle of epidemiological investigation. However, Aim 3 shows that the descriptive, analytical, and experimental types of investigation have applications in health services management. These applications include studies that are disease-specific to determine market penetration and the use of market analysis (marketing) and demographic trends that can promote health education and disease prevention.

This new approach is a must for health service managers in an era of growing interest in preventive health promotion, disease prevention, and self-care, along with the reduced reliance on institutional in-patient care. They should use these techniques to identify new markets and to know what type of services to expand. For instance, the pharmacy at the institution could not only dispense the traditional drugs, but also expand to offer vitamins, minerals, and other health promotion items. Hospitals can provide wellness centers that include aerobic programs, weight-lifting rooms, and jogging or walking tracks in the halls. There is unlimited potential for institutions to innovate in this new era of health promotion and disease prevention.

Types and Methods

The following are three types of epidemiological strategies that involve a variety of associated methods:

1. Descriptive epidemiology is concerned with the occurrence, distribution, size, and progression of health and disease in the population.
2. Analytic epidemiology can involve three main types of studies: retrospective, prospective, and cross-sectional. In a retrospective or case-control study, the epidemiologist collects data in retro-

TABLE 1-7   Aims, Types, and Methods of Epidemiologic Investigations

Aims	Types	Methods
1. To study the occurrence, distribution, size, and progression of health and disease in human populations	Descriptive	Analysis of morbidity and mortality data, collected either routinely or by special studies
2. To provide data that will contribute to the understanding of the etiology of health and disease	Descriptive	Same as above; such descriptive analyses help formulate hypotheses on the etiology of health and disease
	Analytic	■ Retrospective/case-control studies ■ Prospective/cohort studies ■ Cross-sectional/survey/longitudinal studies
	Experimental	Clinical/controlled studies
3. To promote the utilization of the epidemiological concepts to the management of health services	Descriptive	Description of morbidity and mortality data: by service area, by diagnosis-related groups (DRGs)
	Analytic	Determination of patient flow by disease category (DRGs); determination of disease-specific rates; market penetration and market segmentation (age-specific rates)
	Experimental	Identification of potential new health markets, of research areas for expansion, and of demographic trends

spection from two comparable groups of individuals—one with a specific disease or condition and one without—to identify any history or exposure to one or more factors of interest (precursor characteristics). A prospective, cohort, or longitudinal study involves the opposite process. It starts with a group of people (a cohort) characterized by some factor of interest (precursor characteristic) and follows the cohort forward (prospectively) in time (longitudinally) to determine the incidence (i.e., observe the subsequent development) of some disease or condition. A cross-sectional or prevalence study involves the collection of data from a defined specific population at one time. A detailed discussion of research designs used in epidemiology to evaluate evidence-based medicine literature and for the analysis and assessment of community needs will be presented in a later chapter.

3. Experimental epidemiology also tests etiological factors, and involves manipulation of these factors. Evaluation determines effects of introducing, eliminating, or otherwise modifying the hypothesized (suspected) factors on the occurrence or progression of some state of health or disease.

The importance of these methods to the health services manager becomes evident given the new responsibilities that the manager has in the health care environment. Table 1-8 portrays the traditional and future responsibilities for health service managers as applied in the health care management field. Specifically, the table generates the message that the health services manager in the future will be focused on efforts that relate to populations within communities and less on individuals in clinics.

TABLE 1-8 Traditional and Future Role of Health Care Management

Traditional	Future
■ Emphasis on acute inpatient care	■ Emphasis on the continuum of care
■ Emphasis on treating illness	■ Emphasis on maintaining and promoting wellness
■ Responsibility for individual patients	■ Accountability for the health of defined populations
■ All providers are essentially similar	■ Differentiation based on ability to add value
■ Success achieved by increasing market share of inpatient admissions	■ Success achieved by increasing the number of covered lives and keeping people healthy
■ Goal is to fill hospital beds	■ Goal is to provide care at the most appropriate level
■ Hospitals, physicians, and health plans are separate	■ Integrated health delivery system
■ Managers run an organization	■ Managers oversee a market
■ Managers serve as department heads	■ Managers operate service areas across organizational borders
■ Managers coordinate services	■ Managers actively pursue quality and continuous improvement

Source: Adapted from S. M. Shortell and A. D. Kaluzny, eds., *Essentials of Health Care Management* (Albany, N.Y.: Delmar Publishers, 1997).

Summary

The application of epidemiology to health services management is a relatively new approach to the effective and efficient delivery of care. This chapter provides the focus and direction for that link between epidemiology and health services management. The concepts of disease prevention and health promotion as they are aligned with the new framework suggest ways to improve individuals' physical and mental status and encourage them to use services. Institutions can create new dimensions to their delivery of services to reflect the challenge of health promotion and prevention. It suggests that the concept of improved health status be changed from a disease-oriented perspective to a health-oriented perspective.

Of particular importance among the methods of epidemiology is the expanded concept of risk in relationship to disease. This introductory chapter sets the stage for the theme of the book: the application of health promotion and disease prevention techniques, as viewed by epidemiology, to the management of health services.

The determinants of health as endorsed by *Healthy People 2010*—lifestyle, environment, biology, and the delivery of care system—and their application to the management of services must be embraced if the health status of populations and patients is to continue to improve.

References

1. U.S. Department of Health and Human Services, *Healthy People 2010: Understanding and Improving Health* (Washington, D.C.: U.S. Government Printing Office, 2000), foreword.
2. U.S. Department of Health and Human Services, *Healthy People: The Surgeon General's Report on Health Promotion and Disease Prevention* (Washington, D.C.: U.S. Government Printing Office, 1979).
3. U.S. Department of Health and Human Services, *Healthy People 2010*.
4. C. H. Evans, "Finding New Ways to Improve Health," *Health Searchlight* 1, no. 1 (2001):1.
5. U.S. Department of Health and Human Services, *Healthy People 2010*, 7.
6. U.S. Department of Health and Human Services, *Healthy People 2010*, 7.
7. R. G. Rogers et al., *Living and Dying in the USA: Behavioral, Health, and Social Differentials of Adult Mortality* (San Diego: Academic Press, 1995), 3–7.
8. R. Rhyne et al., eds., *Community-Oriented Primary Care: Health Care for the 21st Century* (Washington, D.C.: American Public Health Association, 1998).
9. R. M. Davis, "'Healthy People 2010': National Health Objectives for the United States," *BMJ* 317 (1998):1513–1517.
10. U.S. Department of Health and Human Services, *Healthy People 2010*, 18.
11. U.S. Department of Health and Human Services, *Healthy People 2010*, 18.
12. U.S. Department of Health and Human Services, *Healthy People 2010*, 19.

13. R. H. Friis and T. A. Sellers, *Epidemiology for Public Health Practice* (Gaithersburg, Md.: Aspen Publishers, Inc., 1999), 334–335.
14. Centers for Disease Control and Prevention, "Diagnosis and Management of Foodborne Illnesses: A Primer for Physicians," *MMWR* 50, no. 2 (2001):68.
15. M. J. Schneider, *Introduction to Public Health* (Gaithersburg, Md.: Aspen Publishers, Inc., 2000), 142–162.
16. H. R. Leavell and E. G. Clark, *Preventive Medicine for the Doctor in His Community* (New York: McGraw-Hill Book Company, 1965), 684.
17. M. Lalonde, *A New Perspective on the Health of Canadians* (Ottawa: Office of the Canadian Minister of National Health and Welfare, 1974), 31.
18. G. E. A. Dever, "An Epidemiological Model for Health Policy Analysis," *Social Indicators Research* 2 (1976):455.
19. L. A. Aday et al., *Health Care in the U.S.: Equitable for Whom?* (Beverly Hills, Calif.: Sage, 1980).
20. J. Epp, "Achieving Health for All: A Framework for Health Promotion," *Canadian Journal of Public Health* 77, no. 6 (1986):402.
21. R. G. Evans and G. L. Stoddart, "Producing Health, Consuming Health Care," *Social Science and Medicine* 31 (1990):1347–1363.
22. J. E. Rohrer, *Planning for Community-Oriented Health Systems*, 2d ed. (Washington, D.C.: American Public Health Association, 1999), 17.
23. T. Norris and M. Pittman, "The Healthy Communities Movement and the Coalition for Healthier Cities and Communities," *Public Health Reports* 115, nos. 2 and 3 (2000):118–124.
24. U.S. Department of Health and Human Services, *Healthy People 2010*, 18.
25. Georgia Health Policy Center, Georgia Rural Development Council, *Rural Health in Georgia "A Framework for Success"* (Atlanta: Rural Healthcare Committee, 2001), 18.
26. H. L. Laframboise, "Health Policy: Breaking the Problem Down in More Manageable Segments," *Canadian Medical Association Journal* 108 (1973):388–393.
27. M. Lalonde, *A New Perspective on the Health of Canadians*.
28. G. E. A. Dever, *Community Health Analysis* (Rockville, Md.: Aspen Systems Corporation, 1980), Chapter 10.
29. J. M. McGinnis and W. H. Foege, "Actual Causes of Death in the U.S.," *JAMA* 270, no. 18 (1993):2207–2212.
30. J. Fielding and N. Halfon, "Where Is the Health in Health System Reform?" *JAMA* 272, no. 16 (1994):1292–1296.
31. L. W. Kerr, "Contemporary Epidemiology," *International Journal of Epidemiology* 3, no. 4 (1974):295–296.
32. U.S. Department of Health and Human Services, *Healthy People 2010*.
33. Schneider, *Introduction to Public Health*.
34. I. H. Yen and S. L. Syme, "The Social Environment and Health: A Discussion of the Epidemiologic Literature," *Annual Review of Public Health* 20 (1999):287–308.
35. S. Schwartz et al., "A Future for Epidemiology?" *Annual Review of Public Health* 20 (1999):15–33.
36. G. E. A. Dever, "An Epidemiological Model for Health Policy Analysis," *Social Indicators Research*, 455.

37. U.S. Department of Health, Education, and Welfare, Public Health Service, Centers for Disease Control and Bureau of State Services, Health Analysis and Planning for Preventive Services, *Ten Leading Causes of Death in the United States, 1975* (Washington, D.C. and Atlanta: 1978), 46.

38. Centers for Disease Control and Prevention, "Cigarette Smoking—Attributable Mortality and Years of Potential Life Lost—United States, 1990," *MMWR* 42, no. 33 (1993):645–649.

39. McGinnis and Foege, "Actual Causes of Death in the United States," 2207–2212.

40. Fielding and Halfon, "Where Is the Health in Health System Reform?" 1292–1296.

41. C. Dubnicki, "Bridging Your Own Leadership Gap," *Healthcare Forum Journal* 35, no. 3 (1992):43–65.

42. E. Ginzberg, "U.S. Health Care: A Look Ahead to 2025," *Annual Review of Public Health* 20 (1999):55–66.

43. R. C. Coile, Jr., *New Century Healthcare: Strategies for Providers, Purchasers, and Plans* (Chicago: Health Administration Press, 2000), 225–249.

44. Institute for the Future, *Health and Health Care 2010: The Forecast, the Challenge* (San Francisco: Jossey-Bass Publishers, 2000), insert.

45. R. Coile, *Russ Coile's Health Trends* 13, no. 3 (2001):1–12.

46. Coile, *Russ Coile's Health Trends*, 1–12.

47. Leavell and Clark, *Preventive Medicine for the Doctor in His Community*, 20.

48. Davis, "'Healthy People 2010,'" 1513–1517.

49. S. C. Ratzan et al., "Attaining Global Health: Challenges and Opportunities," *Population Bulletin* 55, no. 1 (1996):13.

50. A. Wildavsky, "Can Health Be Planned?" (lecture delivered at the University of Chicago, April 23, 1976).

51. D. Satcher, "A Message from the Surgeon General," *Health Searchlight* 1, no. 1 (2001):4.

52. S. C. Ratzan, G. L. Filerman, and J. W. LeSar, "Can the World Be Healthy?" in "Attaining Global Health: Challenges and Opportunities," *Population Bulletin* 55, no. 1 (1996):38–47.

53. U.S. Department of Health and Human Services, *Health, United States, 1987* (Hyattsville, Md.: National Center for Health Statistics, 1988), 10–11.

54. U.S. Department of Health and Human Services, *Health, 1987*, 10–11.

55. U.S. Department of Health and Human Services, *Health, United States, 2000* (Hyattsville, Md.: National Center for Health Statistics, 2001), 163.

56. G. E. A. Dever, "The Future of Health Services in Georgia" (paper presented at Armstrong State College, Savannah, Ga., March 1988), 13.

57. G. Vickers, *Human Systems Are Different* (New York: Harper and Row, 1983).

58. U.S. Department of Health and Human Services, *Health, United States, 2000. With Adolescent Health Chartbook* (Hyattsville, Md.: National Center for Health Statistics, 2000), 173.

59. J. J. Dundustadt, "The State of the University—Leadership for the Twenty-First Century," *Michigan Alumnas* (November/December 1988):22–28.

60. J. W. Alley et al., "Social Transformation Model: Human Development and Disease Patterns," Stanford Research International (SRI), Menlo Park, Calif.: Datalog File 87–1153 (October 1986):1–29.

61. Foundation of the American College of Health Care Executives, *Health Care Consumers: Demographic Analysis of the Market for Health Services* (Ann Arbor, Mich.: Health Administration Press, 1985).
62. G. E. A. Dever, "Future Shock and You" (unpublished paper, 1974).
63. U.S. Bureau of the Census, *Statistical Abstract of the United States: 1986*, 106th ed. (Washington, D.C.: U.S. Government Printing Office, 1985), 15.
64. S. Lesse, *The Future of the Health Sciences: Anticipating Tomorrow* (New York: Irvington Publishers, 1981), 100.
65. U.S. Bureau of the Census, *Statistical Abstract of the United States*, 10.
66. P. Selby, *Health in 1980–1990: A Predictive Study Based on an International Inquiry* (New York: S. Karger, 1974), 38.
67. Division of Public Health, *Disease Patterns of the 1980s* (Atlanta: Georgia Department of Human Resources, 1986), 124.
68. Lesse, *Future of the Health Sciences*, 89.
69. Lesse, *Future of the Health Sciences*, 89.
70. Lesse, *Future of the Health Sciences*, 90.
71. Lesse, *Future of the Health Sciences*, 90.
72. R. M. Kreider and J. M. Fields, *Number, Timing, and Duration of Marriages and Divorces: Fall 1996* (Washington, D.C.: U.S. Census Bureau, 2001), 18.
73. U.S. Bureau of the Census, *Statistical Abstract of the United States*, 35.
74. U.S. Bureau of the Census, *Statistical Abstract of the United States*, 185.
75. U.S. Bureau of the Census, *Statistical Abstract of the United States*, 184.
76. Simone de Beauvoir, *The Second Sex* (New York: Alfred A. Knopf, 1952), 28.
77. David E. Bloom, "Women and Work," *American Demographics* (September 1986):25–30.
78. Lesse, *Future of the Health Sciences*, 104.

2

Managerial Epidemiology and Health Policy

Health services managers recognize that a new century of health care is emerging. The model being developed is a shift to risk management from risk avoidance, and the industry is moving from an illness intervention paradigm (secondary and tertiary levels of prevention) to disease prevention and health promotion (primary prevention) while embracing the continuum of disease prevention. Moreover, the new model focuses on the basic premise of promoting good health care for populations within communities and less on the individual patient in a clinical setting. This population-based health care/Medicare perspective requires cooperation with communities where networks, partnerships, and collaboration will dictate the future of the health care services delivered. Thus, hospitals, providers, patients, communities, and insurers must take a long-term approach to establish programs that will meet the needs of all involved through the development of partnerships. To forge these relationships the health services manager must be acutely aware of the service area market in terms of its characteristics—demographics, disease patterns (mortality and morbidity), utilization by diagnostic category, patient origin analysis to define the market area, availability of providers and other health professionals, access issues (distance to facilities), financial stability of the community and the insurers, and the acceptance of the plan (cultural and ethnic diversity). To meet these challenges the health care manager would be wise to embrace the methods and concepts of epidemiology so as to ensure decisions made about the health of the population they serve are rational and based on sound evidence—population or medicine based.

Chapter 1 outlines a basic health policy model that suggests the determinants of health, as specified by the *Healthy People 2010* document: lifestyle, environment, biology, and the health care delivery system. These now classic terms are shown in Figure 1-1 and are displayed in their relationship to the planning and policy functions for the improvement of life expectancy and health status. Of course, the 2010 document far exceeds these two guiding principles and outlines goals and objectives for twenty-eight priority areas and ten leading health indicators, reflecting 468 objectives (Table 2-1).

The health indicators highlight lifestyle, environment, biology, and health care system issues that significantly affect the health of individuals and communities. Noted in *Healthy People 2010* is the importance and influence of income and education on these leading health indicators. Specifically, households with low income are correlated with poor or fair health status because income and education are highly correlated and inequalities in these variables underlie many of the health disparities in the United States.

To achieve equity, a "healthy people" perspective must be adopted by recognizing that community, state, and local/national organizations must support a multidisciplinary approach to improve health status. *Healthy People 2010* strongly states that every person in every community deserves equal access to comprehensive, culturally competent, community-based health care systems. More important, the document puts forth an economic model of managed care that can serve multiple populations within a community.

Managed Care and Epidemiology

Health services managers will be well informed by the *Healthy People 2010* objectives as well as with changes in the financing and delivery of health in a managed care environment. Epidemiology plays a special role in this future because many of the 2010 objectives and the stages of managed care are interconnected and must be measured for performance and results through the patient as well as the community perspective. The National Committee on Quality Assurance incorporated many *Healthy People* target objectives into its Health Plan Employer Data and Information Set (HEDIS) 3.0, a set of standardized measures for health care purchasers and consumers to use in performance assessment of managed care organizations in the area of immunizations, mammography, screening, and other preventive services. Health services managers and providers can encourage patients to pursue healthier lifestyles and to participate in community-based programs that promote healthy communities. The importance of epidemiology in health services management is in the use of these objectives as benchmarks for their network plans by building an agenda for community health improvements and to monitor the results and outcomes over time.

TABLE 2-2 Stages of Managed Care and Epidemiology in Health Services Management

Stage	Characteristics	Strategies Requiring Epidemiological Measurement	
		Strategies	Epidemiological Measurements
1	HMO penetration <5%	▪ MDs begin to compete with freestanding centers ▪ Respond to JCAHO, regulation ▪ Build working relationships with existing and emerging medical groups ▪ Cooperate or affiliate regional managed care networks with larger providers	▪ Perform service area analysis ▪ Obtain baseline measurement ▪ Perform monitoring and evaluation ▪ Establish prevention priorities ▪ Assess population in communities
2	HMO penetration 5–14%	▪ Organize networks for regional contracts ▪ Expand networks, manage weak facilities ▪ Initiate benchmarking with local providers ▪ Develop a regional network of preferred hospitals for managed care contracting ▪ Upgrade information systems for contract management and quality monitoring	▪ Develop networks using Geographical Information Systems (GIS) ▪ Utilize *Healthy People 2010* and HEDIS (3.0) ▪ Assess physician workforce by location, specialty, and demographics ▪ Develop total quality management tools for use in assessing improvement in process, structure, and outcome

TABLE 2-2 Stages of Managed Care and Epidemiology in Health Services Management (*continued*)

		Strategies Requiring Epidemiological Measurement	
Stage	Characteristics	Strategies	Epidemiological Measurements
3	HMO penetration 15–24%	■ Build regional network of ambulatory centers ■ Re-engineer high-cost clinical processes ■ Monitor "dashboard" of clinical indicators ■ Begin a regional branding campaign with marketing and advertising ■ Provide performance data on costs and clinical outcomes to all doctors ■ Complete the development of clinical paths for the top 20 inpatient and ambulatory procedures ■ Develop a flexible staffing model for changes in utilization	■ Monitor and survey of clinical indicators ■ Market products using basic demographics of institutional and community-based populations ■ Perform cost profiles and performance measurement using basic descriptive epidemiological measures ■ Analyze morbidity patterns ■ Assess mortality ■ Assess utilization patterns
4	HMO penetration 25–39%	■ Build "bedless hospitals" in growth markets ■ Publicize outcomes, patient satisfaction ■ Build a new organizational culture across the network among mid-level managers, physicians, leaders, and board trustees ■ Initiate consolidation planning among network hospitals to regionalize services and reduce infrastructure costs (e.g., home health, post-acute)	■ Assess market for best locations ■ Access evaluation ■ Profile institution—benchmark to 2010 objectives or national HEDIS (3.0) indicators ■ Assess diversity ■ Employ strategic planning to utilize GIS to optimize services ■ Develop clinical preventive services guidelines

TABLE 2-2 Stages of Managed Care and Epidemiology in Health Services Management (*continued*)

Stage	Characteristics	Strategies Requiring Epidemiological Measurement	
		Strategies	Epidemiological Measurements
4	HMO penetration 25–39%	■ Complete the development of patient-centered care paths and clinical protocols	
5	HMO penetration >40%	■ Add incentives for quality and prevention	■ Assess for quality—develop prevention programs
		■ Compete on outcomes, patient ratings	■ Perform hospital physician profiling satisfaction surveys
		■ Develop the ability to clearly identify target customers and understand requirements of each customer segment	■ Assess populations in communities using standard demographics and epidemiological techniques
		■ Develop the ability to identify target populations (e.g., hypertensive patients) that can be served by the health care organization	■ Analyze markets by DRGs
			■ Perform community needs assessment
		■ Gather the resources to replace facilities-based services with new forms of medical care (e.g., inhome monitoring)	■ Assess resources and develop strategies
			■ Identify new markets
		■ Develop the ability to expand market strategies and programs to meet target customers' needs (e.g., ambulatory care, complementary medicine)	■ Assess consumer needs
			■ Prepare hospital profiles and ratings based on variety of outcomes that are disease-based and customer satisfaction driven
		■ Develop the ability to become competent at reporting outcomes and satisfaction to demonstrate the organization's value to its customers	

Source: Adapted from R. C. Coile, *New Century Healthcare: Strategies for Providers, Purchasers, and Plans* (Chicago: Health Administration Press, 2000), 1–20.

Coile introduced this sixth stage of managed care and noted, "[It] is not just higher HMO market penetration. Stage Six markets work differently. . . . There is more communication, . . . more trust, in the relationships between providers, planners, purchasers, and patients [and communities]."[5] What will be the factors that contribute to this movement—this sixth stage of managed care evolution? Partnerships are critical.[6] Several factors and shifts in the health care system are making the medical and public health systems become more dependent on one another.

Today the institutions, the providers, the plans, the patients, and the communities need each other to address not only patients in the clinics but also populations in communities in order to promote professional/institutional health in addition to disease prevention and health promotion for the community as a whole.

Table 2-3 illustrates at least ten strategies to bring medicine and the communities together for overall improvement in the health status of a population. Associated with these ten strategies for the twenty-first century are the basic epidemiological measurement issues that a health services manager must be familiar with to ensure an analytical approach to improving the health status of the community. By applying these concepts and methods of epidemiology, the health services manager will be able to add to the understanding of the etiology of health and disease; the planning, administration, and evaluation of health services; the forecasting of the health needs of population groups; the supply of the health professional workforce; and the assessment of the outcomes of various diagnoses in clinical and population-based settings (e.g., disease management, HEDIS 3.0, *Healthy People 2010*). Further, institutions need to understand performance data and identify benchmarks, which many times may need to be retrieved from large claim databases. These efforts must be geography-specific and utilize the basis of the epidemiology of medical care, including small-area analysis of variations in outcomes.[7]

The evolution of managed care to this new level is not driven by HMO penetration but by the importance of and increasing emphasis on partnerships and collaboration, thereby promoting an increased focus on identifying problems and practices and improving health status by applying the levels of prevention. Thus now more than ever, planning, evaluation, administration, and analysis must shift from individuals in clinics to populations in communities. This shift will allow continuous monitoring, surveillance, and evaluation of the health care community where the concern is not only for those who utilize the institutional facilities but also for the population that is within the overall service area of the facility. As Ibrahim states:

> If health care is ever to develop a true population rather than an individual patient perspective . . . then epidemiology and public health [medicine] research must be charged with finding ways to better understand and resolve the huge differences in health, health behaviors [lifestyles], health care [system] . . . among communities and the population groups

TABLE 2-3 Managed Care and Epidemiological Measurement Issues
Evolutionary Model for the Twenty-first Century

Transition Strategies for the Twenty-first Century Managed Care Model	*Epidemiological Management Issues Related to Strategies*
1. Long-Term Agreements	■ Increased employee or disease prevention and health promotion ■ Quality improvement and outcome measures
2. Strategic Business Relationships	■ Community-based health plans
3. Empower Consumers	■ Internet epidemiology—addressing lifestyle, environment, biology, and health care delivery ■ Issues by the individual, "information therapy"
4. Risk Sharing	■ Population in communities (population-based medicine) allows for risk sharing ■ HEDIS and 2010 objective measurements and outcomes
5. Information-Enabled Processes	■ "Health Information Sharing" Web site—health services managers will monitor utilization, disease management ■ Data warehouses will service communities, patients, physicians, hospitals, and managers
6. Risk Management/ Disease Management	■ Disease management stressing profiles of hospitals by top 100 best to treat specific diseases ■ Set of outcome measurements of physicians by profitability ■ Primary care as a level of prevention
7. Health Improvement	■ Engagement in health prevention and disease prevention ■ Clinical Preventive Services Guidelines—HEDIS Indicators and *Healthy People 2010* objectives
8. Competency or Quality	■ Selecting best hospitals and best plans—needs epidemiological measurement of adjustments, rates, and rankings ■ Benchmarks for performance-based measurement
9. Community Health	■ Health needs assessment, assessment of priorities ■ Identification of priorities—holistic health planning

TABLE 2-3 Managed Care and Epidemiological Measurement Issues
Evolutionary Model for the Twenty-first Century *(continued)*

Transition Strategies for the Twenty-first Century Managed Care Model	Epidemiological Management Issues Related to Strategies
9. Community Health	▪ *Healthy People 2010* objectives of lifestyle, environment, biology, and the health care delivery system ▪ Investment in a healthier population and fewer risks
10. Universal Coverage	▪ Unlikely probabilities related to achievement—analyzing populations (improving health status—high probability) and eliminating health disparities ▪ Assessing disease patterns, levels of prevention

Source: Adapted from *New Century Healthcare: Strategies for Providers, Purchasers, and Plans* by R. C. Coile, Jr. (Chicago: Health Administration Press, 2000), 225–249.

within them. Epidemiology, the core discipline of public health research, relates the health problems and use of health care resources to defined populations. It identifies groups that do not present themselves for health care, as well as those that do. Thus epidemiology can assess the health problems and the provision of health care for the total population [the evolutionary stage of managed care—the sixth stage] rather than just those who are in contact with health services. . . . The effect of health care measures on the entire population are important factors in formulating health policy, organizing health services, and allocating limited resources.[8]

Epidemiological Consideration

As noted in Chapter 1, epidemiology has three main aims: to study the occurrence, distribution, size, and progression of health and disease in human populations; to contribute to the comprehension of the etiology of health and disease; and to promote the utilization of epidemiological concepts in the management of health services. These aims relate to and, in fact, become intertwined in the pursuit of health policy's ultimate goal: the promotion and preservation of the population's health.

As was also discussed, disease patterns switched over time from infectious to noninfectious chronic ailments. The greatest potential for the promotion and preservation of the public's health still lies in prevention. As it did for infectious diseases, epidemiology makes an important contribution to understanding the causes and means to prevent noninfectious ailments.

It is significant that the concepts and methods of epidemiology have not only been used to add to the understanding of the etiology of disease, but are also used in the areas such as evaluation of health services and systems; planning, administering, assessing, forecasting, and projecting the health needs of population groups; the supply and distribution of the health workforce; and assessing outcomes of treatment in clinical settings (i.e., assessing individual patients in a clinical setting).[9]

Ford describes three stages in the control of a disease: the popular, the scientific, and the application phases.[10] The popular phase consists of the gathering of knowledge "from its early roots in folk wisdom and common sense observation." The scientific phase is the transformation of this commonsense knowledge into scientific understanding. The application phase translates this scientific understanding into effective prevention.

Descriptive epidemiology parallels the popular phase, while analytic and experimental (as well as descriptive) epidemiology contributes to the scientific understanding of disease. In the application phase, the epidemiological data is translated into meaningful and natural public policy decisions. This is what Gordis calls the "societal responsibility" of epidemiologists,[11] and this is where they are in the handling of most leading causes of death. Epidemiological research has already identified the major risk factors in heart diseases, in most cancers, in cerebrovascular diseases, and in most other leading causes of death.[12] This knowledge, however, has yet to be translated fully into health policy.

The fact that health policy is determined by many factors other than epidemiology partially explains the nonapplication of epidemiological knowledge. In addition, as Ford points out, the major decision makers of health policy (namely, average citizens, physicians, health care managers, and public health experts) have different and distinct points of view on health and illness.[13]

Epidemiology and public health involve knowledge and consideration of both a numerator (number of cases, deaths, services, and so forth) and a denominator (the general population from which the numerator is taken). Average citizens are aware that they are part of the denominator but have only limited knowledge of the numerator or the extent of the populace. In contrast, physicians are centered on, and value, the individual patient-doctor relationship. Physicians know quite a bit about the numerator but little about the denominator. Finally, health care managers usually are very much aware of the general population but too often in economic terms rather than by concern for unmet needs, prevention of illness, and health maintenance and promotion.

There are no easy pathways to society's goal of health for all. However, the widespread adoption of the epidemiological perspective may facilitate a reduction in the impact of the major cripplers and killers. Gordis writes: "In the last analysis, these [policy] decisions are societal and as active and concerned members of society, each of us should be a participant in this process and should not abdicate this community responsibility."[14]

The epidemiologist-public health expert should become more vocal and more involved in policy making. As many authors advocate, physician training should incorporate a widened epidemiological perspective when considering patients' health.[15,16,17,18] The average citizen also must become involved through greater awareness of the determinants of health and illness and through increased participation in the formulation of policy.

Health care management should become population based. Health organizations must be aware of the needs and problems of the population they are serving. They also must get involved in the maintenance and promotion of the public's health.

Epidemiological Models of Health Policy

As a consequence of the changes in managed care and the ever pressing need to analyze problems using the epidemiological perspective, there have been several approaches used to develop health policy. In today's environment many changes, including changing demographics, increased diversity, shifting perspectives of population-based medicine (clinical versus community/patients versus population), changes in managed care financing structures (as discussed in Chapter 1), institutional performance pressures, measure results related to individuals and communities, and the shift in health policy from the independence to the partnership focus, have all contributed to the need for several approaches to develop health policy from an epidemiological perspective.[19]

Health Field Concept

It is not necessary to dwell on this model, as no doubt many readers will recognize this model, developed in the late 1970s.[20] However, with the release of *Healthy People 2010* it is apparent that the four major components that still contribute to the improvement in health status and are major determinants for establishing health policy are lifestyle, environment, health care delivery system, and biology. No matter how it is stated, evidence still persists that points to the importance of embracing this holistic approach to policy and the management of health care services.

Although this conceptualization of health in four primary divisions (lifestyle, environment, human biology, and system of health care organization) was proposed initially as a disease-causation model,[21] it became popular when applied to health policy in Canada.[22,23] This epidemiological model provides a more balanced approach to the development of health policy when compared with the limiting, traditional divisions of prevention, diagnosis, therapy, and rehabilitation, or with public health, mental health, and clinical medicine.[24] Figure 1-3 shows the primary divisions of this epidemiological model for health policy analysis.

Lifestyle

Lifestyles or, more accurately, self-created risks can be divided into three elements: (1) leisure activity risks, (2) consumption patterns, and (3) employment participation and occupational risks. This division of the epidemiological model involves the aggregation of decisions by individuals affecting their health and over which they have more or less control.[25] Bad or incorrect decisions result in destructive modes of health that contribute to an increased level of illness or premature death.

Environment

The environment in the epidemiological model is defined as events external to the body over which the individual has little or no control. This element can be subdivided into physical, social, and psychological dimensions.[26]

Human Biology

This element, focusing on the human body, concerns basic human biologic and organic makeup of each individual. Thus, a person's genetic inheritance creates genetic disorders, congenital malformations, and mental retardation. The maturation and aging process is a contributing factor in arthritis, diabetes, atherosclerosis, and cancer. Obvious disorders of the skeletal, muscular, cardiovascular, endocrine, and digestive systems are subcomponents of complex internal systems.

Disease categories that involve human biology must be weighted in accordance with the other divisions of the epidemiological model. Genetic counseling of parents whose children may have Tay-Sachs disease is a step in the right direction. If the problems that result from human biology can be overcome, it should be possible to save many lives, decrease misery, and reduce the cost of treatment services. For health care providers, this is an obligation to their patients.

Health Care Delivery System

The final division of the epidemiological model is the health care delivery system of medical care. This can be subdivided into three elements: curative, restorative, and preventive. The system itself consists of the availability, quality, and quantity of resources to provide health care. Its restorative elements include hospital, nursing home, and ambulance services. Its curative elements involve medical drugs, dental treatments, and health care professionals. The system has very limited preventive elements.

Efforts and expenditures to improve health in the United States have been directed almost totally toward the system of medical care organization. Yet the morbidity and mortality disease patterns of today are deeply entrenched in the three other divisions of the epidemiological model. The huge sums spent for restoring health and curing disease could be used far more effectively if they could be earmarked for prevention of disease. Rather than concentrate on the failures of the system of medical care organization, it would be more advantageous to promote the positive points of the three other divisions—lifestyle, environment, and human biology.

Advantages of the Model

The combination of the four divisions—system of medical care organization, lifestyle, environment, and human biology—into an epidemiological model for health policy analysis has many advantages. Lalonde cites the following:

1. This model raises lifestyle, environment, and human biology to a level of categorical importance equal to that of the system of medical care organization.
2. The model is comprehensive. Any health problem can be traced to one or a combination of the four divisions.
3. The model allows a system of analysis by which a disease or pattern can be examined under the four divisions in order to assess relative significance and interaction (i.e., what percentage or proportion of lifestyle, environment, human biology, and system of medical care organization contributes to suicide?).
4. This model permits further subdivision of the four major factors: for example, environment is subdivided into physical, social, and psychological.
5. This model provides a new perspective on health that creates a recognition and exploration of previously neglected fields that is still viable in the health policy field today.[27]

Applications of the Model to Health Policy

The application of this model involves four steps:

1. The selection of diseases that are of high risk and that contribute substantially to overall mortality and morbidity
2. The proportionate allocation of the contributing factors of the disease to the four elements of the epidemiological model
3. The proportionate allocation of total health expenditures to the four elements of the epidemiological model

4. The determination of the difference in proportions between (2) and (3)

This is essentially what the Canadian government did, as a basis for its federal health policy, as Lalonde writes in *A New Perspective on the Health of Canadians*. The use of the model in studying disease patterns in Georgia and in other U.S. states has been examined by several authors (Table 1-3).

It is clear that present policies do not support methods most likely to improve health status. If, however, the epidemiological model is applied to health status (disease-specific), it will provide a basic framework for specifying goals and objectives. This will lead to recommendations for public and private institutions to program actions at state and area levels to improve health status. The goals developed would relate to both health status and health system, the latter as a description of the desired system and with considerable attention to services to promote health and prevent disease.

Collaboratives and Partnerships

In contrast with the "managed care" model of health care delivery at the end of the twentieth century, the "collaborative care" model has emerged in the twenty-first century. The collaborative care model of health care delivery is based on the premise that a basic purpose of the health care system is to achieve measurable improvements in the health of individuals and communities in ways that are cost-conscious; quality-driven; evidence-based; oriented to more patients, families, and communities; and more reliant on teams of caregivers.[28] The most promising aspect of this model is its grounding in principles of collaboration (i.e., between doctor and patient, between generalist and specialist, between physician and hospital, between doctors and other health professionals, between hospitals and community-based facilities, between faculty and community-based practitioners, and between and among participating health systems).[29,30]

Thus, much of health policy in this early part of this century will be made by networks that support collaborations and partnerships. The previous chapter showed the new approaches to health policy formulation have clearly evolved into the development of regional networks that embrace the concepts of holism and are population-based focusing on populations in communities. A second application of the epidemiological approach to health policy is outlined by the Lasker report *Medicine & Public Health: The Power of Collaboration*.[31] In the late 1990s a survey conducted by the Committee on Medicine and Public Health sought to determine the extent of cross-cultural collaboration by examining organizations across the country (Figure 2-1). The organizations represent diverse regions of the country, including urban and rural communities. Although the document describes in great detail the dimensions of the evolved relationships in the communities, the intent here is to provide the summary results and the

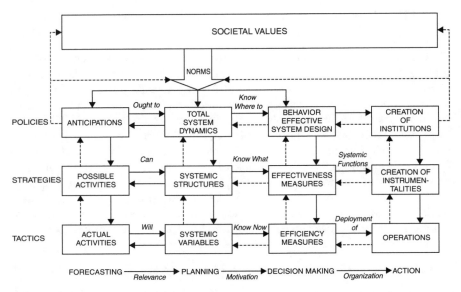

FIGURE 2-1 Geographic Distribution of Cases. *Source:* R. D. Lasker and the Committee on Medicine and Public Health, *Medicine & Health: The Power of Collaboration* (New York: New York Academy of Medicine, 1997), 49.

models that express those relationships. Three broad-based models are identified that have significant epidemiological and health policy attributes. The three models can be classified by type of analysis or by focus of the program. The models are as follows:

- Individuals in clinics
- Populations in communities
- Populations in communities and individuals in clinics

Each of the models reflect two collaborative objectives, which in turn show what health services managers must do to meet those objectives utilizing basic epidemiological methods (Table 2-4). As an example, Model A (population in communities) poses a collaborative strategy of strengthening health promotion and health prevention by mobilizing community campaigns. To meet this challenge health services managers using epidemiological methods would conduct a community health needs assessment of the demographics, disease patterns, health workforce resources, and social and economic conditions to determine the level, effort, direction, and geographic targeting for health education campaigns. For this to happen, the levels of prevention specific to the problems would result in preventive medicine objectives for the development of community-wide campaigns that target opportunities based on the community-needs assessment. This

TABLE 2-4 Health Policy Models of Collaboration—Health Services
Management Medicine and Public Health

Models	Health Services Management and Epidemiological Methods
Populations in Communities	

Strengthening health promotion and health protection by mobilizing community campaigns	A. Conduct community health assessments
	B. Mount health education campaigns
	C. Advocate health-related laws and regulations
	D. Engage in community-wide campaigns to
	   ■ achieve health promotion
	   ■ objectives
	E. Launch "Healthy Communities" initiatives

Shaping the future direction of the health system by collaborating around policy, training, and research	A. Influence health system policy B. Engage in cross-sectoral education and training C. Conduct cross-sectoral research
Individuals in Clinics	
Improving health care by coordinating services for individuals	A. Bring new personnel and services to existing practice sites B. Establish "one-stop" centers C. Coordinate services provided at different sites
Improving access to care by establishing frameworks to provide care for the uninsured	A. Establish free clinics B. Establish referral networks C. Enhance clinical staffing at public health facilities D. Shift indigent patients to mainstream medical settings
Populations in Communities/Individuals in Clinics	
Improving the quality and cost-effectiveness of care by applying a population perspective to medical practice	A. Use population-based information to enhance clinical decision making B. Use population-based strategies to "funnel" patients to medical care C. Use population-based analytic tools to enhance practice management

TABLE 2-4 Health Policy Models of Collaboration—Health Services Management Medicine and Public Health *(continued)*

Models	Health Services Management and Epidemiological Methods
Populations in Communities/Individuals in Clinics	
Use clinical practice to identify and address community health problems	A. Use clinical encounters to build community-wide databases B. Use clinical opportunities to identify and address underlying causes of health problems C. Collaborate to achieve clinically oriented community health objectives

Source: Adapted from *Medicine and Public Health: The Power of Collaboration* by R. D. Lasker (Chicago: Health Administration Press, 1997), 51.

effort results in potentially launching a "Healthy Communities" initiative or a similar program that partners the entire community to focus on the improvement in health status.

These types of collaborative health policy models do not follow or fit an objective methodology that is as precise as the health field concept. That is not to say that anyone of these collaborative models would not use the health field concept if deemed appropriate. What the health policy models do reveal is that the formulation of health policy must be fluid and the players are negotiators and have the ability to compromise in order to pursue the common theme of improving health status. However, once the objectives are decided by the partnership, there must be some acknowledgment that epidemiology drives the process so there can be appropriate allocation of resources toward the target populations. As usual, the problem emerges as to how to allocate minimal resources to maximize the potential to improve the outcomes and is health care more concerned with preventative or curative programs? As noted previously, the movement in medicine, public health, and government is toward creating an increased life expectancy and eliminating health disparities by focusing on prevention, particularly on the determinants of health: lifestyle, environment, biology, and the health care delivery system. This is the basic tenet of *Healthy People 2010*.

Preventive Services—Policy Models

In this new century, preventive services and the practice guidelines are touted as fundamental to the practice of medicine and policy of health care decisions. Embedded in these decisions are the epidemiologic principles that help (1) to influence the appropriateness of preventive services, (2) to understand the concepts that help determine the usefulness of screening tests, and (3) to aid in the examination of prevention programs at the individual and community level. The basic epidemiologic principles used to develop preventive services guidelines also provide the context in which to consider these general recommendations and their policy relevance to populations, communities, and patients.[32]

To fully appreciate and understand the importance of the preventive services guideline, the health services manager must be equally cognizant of basic descriptive epidemiological principles. In subsequent chapters these principles will be described and applied to specific relevant problems. Policy-relevant preventive services for implementation are outlined and detailed at the population/community level and at the individual level.

Canadian Task Force on Preventive Services

In this application of the epidemiological approach and techniques in the formulation of health policy, a Canadian task force in 1979 reported on periodic health examinations and developed health protection packages.[33] The panel identified nearly eighty major disabling and/or fatal conditions and unhealthy states and behaviors that affect Canadians as potentially preventable. It explained, "Such states and behaviours are those that, when discovered, indicate that a person is at a degree of risk for a subsequent disease or disorder."[34]

Each of these potentially preventable conditions was studied extensively in the medical world literature and in assessment of the scientific evidence, mostly epidemiologic, on the benefits of early detection or prevention. For each of the conditions then judged preventable, recommendations were developed on the procedure and frequency of the desirable specific test or maneuver. These individual maneuvers then were grouped into packages of examinations to be carried out at specific ages. The result was a proposal for a lifetime program of periodic health assessments or health protection packages for all Canadians.

The most interesting aspect of this model lies in the use of the epidemiological approach to arrive at a highly concrete, selective, and efficient health policy. Instead of the conventional, routine, nondirected method, this series of health protection packages provides a selective approach to prevention, health maintenance, and health promotion. The task force comments:

> This will help health professionals and the health service system to concentrate on the identification and early management of conditions that are potentially preventable. This selective approach restricts detections manoeuvres to those for which there is evidence of benefit through casefinding or screening.[35]

An abridged health protection package (for women and men ages 16 to 44 years) is reproduced in Table 2-5.

TABLE 2-5 Health Protection Package: Women and Men 16 to 44 Years

Target Condition	Maneuver	Optimal Frequency or Maneuver	Remarks
Tetanus and diphtheria	Immunization	Booster every ten years (optional for diphtheria)	Only persons in good health should be immunized
Alcoholism, smoking, motor vehicle accidents	Elicit information on patient's history; counsel; provide effective contraceptive services to alcoholic sexually active women; control underlying medical conditions	At first encounter and at regular and appropriate intervals thereafter	Research priority: to establish the effectiveness of counseling
Family dysfunction, marital and sexual problems	Elicit history; counsel	Appropriate intervals based on clinical judgment	Research priority: to determine the effectiveness of preventive maneuvers
Hearing impairment	Elicit history and conduct clinical examination	During visits for other reasons	Research priority: to determine the value of early detection and of the detection strategies available
Hypertension	Blood pressure measurement	At least every five years	At every visit made for other reasons
Cancer of the cervix	Papanicolaou smear	When first sexually active, but recheck within a year, then every 3 years to age 35 and every 5 years thereafter	For subjects at high risk: annual smears, particularly when early age of onset of sexual activity and multiplicity of sexual partners. Research priority: to determine the optimal age and frequency for taking smears

TABLE 2-5 Health Protection Package: Women and Men 16 to 44 Years *(continued)*

Target Condition	Maneuver	Optimal Frequency or Maneuver	Remarks
Gonorrhea	Smears of cervix and/or urethra; cultures of cervical and/or urethral secretions and of first-voided urine	At appropriate intervals on the basis of clinical judgment	Pregnant women should be tested; incidence higher in persons with history of multiple sexual partners
Syphilis	Serologic testing	At appropriate intervals on the basis of clinical judgment	Pregnant women should be tested; incidence higher in persons with history of multiple sexual partners
Iron-deficiency anemia and malnutrition	History taking; determination of serum protein and hemoglobin concentrations; measurement of height and weight	At appropriate intervals on the basis of clinical judgment	Women in low socioeconomic circumstances; Indians and Inuit; food faddists
Cancer of the skin	Inspection; counseling	At appropriate intervals on the basis of clinical judgment	High-risk groups: persons who work outdoors or are in contact with polycyclic aromatic hydrocarbons

Source: Adapted from *Periodic Health Examination Monograph* (report of a task force to the Conference of Deputy Ministers with permission of Health and Welfare Canada, 1980), 114–115.

Thus the 1979 report arrived at an important central recommendation, namely that the "undefined annual check-up" should be abandoned and replaced with a series of age-specific "health protection packages." From 1979 to 1994 the task force published nine updates and in 1994 the *Canadian Guide to Clinical Preventive Health Care* was published making recommendations for eighty-one conditions. Since 1994 they have published five updates in the *Canadian Medical Association Journal (CMAJ)*. In order to make specific recommendations they graded the strength of the recommendations by focusing on the quality of published medical evidence—evidence-based medicine. They placed a significant weight on the features of the study designs and the analysis to recognize the potential of biased results. The grades of recommendations and the quality of the published evidence were used to make recommendations and are presented in Tables 2-6 and 2-7. Table 2-8 is an abridged set of recommendations for

---

TABLE 2-6   Grades of Recommendations

A   Good evidence to support the recommendation that the condition be specifically considered in a Periodic Health Examination (PHE).

B   Fair evidence to support the recommendation that the condition be specifically considered in a PHE.

C   Poor evidence regarding inclusion or exclusion of a condition in a PHE, but recommendations can be made on other grounds.

D   Fair evidence to support the recommendation that the condition be specifically excluded from consideration in a PHE.

E   Good evidence to support the recommendation that the condition be specifically excluded from consideration in a PHE.

Source: Canadian Task Force on Preventive Health Care (CTFPHC History/Methodology. http://www.ctfphc.org/ctfphc&methods.htm).

TABLE 2-7   Quality of Published Evidence

I   Evidence from at least one properly randomized controlled trial (RCT).

II-1   Evidence from well-designed controlled trials without randomization.

II-2   Evidence from well-designed cohort or case-control analytic studies, preferably from more than one center or research group.

II-3   Evidence from comparisons between times or places with or without the intervention. Dramatic results in uncontrolled experiments could also be included here.

III   Opinions of respected authorities, based on clinical experience, descriptive studies, or reports of expert committees.

Source: Canadian Task Force on Preventive Health Care (CTFPHC History/Methodology, http://www.ctfphc.org/ctfphc&methods.htm).

TABLE 2-8 Men 21 to 64 Years Quick Table: All Relevant Recommendations

Condition	Maneuver	Population
"A" Recommendations		
Colorectal Cancer	Multiphase screening with the Hemoccult test	Average-risk adults > age 50
Dental caries	Community fluoridation, fluoride toothpaste or supplement	General population
Hypertension	Pharmacologic treatment	Adults ages 21 to 64 years with DBP > 90 mmHg
Pneumococcal pneumonia	Single dose of 23-valent pneumococcal vaccine	Immunocompetent patients ≥ age 55 years in institutions
Tobacco-caused disease	Counseling, smoking cessation, nicotine replacement therapy	Smokers
"B" Recommendations		
All-cause mortality and morbidity	Moderate physical activity	General population
Colorectal cancer	Sigmoidoscopy	Average-risk adults > 50 years
Colorectal cancer	Flexible sigmoidoscopy beginning at puberty, genetic testing	High-risk adults with FAP
Colorectal cancer	Colonoscopy	High-risk adults with HNPCC
Coronary heart disease	Diet/drug treatment	Males 30 to 59 years with elevated cholesterol or LDL-C
Coronary heart disease	General dietary advice on fat and cholesterol	Males 30 to 69 years
Lung cancer	Dietary advice on green leafy vegetables and fruit	Smokers
MVA injury	Counseling on restraint, use, and avoidance of drinking and driving	General population

TABLE 2-8 Men 21 to 64 Years Quick Table: All Relevant Recommendations (*continued*)

Condition	Maneuver	Population
	"B" Recommendations	
Obesity	BMI measurement	Obese adults with obesity-related disease
Obesity	Weight-reduction therapy	Obese adults with obesity-related disease
Skin cancer	Counseling, reduced sun exposure, clothing	General population
Tobacco-caused disease	Referral to validated cessation program	Smokers
	"C" Recommendations	
Abdominal aortic aneurysm	Abdominal palpation	General population
Abdominal aortic aneurysm	Abdominal ultrasound	General population
All-cause mortality and morbidity	Counseling, physical activity; prevent obesity	General population
All-cause mortality and morbidity	Measure body mass index and treat obesity	General population
Colorectal cancer	Hemoccult/sigmoidoscopy in combination	Average-risk adults > 50 years
Colorectal cancer	Colonoscopy	Average-risk adults, high-risk adults with family history of polyps/CRC
Coronary artery disease events	Vitamin therapy (folic acid alone or with vitamin B12) to lower total plasma homocysteine levels	All populations
Coronary heart disease	General dietary advice on fat and cholesterol	General population except males 30 to 69 years
HIV/AIDS	History, sexual and drug use counseling	General population
Household and recreational injury	Public education/legislation, gun control, use of Heimlich maneuver	General population

TABLE 2-8   Men 21 to 64 Years Quick Table: All Relevant Recommendations (*continued*)

Condition	Maneuver	Population
	"C" Recommendations	
Iron deficiency anemia	Routine hemoglobin	General population
Obesity	Community-based obesity prevention programs	General population
Prostate cancer	Digital rectal examination	Males > 50 years
Skin cancer	Counseling, skin self-examination	General population
Skin cancer	Counseling, sun block	General population
Testicular cancer	Physical exam or self-examination	Men
	"D" Recommendations	
Bladder cancer	Urine dipstick or cytology	General population
Cystic fibrosis	DNA analysis for carrier status	General population
Depression	General health questionnaire or Zung self-rating depression scale	General population
Diabetes mellitus	Blood glucose, fasting	Non-pregnant general population
Periodontal disease	Brushing with electric toothbrush	General population
Prostate cancer	Prostate specific antigen	Males > 50 years
	"E" Recommendations	
Lung cancer	Sputum cytology	General population
Tuberculosis	Mantoux tuberculin skin test	General population

Source: Canadian Task Force on Preventive Health Care (CTFPHC History/Methodology. http://www.ctfphc.org/ctfphc&methods.htm).

men 21 to 64 years of age. Each condition is listed by level of recommendation, the maneuver to be accomplished, and the population to which it applies.

U.S. Task Force on Preventive Services

In the 1980s, the Canadian Task Force Methodology was utilized by the U.S. Preventive Services Task Force with minimal modification. Presently it applied successfully by both task forces to evaluate the preventability of over two hundred conditions. These efforts have achieved international recognition as a basis to develop guidelines for clinical practice and public health policy for health services managers. The original U.S. Task Force document was published in 1989[36] and the second edition was published in 1996[37,38] while new updates are released periodically as recently as 2002. An example of the preventive services recommendations for ages 25 to 64 are presented in Table 2-9 and Table 2-10. Notably the leading causes of death are linked for the age group along with instructions for the general population, which includes screening, counseling, immunization, and chemoprophylaxis. Additionally, intervention for high-risk populations in the age group are also outlined. The rating system or the quality of the scientific evidence to be included in the preventive services recommendations is identical to the one used by the Canadian Task Force (Table 2-8). Also, Table 2-7 from the Canadian Task Force outlines the grades of recommendation, which are the same guides used by the U.S. Task Force.

For health services managers who meet or deal with health policy issues that are based on epidemiological measurement and risk factors, the *Clinicians Book of Preventive Services* provides specific prevention services to be implemented based on risk factors. Health services managers who wish to expand services must be aware or should consider the need to offer particular preventive services based on the knowledge of the individual's risk factors and understand the community population to know the magnitude and frequency of such risk factors in a community. The guidebook notes the detections of various risk factors (primary prevention) on preclinical conditions—screening (secondary prevention) so the management, policy, and, (it is hoped) the health outcomes, can be modified. Basically, these tables detail risk factors, grouped or targeted by specific epidemiological conditions. For example, age, gender, social conditions and living conditions, geographic, ethnic, occupational, recreational, environmental, residential,

TABLE 2-9 U.S. Preventive Services Task Force Recommendations for Ages 25 to 64—Intervention for the General Population

Screening	
	■ Blood pressure
	■ Height and weight
	■ Total blood cholesterol (men ages 35–65, women ages 45–65)
	■ Papanicolaou (Pap) test (women)*
	■ Fecal occult blood test** and/or sigmoidoscopy (≥ 50 years)
	■ Mammogram +/- clinical breast exam*** (women ages 50–69 years)
	■ Assess for problem drinking
	■ Rubella serology or vaccination hx**** (women of child-bearing age)

Counseling	
Substance Abuse	■ Tobacco cessation
	■ Avoid alcohol/drug use while driving, swimming, boating, etc.
Diet and Exercise	■ Limit fat and cholesterol; maintain caloric balance; emphasize grains, fruits, vegetables
	■ Adequate calcium intake (women)
	■ Regular physical activity‡
Injury Prevention	■ Lap/shoulder belts
	■ Motorcycle/bicycle/ATV helmets
	■ Smoke detector‡
	■ Safe storage/removal of firearms‡
Sexual Behavior	■ STD prevention: avoid high-risk behavior,‡ condoms/female barrier with spermicide‡
	■ Unintended pregnancy: contraception
Dental	■ Regular visits to dental care provider
	■ Floss, brush with fluoride toothpaste daily‡
Immunizations	■ Tetanus-diphtheria (Td) boosters
	■ Rubella**** (women of childbearing age)
Chemoprophylaxis	■ Multivitamin with folic acid (women planning or capable of pregnancy)

Source: Adapted from U.S. Preventive Services Task Force (Table 3. Ages 25–64 Years. http://hstat.nlm.nih.gov/hq/Hquest/screen/TextBrowse/t/1018901745700/s/44605).

*Women who are or have been sexually active and who have a cervix: q ≤ 3 years

**Annually

***Mammogram q1–2 years, or mammogram q1–2 years with annual clinical breast examination

****Serologic testing, documented vaccination history, and routine vaccination (preferably with MMR) are equally acceptable alternatives

‡The ability of clinician counseling to influence this behavior is unproven

TABLE 2-10 U.S. Preventive Services Task Force Recommendations for Ages 25 to 64—Intervention for High-Risk Populations

Population	Potential Interventions
High-risk sexual behavior	RPR/VDRL,[HR1] screen for gonorrhea (female),[HR2] HIV,[HR3] chlamydia (female),[HR4] hepatitis B vaccine,[HR5] hepatitis A vaccine[HR6]
Injection or street drug use	RPR/VDRL,[HR1] HIV screen,[HR3] hepatitis B vaccine,[HR5] hepatitis A vaccine,[HR6] PPD,[HR7] advice to reduce infection risk[HR8]
Low-income TB contacts, immigrants, alcoholics	PPD[HR7]
Native Americans/Alaska Natives	Hepatitis A vaccine,[HR6] PPD,[HR7] pneumococcal vaccine[HR9]
Travelers to developing countries	Hepatitis B vaccine,[HR5] hepatitis A vaccine[HR6]
Certain chronic medical conditions	PPD,[HR7] pneumococcal vaccine,[HR9] influenza vaccine[HR10]
Blood product recipients	HIV screen,[HR3] hepatitis B vaccine[HR5]
Susceptible to measles, mumps, or varicella	MMR,[HR11] varicella vaccine[HR12]
Institutionalized persons	Hepatitis A vaccine,[HR6] PPD,[HR7] pneumococcal vaccine,[HR9] influenza vaccine[HR10]
Health care/lab workers	Hepatitis B vaccine,[HR5] hepatitis A vaccine,[HR6] PPD,[HR7] influenza vaccine[HR10]
Family h/o skin cancer, fair skin, eyes, hair	Avoid excess/midday sun, use protective clothing[‡HR13]
Previous pregnancy with neural tube defect	Folic acid 4.0 mg[HR14]

	High-Risk Definitions
HR1	Persons who exchange sex for money or drugs, and sex partners with other STDs (including HIV) and sexual contacts of persons with active syphilis. Clinicians should also consider local epidemiology.
HR2	Women who exchange sex for money or drugs, or who have had repeated episodes of gonorrhea. Clinicians should also consider local epidemiology.
HR3	Men who had sex with men after 1975, past or present injection drug use, persons who exchange sex for money or drugs and their sex partners, injection drug-using, bisexual, or HIV-positive sex partner currently or in the past, blood transfusion during 1978–1985, persons seeking treatment for STDs. Clinicians should also consider local epidemiology.

TABLE 2-10 U.S. Preventive Services Task Force Recommendations for Ages 25 to 64—Intervention for High-Risk Populations *(continued)*

Population	Potential Interventions
High-Risk Definitions (continued)	
HR4	Sexually active women with multiple risk factors including: history of STD, new or multiple sex partners, nonuse or inconsistent use of barrier contraceptives, cervical ectopy. Clinicians should also consider local epidemiology.
HR5	Blood product recipients (including hemodialysis patients), persons with frequent occupational exposure to blood or blood products, men who have sex with men, injection drug users and their sex partners, persons with multiple recent sex partners, persons with other STDs (including HIV), travelers to countries with endemic hepatitis B.
HR6	Persons living in, traveling to, or working in areas where the disease is endemic and where periodic outbreaks occur (e.g., countries with high or intermediate endemicity, certain Alaska Native, Pacific Island, Native American, and religious communities), men who have sex with men, injection or street drug users. Consider institutionalized persons and workers in these institutions, military personnel, and day-care, hospital, and laboratory workers. Clinicians should also consider local epidemiology.
HR7	HIV positive, close contacts of persons with known or suspected TB, health care workers, persons with medical factors associated with TB, immigrants from countries with high TB prevalence, medically underserved low-income populations (including homeless), alcoholics, injection drug users, and residents of long-term care facilities.
HR8	Persons who continue to inject drugs.
HR9	Immunocompetent institutionalized persons aged ≥50 years and immunocompetent persons with certain medical conditions, including chronic cardiac or pulmonary disease, diabetes mellitus, and anatomic asplenia. Immunocompetent persons who live in high-risk environments or social settings (e.g., certain Native American and Alaska Native populations).

TABLE 2-10 U.S. Preventive Services Task Force Recommendations for Ages 25 to 64—Intervention for High-Risk Populations *(continued)*

Population	Potential Interventions
High-Risk Definitions (continued)	
HR10	Annual vaccinations of residents of chronic care facilities persons with chronic cardiopulmonary disorders, metabolic diseases (including diabetes mellitus), hemoglobinopathies, immunosuppression, or renal dysfunction, and health care providers for high-risk patients.
HR11	Persons born after 1956 who lack evidence of immunity to measles or mumps (e.g., documented receipt of live vaccine on or after the first birthday, laboratory evidence of immunity, or a history of physician-diagnosed measles or mumps).
HR12	Healthy adults without a history of chicken pox or previous immunization. Consider serologic testing for presumed susceptible adults.
HR13	Persons with a family or personal history of skin cancer, a large number of moles, atypical moles, poor tanning ability, or light skin, hair, and eye color.
HR14	Women with previous pregnancy affected by neural tube defect who are planning pregnancy.

Source: Adapted from U.S. Preventive Services Task Force (Table 3. Ages 25–64 Years. http://hstat.nlm.nih.gov/hq/Hquest/screen/TextBrowse/t/1018901745700/s/44605).

‡The ability of clinician counseling to influence this behavior is unproven

substance abuse, personal medical history, family history, sexual history, and reproductive history. Clearly, these multiple target conditions can be classified by the health field concept model of lifestyle, environment, biology, and the health care delivery system. Table 2-11 gives examples using the risk factors, categories of geography and ethnic background for all ages by target condition, preventive service, and/or referral and the health policy strategy.[39]

TABLE 2-11 Risk Factor Category: Geographic and Ethnic Background—All Ages

Risk Factor	Prevention Target Condition	Preventive Service and/or Referral	Health Policy Strategy
African, African-American, Southeast Asian, Middle Eastern, or Mediterranean ethnicity	Hemoglobinopathy (pregnant women)	Hemoglobin electrophoresis	Health Care Delivery System
African-American, Mexican-American, American Indian, Alaska Native ethnicity, immigrants from developing countries	Lead poisoning (children 1 to 5 years)	Blood lead level; residential lead hazard control	Environmental
African-American, Hispanic, Pacific Island ethnicity (also see low-income)	Tuberculosis	PPD	Lifestyle
American Indian, Hispanic, African-American ethnicity	Diabetes mellitus	Fasting glucose; obesity screening; nutritional counseling; exercise counseling	Lifestyle Biology
Immigrants from areas with high prevalence of tuberculosis, hepatitis B, or HIV (includes most countries in Africa, Asia, or Latin America)	Tuberculosis; hepatitis B; STD/HIV	PPD; hepatitis B vaccine; STD/HIV counseling; STD/HIV screening	Environment Lifestyle
African-American ethnicity	Glaucoma (≥40 years); prostate cancer	Ophthalmology referral for screening; digital rectal exam[*]; prostate specific antigen[*]	Biology Lifestyle Environment

TABLE 2-11 Risk Factor Category: Geographic and Ethnic Background—All Ages (continued)

Risk Factor	Prevention Target Condition	Preventive Service and/or Referral	Health Policy Strategy
Asian Indians who use chewing tobacco or betel nut	Oral cancer	Oral exam; cessation counseling; regular dental exam	Lifestyle
Caucasian females	Post-menopausal osteoporosis	Nutritional counseling; exercise counseling; smoking cessation counseling; post-menopausal hormone replacement therapy	Lifestyle Biology

Source: Adapted from *Clinician's Handbook of Preventive Services*, 2d ed. (Washington, D.C.: Office of Disease Prevention and Health Promotion, Agency for Health Care and Quality, U.S. Preventive Services Task Force Put Prevention into Practice, 1998), 474.

*Whether these procedures diminish the morbidity and mortality associated with prostate cancer is controversial.

Summary

This chapter examined the role of epidemiology in health policy. It argued that the adoption of the epidemiological perspective by all involved in health policy making—including health care managers—would lead to a reduction in today's major cripplers and killers.

This impact on the population's health will come through careful analysis of prevalent health problems. The analysis should be supported by an inherently prevention-oriented conceptualization (or framework) of health and illness. Three examples or models of such an approach were reviewed in this chapter.

References

1. R. C. Coile, Jr., *New Century Healthcare: Strategies for Providers, Purchasers, and Plans* (Chicago: Health Administration Press, 2000), 225–249.
2. C. S. Lesser and P. B. Ginsburg, "Back to the Future? New Cost and Access Challenges Emerge: Initial Findings from HSC's Recent Site Visits," *Issue Brief Findings from HSC*, no. 35 (February 2001):4.
3. J. Harkey, "Industry Focus, Is the HMO Concept out of Steam? Recent Enrollment Trends in Four Southeastern States," *Georgia Managed Care* 8, no. 4 (2000):2.
4. P. K. Halverson et al., *Managed Care & Public Health* (Gaithersburg, Md.: Aspen Publishers, Inc., 1998), 48.
5. Coile, *New Century Healthcare*, 227.
6. S. T. Roussos and S. B. Fawcett, *A Review of Collaborative Partnerships as a Strategy for Improving Community Health: Annual Review Public Health* 21 (2000):369–402.
7. H. A. Sultz and K. M. Young, *Health Care USA: Understanding Its Organization and Delivery*, 2d ed. (Gaithersburg, Md.: Aspen Publishers, Inc., 1999).
8. M. A. Ibrahim, *Epidemiology and Health Policy* (Gaithersburg, Md.: Aspen Publishers, Inc., 1985), 6.
9. Sultz and Young, *Health Care USA*, 372–375.
10. A. B. Ford, "Epidemiological Priorities as a Basis for Health Policy," *Bulletin of the New York Academy of Medicine* 54, no. 1 (1978):10–22.
11. L. Gordis, "Challenges to Epidemiology in the Coming Decade," *American Journal of Epidemiology* 112, no. 2 (1980):319.
12. M. Terris, "Epidemiology as a Guide to Health Policy," *Annual Review of Public Health, 1980* (1980):323–344.
13. Ford, "Epidemiological Priorities as a Basis for Health Policy," 10–13.
14. Gordis, "Challenges to Epidemiology in the Coming Decade," 319.
15. K. L. White, "Teaching Epidemiologic Concepts as the Scientific Basis for Understanding Problems of Organizing and Evaluating Health Services," *International Journal of Health Services* 2, no. 4 (1972):525–529.

16. M. Jenicek and R. H. Fletcher, "Epidemiology for Canadian Medical Students—Desirable Attitudes, Knowledge, and Skills," *International Journal of Epidemiology* 6, no. 1 (1977):69–72.

17. C. W. Blair, "Teaching Community Diagnosis to Medical Students," *Journal of Community Health* 6, no. 1 (1980):54–64.

18. M. A. Faghih, "Epidemiology and the Training of Physicians," *International Journal of Epidemiology* 6, no. 4 (1977):331–333.

19. S. Glouberman, and J. Millar, "Evolution of the Determinants of Health, Health Policy, and Health Information Systems in Canada," *American Journal of Public Health* 93, no. 3 (2003):388–392.

20. G. E. A. Dever, *Epidemiology in Health Services Management* (Gaithersburg, Md.: Aspen Publishers, Inc., 1984):2–5, 27–38.

21. H. L. Blum et al., *Notes on Comprehensive Planning for Health* (San Francisco: American Public Health Association, Western Regional Office, 1968).

22. H. L. Laframboise, "Health Policy: Breaking the Problem Down in More Manageable Segments," *Canadian Medical Association Journal* 108 (February 3, 1973):388–393.

23. M. Lalonde, *A New Perspective on the Health of Canadians* (Ottawa: Health and Welfare Canada, 1974), 76.

24. Laframboise, "Health Policy," 388.

25. Lalonde, *A New Perspective on the Health of Canadians*, 76.

26. G. E. A. Dever, "Dimensions of Environmental Health" (Paper presented at the annual convention of the Georgia Public Health Association: Macon, Ga., 1974), 11.

27. Lalonde, *A New Perspective on the Health of Canadians*, 76.

28. J. J. Cohen, "Collaborative Care: A New Model for a New Century," *Academic Medicine* 75, no. 2 (2000):107–112.

29. Cohen, "Collaborative Care," 107–112.

30. R. A. Harvan, *Faculty Development: Facilitating Cross-Professional Collaboration in Education, Research and Clinical Service* (Washington, D.C.: Association of Academic Health Centers, 2001), 7.

31. R. D. Lasker, *Medicine & Public Health: The Power of Collaboration* (Chicago: Health Administration Press, 1997).

32. American Academy of Family Practice, *Clinician's Handbook of Preventive Services: Put Prevention into Practice*, 2d ed. (McLean, Va.: U.S. Public Health Services, International Medical Publishing, Inc., 1997), 524.

33. Health and Welfare Canada, *The Periodic Health Examination Monogram* (report of a task force to the Conference of Deputy Ministers of Health, Ottawa, 1980).

34. Health and Welfare Canada, *The Periodic Health Examination Monogram*, 15.

35. Health and Welfare Canada, *The Periodic Health Examination Monogram*, 96.

36. U.S. Preventive Services Task Force, *Guide to Clinical Preventive Services*, 1st ed. (Washington, D.C.: Office of Disease Prevention and Health Promotion, 1989).

37. U.S. Preventive Services Task Force, *Guide to Clinical Preventive Services*, 2d ed. (Washington, D.C.: Office of Disease Prevention and Health Promotion, U.S. Government Printing Office, 1996).

38. U.S. Preventive Services Task Force Put Prevention into Practice, *Clinician's Handbook of Preventive Services*, 2d ed. (Washington, D.C.: Office of Disease Prevention and Health Promotion, Agency for Healthcare and Quality, 1998).

39. U.S. Preventive Services Task Force Put Prevention into Practice, *Clinician's Handbook of Preventive Services*, 474.

3

Epidemiology—
Population Health
in Health Services
Management

Uses of Epidemiology

Epidemiology is a discipline that has evolved into relatively specialized methods to investigate disease causation and brings to bear, according to the needs of the moment, specific knowledge and special skills from many other sciences. With some justice, epidemiology is called a method rather than an independent science.[1]

Epidemiologic principles and methods can be applied to a wide range of problems in many fields. These principles and methods relate to the description of human populations, to the investigation of the processes beneath the surface, to the interpretation and analysis of such information, and to the uses to which this data can be put. Epidemiology has also been defined as "a means of learning, or asking questions . . . and getting answers that lead to further questions."[2] Whereas the study of disease distribution and causation remains central to epidemiology, the techniques of epidemiology have a wider application that also relates to wellness and health services. In the health field, epidemiology has three main uses: etiological, clinical, and administrative.[3]

Etiological Use

"Classical" epidemiology primarily concerns the search for causes and risk factors that contribute to health and disease patterns. In cooperation with the other medical sciences—such as biochemistry, physiology, microbiology, and pathology—epidemiology contributes to the understanding of the natural history of diseases and of their determinants and deterrents. It also informs many social sciences that contribute to the knowledge and nature of the health of populations and the determinants of disease. As discussed in Chapter 1, an expanded and multifaceted concept of causality allows epidemiologists to determine risk factors; that is, to estimate individuals' risks and chances of developing a state of wellness or disease.

Clinical Use

Epidemiology is used, in the words of Morris, to help complete the picture in a clinical setting and to aid in the clarification of clinical syndromes.[4] As the International Epidemiological Association puts it:

> A [medical] student's understanding of anatomy, physiology, and biochemistry will be seriously deficient if he does not appreciate the variability of physical, physiological, biochemical, immunological, and other attributes in the general population and understand that it is rarely possible to draw a clear line between the normal and the pathological. In the clinical disciplines, knowledge of prevalence, etiology, and prognosis derived from epidemiological research has obvious implications for the diagnosis and management of individual patients and of their families.[5]

Recently, health professionals and in particular health services managers recognized the importance of a broader perspective, which includes populations in communities. Such efforts are presented as population-based health, and managers need to embrace this approach to be effective and compete in the marketplace.

Administrative Use

Epidemiology can and should be used for purposes of health services management. It contributes to diagnoses within a community about the presence, nature, and distribution of health and disease. It provides a means to monitor the health of a population as well as chart changes over time and among places.

Fos and Fine, Morris, and Park identified several additional uses of epidemiology,[6,7,8] five of which extend epidemiology beyond the search for causes of disease and bring it closer to the day-to-day concerns of health services management and policy. For example, the evaluation of risk, identification of syndromes, understanding of the natural history of disease, and identification of causes as they relate to the disease process are distinct uses of epidemiology. Other uses that health services managers are more likely to be concerned about are the change in disease patterns and population change, a community diagnosis, plans, and evaluation.

Changes in Diseases and Population Patterns

Winston Churchill said, "The farther back you look, the farther forward you can see." The use of epidemiology relates to the aspect of the study of disease in human population. These are fluctuations in the health and disease patterns in a community over long and short periods of time. For example, the first contribution of epidemiology to the study of coronary heart disease was that it was an "epidemic." As old diseases (e.g., small pox) are conquered, new ones (e.g., Legionnaires' disease, Lassa fever, AIDS) are identified, in which epidemiology plays a major role. The study of trends of diseases could lead to identification of emergent health problems and their correlates.

Community Diagnosis

Community diagnosis generally refers to the identification and quantification of health problems in a community in terms of mortality and morbidity rates and ratios and the identification of their correlates for the purpose of defining those individuals or groups at risk or those in need of health care, and it establishes priorities for disease control and prevention. Quantification of morbidity and mortality can serve as benchmarks for the evaluation of health services for the future. This could be a source of new knowledge about disease distribution, causation, and prevention. Epidemiology therefore is described as a "diagnostic tool" of community medicine.

Planning and Evaluation

Planning is essential for a rational allocation of limited resources. For example, in developing countries, too many hospitals are built and equipped without knowledge of the particular disease problems in the community. Some solutions to this include mapping out the facilities for medical care (e.g., number of hospital beds required for patients with specific diseases, with appropriate health workforce allocation); built-in facilities for preventive services (e.g., screening programs, immunization campaigns, provision of sanitary services); and laboratory resources for research. Evaluation is an important tool in epidemiology, as any measures taken to control and prevent a disease must be followed by an appraisal for effectiveness.

Through the use of epidemiological principles and methods, health services managers can determine which diseases are of major importance in their population. Furthermore, using the causal data available from classical epidemiological studies, they can identify individuals at risk—their potential market or target population. Epidemiology thus supplies many of the facts needed for the management and planning of population health services and for their evaluation.

Thus, epidemiology information by public health planners and health care managers can be a guide for services and programs. Of particular importance to the population-based perspective of health services management is the analysis of populations in communities while still marketing the individual components of a patient's admission to a hospital or clinic. Fos and Fine note also that epidemiological data can be used to measure or analyze the following managerial problems: planning, policy formulation, managed care, health promotion, marketing, public health intervention, insurance, health education, quality measurement, survey methods, and effectiveness measures.[9]

Health Services Management

Health care comprises collective and organized action and involves the coordination of interrelated parts of an organization to achieve the objectives embodied in providing care.[10] Management is the process that oversees the production of services—in this case, health.[11]

The "Functional Approach"

Management is a subject of controversy. Most management textbooks, and most classical organizational theorists, adopt a functional approach to defining the process. Five functions that are typically listed to examine the work of managers in terms of functions or areas of activity are planning, organization, directing, coordinating, and controlling.[12,13,14]

Planning   Planning is a primary function of management. Decisions taken well in advance smoothly expedite the process. The aim of planning is to achieve a coordinated and consistent set of operations toward desired objectives.

Organizing   This combines people and resources into a unit capable of direction toward organizational objectives. The basic objective of organization is the development of a framework called the formal organizational structure.

Directing   Once the planning is done and the organization is created to put things into effect, the next function of management is to perform the required work: personnel functions, supervision, leadership, motivation, and communications.

Coordinating   This is the assembly of people in a synchronous manner so that they function harmoniously in the attainment of organization objectives.

Controlling   This is defined as regulation of activities in accordance with the requirement of plans. It is a form of surveillance as it corrects activities of people and things in an organization to ensure that objectives and plans are accomplished.

The "Process" Approach

Management can be subdivided into component processes: technical, administrative, and political.[15] The technical process specifies the actions that will be accomplished. The administrative process enables the actions to be taken and is concerned with the methods of carrying them out. The political process involves doing whatever is necessary to achieve the objectives of the organization by mobilizing support for the actions. Progress toward an action blends the necessary objective or technical evidence with the equally essential administrative and political elements.[16] The process-oriented approach to the analysis of management has several advantages:

- It reflects the dynamic and political nature of management much more than does the functional approach, involving managers continually in a negotiation process with the organization's internal and external influencers.[17]

- It allows the examination of any level of management, which extends from a country's government to the smallest organization. At any level, organized action results from a blend of the technical, administrative, and political process.

- It remains consistent with a comprehensive, systemic analysis of a given action. Management and planning for health programs or institutions without full consideration of their interdependencies with other parts of society ignore the fact that the programs or facilities are a part of a larger system.

Epidemiology and Decision Making

Regardless which approach is adopted, what ties together the functions or the subprocesses is decision making, the essence of management. Furthermore, decisions will always be made on the basis of some "information." Managers within any system function as receivers and perceivers of information or signals from the environment, as decoders of this information, as deciders of courses of action, and as composers and transmitters of messages designed to influence others in the system to act according to these decisions.[18] This information might be "hard" (formal) or "soft" (more or less subjective). In either case, the managers will process some kind of information on which to base their decisions. The courses of action they determine from those decisions are translated into some organized action. The use of epidemiology in health services management is to supply some of this "hard" information as a basis for decision making.

The rest of this chapter explains how an expanded comprehensive planning process provides a framework for managerial decisions. The management process, examined from either the functional or the process approach, operates within the overall framework of the plan. It is through the planning process that the contributions of epidemiology to health services management are analyzed.

The Planning Process

In its usual, everyday meaning, planning refers to the design of a desired future and of effective ways to bring it about.[19] The contention here, however, is that planning can be considered in a much broader perspective so as to incorporate policy making at the societal level as well as program management in an organizational setting. Planning is the guidance of change within a social system,[20] the process by which present decisions are related to future desired results.[21] It aims to enrich decision making. Its fundamental purposes are to extend the depth of knowledge and to broaden the vision of those responsible for decision making at any level. Defined in this way, planning is an action-oriented process by which the institution adapts to changes in both its internal constituency and its external environment.

As stated previously, decision making is the essence of management, but it takes place in an arena of uncertainty. As organizational theorists demonstrate convincingly, the decision-making process rarely corresponds to the classical, rational model. To the contrary, it essentially is a process of "short-run adaptive reactions,"[22] "satisficing" instead of "maximizing,"[23] a "muddling through,"[24] or "disjointed incrementalism."[25] Decision making is highly "reactive-adaptive." It is the paradox of decision making that effective action is born of reaction. Only when organizations as open systems take in information from the environment and react to changing conditions can they act on that same environment to reduce uncertainty and increase discretionary flexibility.[26] Planning, as conceived here, is a process of information collection from the environment and putting it to use in the development and elaboration of the organization's actions and activities. For a health-related institution, epidemiology provides a method, within the planning process, to collect this information and guide the implementation of the activities or programs.

Levels of Planning

This analysis is based on the concept of three levels of planning: 1.) normative or policy planning, 2.) strategic or comprehensive planning, and 3.) tactical/operational or program planning. Figure 3-1 illustrates the interrelation of these three planning levels. Chapter 2 dealt with policy planning, so the focus here turns more particularly to strategic and tactical planning, with which health managers are directly concerned. More material on policy planning is available from other sources.[27,28,29,30]

Strategic Planning   Strategic planning provides a general framework for organizational action. This process aims to establish the entity's principal objectives and priorities. At the strategic level, long-range goals are set and possible means of achieving them are considered.

  As indicated in Figure 3-1, strategic planning deals with the examination of possible activities to carry out the anticipations of society. Specific system structures are established, effective outcome indicators are defined, and instrumentals or means to operate institutions are created. The emphasis is on predicting the future behavior of external variables and the formulation of alternative courses of action in light of expected events.[31]

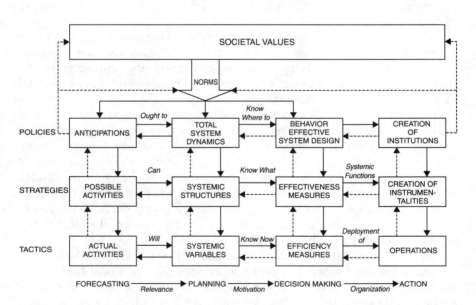

FIGURE 3-1   A Paradigm for Planning. *Source:* Adapted from *Technological Planning and Social Futures* by Erich Jantsch (London: Associated Business Programmes, 1972), 16.

Strategic planning models quite commonly focus on similar approaches and recent contributions tend to recognize the necessity of such planning but also realize it is not the end point of an organization's function.[32,33,34]

Operational Planning   This final level develops the detailed plans to carry out the strategies for some of the priorities that were considered at the previous planning level. Operational planning describes an iterative process in which expectations about when, where, and how activities will occur are set and in which results are monitored, measured, and redirected when deviations from the expressed targets are detected.

The important point is that the operational plan must be implemented. To be capable of implementation, it must fit within the operational (production) framework of the organization and it must influence how its resources are assigned. "The acid test for the success of health planning is its ability to influence the allocation of resources so that what is planned for comes to pass."[35,36]

Planning for Health

Planning, at whatever level, is not carried out in a vacuum. At all points it is permeated by social values and by the prevalent paradigm or framework of health. This is illustrated in Figures 3-2 and 3-3.

Figure 3-2, the traditional planning model for medical care, pays no attention to societal values. "Norms" and "Anticipations" depend only upon the technological ability to accomplish something. Furthermore, the concept of health system activities ignores lifestyle and environmental "aspects" of health and disease.

In contrast, Figure 3-3, based on the holistic (ecological) framework of health described previously, indicates that people value a high quality of life, the opportunity to be productive, wellness, and freedom from sickness. The associated norms of reduced morbidity, disability, and mortality and of increased levels of wellness become expectations, as shown in the model. At the policy level, anticipations of high-level wellness proceed dynamically through appropriate functions toward being, and the achievement of a healthier society. This holistic design leads to the creation of an institution called a community health care system.

In the second phase of planning, strategies that closely parallel the policy phase are determined. For example, anticipations of a healthier society evolve to strategies of physical exercise, nutritional awareness, stress management, and self-responsibility. At that operational phase of the planning process, the activities include running, swimming, cycling, consuming healthful foods and vitamins, and developing coping skills. These put high-level wellness into day-to-day life and point out the need for individ-

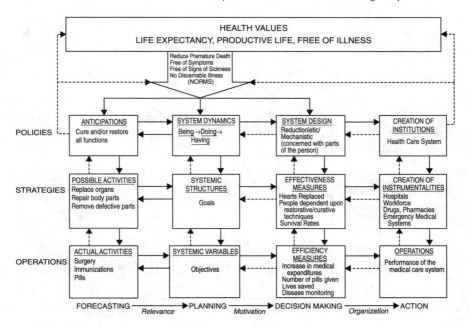

FIGURE 3-2 The Traditional Model for Medical Care. *Source:* Adapted from *Technological Planning and Social Futures* by Erich Jantsch (London: Associated Business Programmes, 1972), 16.

uals' responsibility and authority in the management of their health. Development of a health care system that reflects these values generates greater potential to meet the needs of society.

Population-Based Health—A Planning Blueprint

To implement population-based health planning, a blueprint has been developed by Canadian researchers and government agencies.[37,38,39] They outline six core components for the plans and actions of population-based health planning.[40,41] The six core components are 1.) Theory, 2.) Policy, 3.) Evidence, 4.) Marketing, 5.) Mobilization, and 6.) Institutionalization. This blueprint model is shown in Figure 3-4, which highlights the six components and identifies short-term, mid-term, and long-term outcomes, respectively labeled "building blocks," "outreach," and "pay-off." To the health

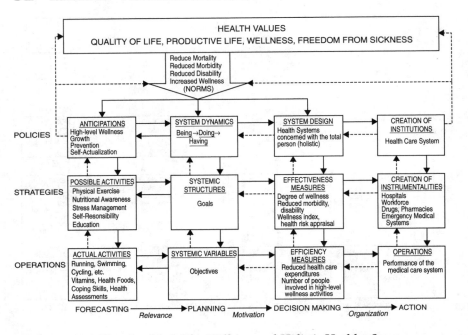

FIGURE 3-3 A Planning Model for Wellness and Holistic Health. *Source:* Adapted from *Technological Planning and Social Futures* by Erich Jantsch (London: Associated Business Programmes, 1972), 16.

services manager all three time frames are critical; however, the utilization of basic epidemiological measurement is most apparent at the building blocks stage (i.e., short-term objectives). These short-term objectives are tied to the six components, which reveal the needs, skill, and knowledge necessary to implement the blueprint for population health. Thus, the managerial epidemiologists and the marketing and planning staff can gain by utilizing this blueprint and applying it to their organizational structure. For instance, theory will increase the basic knowledge of the determinants of health through the research methods typical of epidemiological analysis: case reports, case series, ecological studies, cross-sections, case-control, cohorts, and randomized clinical trials.

The order of these methods suggests an hierarchal structure of weak to strong evidence-based studies. Policy analysis is basic to "how to use the population health approach." Evidence-based population health planning

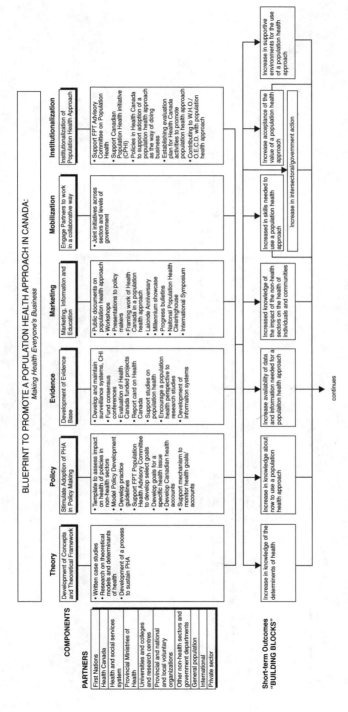

FIGURE 3-4 Blueprint to Promote a Population Health Approach in Canada. *Source:* Health Canada, Population Health Directorate, Population and Public Health, "Taking Action on Population Health," Monograph (Ottawa, 1999), 26.

FIGURE 3-4 (continued)

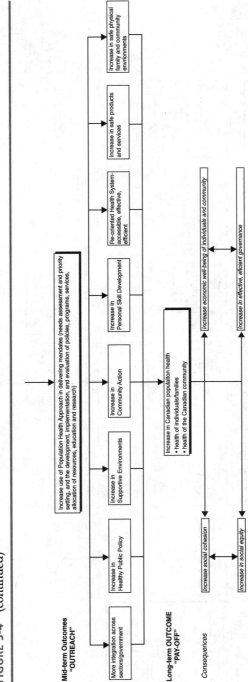

is absolutely critical and thus is discussed in a subsequent chapter. At present, it is sufficient to understand that the health services managers must recognize the need for data and information to make informal but sound statistical, program, planning, and policy decisions.

Marketing, discussed in a subsequent chapter, is the conduit to improve positioning in the competitive marketplace. To foster these first four components, the fifth component—mobilization (engage partners to work collaboratively)—is the basic building block of a successful implementation for planning the health blueprint model. Managers must acquire the knowledge and train all levels of staff in the skills required to implement the process. Finally, institutionalization of the process to increase the acceptance of the approach and implementation allows for the development of supportive environments.

These short-term goals, if successful, result in mandates for doing needs assessments, establishing priorities, and developing and implementing the evaluation of programs, services, and policies. The eventual outcome is the appropriate and fair allocation of resources and realizing the needs for further evaluation and research. The goal called "pay off" is the improved health status of the population. The individuals in the clinics will also benefit, but the main thrust will be to improve the population within the communities that the institutions serve. This is what health services managers must initiate if they are to be effective in program delivery and competitive in allocating resources to the appropriate problems.

Population Health and Health Services Management

A recurring theme of this book is the emphasis on populations in communities and the shift in focus away from individuals in clinics. This theme is known as population-based health or population-based medicine. Given the shifts in other aspects of health care—tertiary prevention to primary and secondary prevention, fragmented care to continuity in care, physician provider to team provider, in-patient care to ambulatory home care, and anecdotal decisions to evidence-based (public health and medicine) decisions—a population health perspective is essential to analyze management and health services utilization problems and issues.

The population health approach is composed of several key elements and is built on the long-standing concepts of traditional public health, community-oriented primary care, health promotion, disease prevention, and basic community health. Like many of the concepts detailed in previous chapters, the population health approach recognizes that many variables, factors, and conditions contribute to a health/holistic/wellness perspective. As typical of the models of health policy and prevention, the focus is on improving the health status of the population so as to influence a reduction in the inequities in health care among population groups. Today health services managers see more the need for such an approach to analyze the issues and problems related to their responsibilities and to the institution's viability. Therefore, to meet these requirements, the population key planning elements are outlined in Figure 3-3.[42] This approach can be utilized and applied by managers to help in making policy and developing program plans. Other uses include a blueprint for training staff to reinforce the population health approach and further, for evaluations to provide a benchmark by which other population health measures can be assessed. Such a model utilizes many of the basics of an epidemiological perspective, and the health services manager will recognize that epidemiology interfaces with many of the key elements and the associated actions. The eight key elements are as follows:

1. **Focus on the health of populations.** *Population health assesses health status inequities over the life span at the population level.* This element introduces the issue or concern, explaining its connection to health and the population(s) primarily affected by it.[43]

2. **Address the determinants of health and their interactions.** *Population health measures and analyzes the full spectrum of factors—and their interactions—known to influence and contribute to health.* Commonly referred to as the determinants of health, these factors include social, economic, and physical environments, childhood development, personal health practices, individual capacity and coping skills, human biology, and health services. This element "frames" the health issue in terms of how it came about—what factors or determinants contributed to its emergence or worsening, and how far upstream these are located. This forms the basis for developing population health interventions.[44]

3. **Base decisions on evidence.** *Population health uses "evidence-based decision making." Evidence on health status, the determinants of health, and the effectiveness of interventions is used to assess health, identify priorities, and develop strategies to improve health.* This element defines evidence-based decision making and outlines the need to support findings and recommendations with systematic, empirical evidence and/or cogent argument. It includes information about the types of evidence available and their strength, relevance, and possible weaknesses.[45]

4. **Increase upstream investments.** *The potential for improved population health is maximized by directing increased efforts and investments "upstream" to maintain health and address the root causes of health and illness. This will help to create a more balanced and sustainable health system.* This element explains the options for interventions considered and how choices are made both in terms of addressing the more immediate causes and at deeper levels (broad determinants) over the long term—for example, in upstream investments (protection, prevention, health promotion, and action on the determinants of health) and downstream investments (treatment, rehabilitation).[46]

5. **Apply multiple strategies.** *Population health integrates activities across the wide range of interventions that makes up the health continuum: from health care to prevention, protection, promotion, and action on the determinants of health.* This element answers the question, "How much should we take on?" It then frames the selected actions/strategies and describes in what combinations, at which levels, by whom, at what sites, and over what time frame they will be implemented.[47]

6. **Collaborate across sectors and levels.** *Population health calls for shared responsibility and accountability for health outcomes with multiple sectors and levels whose activities directly or indirectly impact health or the factors known to influence it.* This element describes the partnership-building process and what it takes to make it work. It includes who is represented at the table and how they contribute. It also explains how the group is structured and organized and people's roles, responsibilities, and relationships. This includes leadership, management/coordination, processes, mechanisms, and communication modes.[48]

7. **Employ mechanisms for public involvement.** *Population health promotes citizen participation in health improvement. Citizens are provided opportunities to contribute meaningfully to the development of health priorities and strategies and the review of health-related outcomes.* This element outlines how the public is involved at different stages of the initiative (e.g., needs identification, planning, delivery, evaluation), including their roles (e.g., advisory committee members, peer helpers) and the processes by which they are engaged (e.g., surveys, focus groups, community forums).[49]

8. **Demonstrate accountability for health outcomes.** *Population health focuses on health outcomes and determining the degree of*

change that can actually be attributed to interventions. This element identifies the accountability tools needed to capture and report on changes (both intended/actual and unintended) in the health status of populations and in the determinants of health.[50]

A comprehensive and thorough discussion of these eight elements is included in a significant treatise on population health.[51] Table 3-1 summarizes these eight key elements for initiating and applying the population health model in a health services setting.

TABLE 3-1 Summary Table of Population Health Key Elements

Key Element	Actions
1. **Focus on the Health of Populations**	■ Determine indicators to measure health status ■ Measure and analyze population health status and health status inequities to identify health issues ■ Assess contextual conditions, characteristics, and trends
2. **Address the Determinants of Health and Their Interactions**	■ Determine indicators to measure the determinants of health ■ Measure and analyze the determinants of health, and their interactions, to link health issues to their determinants
3. **Base Decisions on Evidence**	■ Use best evidence at all stages of policy and program development ■ Explain criteria for including or excluding evidence ■ Draw on a variety of data ■ Generate data through mixed research methods ■ Identify and assess effective interventions ■ Disseminate research findings and facilitate policy uptake
4. **Increase Upstream Investments**	■ Apply criteria to select priorities for investment ■ Balance short- and long-term investments ■ Influence investments in other sectors
5. **Apply Multiple Strategies**	■ Identify scope of action for interventions ■ Take action on the determinants of health and their interactions ■ Implement strategies to reduce inequities in health status between population groups ■ Apply a comprehensive mix of interventions and strategies ■ Apply interventions that address health issues in an integrated way

TABLE 3-1   Summary Table of Population Health Key Elements *(continued)*

Key Element	Actions
5. **Apply Multiple Strategies**	■ Apply methods to improve health over the life span ■ Act in multiple settings ■ Establish a coordinating mechanism to guide interventions
6. **Collaborate across Sectors and Levels**	■ Engage partners early on to establish shared values and alignment of purpose ■ Establish concrete objectives and focus on visible results ■ Identify and support a champion ■ Invest in the alliance-building process ■ Generate political support and build on positive factors in the policy environment ■ Share leadership, accountability, and rewards among partners
7. **Employ Mechanisms for Public Involvement**	■ Capture the public's interest ■ Contribute to health literacy ■ Apply public involvement strategies that link to overarching purpose
8. **Demonstrate Accountability for Health Outcomes**	■ Construct a results-based accountability framework ■ Ascertain baseline measures and set targets for health improvement ■ Institutionalize effective evaluation systems ■ Promote the use of health impact assessment tools ■ Publicly report results

Source: Health Canada, Population and Public Health Branch, Strategic Policy Directorate, 2001 draft. "The Population Health Template: Key Elements and Actions That Define a Population Health Approach," monograph, 7.

The health services manager, by using this population health model for planning, can next embrace typical management issues that focus on epidemiological problems and correlate them to the population health model. Building the population health approach into the management of health services will require a thorough understanding of the eight population health key elements and the realization that these elements are keyed to several significant management issue questions. To manage health services the "population health way," it is essential to outline the six steps in management issues that reflect epidemiological consideration. Table 3-2 provides a fairly detailed overview of the relationship of the steps in issues related to health services management and the corresponding population considerations.[52]

TABLE 3-2 Key Considerations in Managing Health Services the "Population Health Way": An Epidemiological Perspective

Epidemiological Perspective Management Issues	Population Health Considerations
1. **Identifying problems or opportunities** *"What would we need to move on or respond to?"*	▪ Collect population health data ▪ Analyze data considering wider range of risk factors and conditions, not just those that immediately present themselves
2. **Defining the population health issues** *"What is the issue?"*	▪ Describe how the health issue is distributed in the population (time, place, and person) ▪ Identify: 　▪ Determinants/causes of health issue 　▪ The risk factors/conditions for the population 　▪ How general health can be promoted 　▪ Whether or not health problems can be prevented 　▪ Needs of people/families with health problem ▪ Assess capacity to change (within government agencies and with partners) ▪ Identify need for taking action (and role of government agencies and existing/potential partners)
3. **Assessing significance** *"Is the issue significant enough to merit further work?"*	▪ Work with and consult stakeholders—draw on their knowledge and expertise ▪ Analyze population health data
4. **Analyzing existing intervention strategies and identifying options for additional/new strategies**	▪ Work with and consult stakeholders—effective population health depends on including perspectives from many disciplines and fields ▪ Gather and assess information on the community's situation and strengths (individual, family, local community, provincial, national)
"Is the issue being addressed sufficiently and appropriately by existing strategies?" and	▪ Review evidence of "what works" ▪ Identify possible strategies such as health promotion, health protection, health care, and those based in nonhealth sectors
"What alternative or additional strategies would be appropriate?"	▪ Consider strategies directed at individuals/family/community and systems/sectors/society ▪ Select strategies based on best possible impact on health of the population ▪ Develop an evaluation framework for selected strategies to ensure effective evaluation of strategies and to contribute to a broader knowledge base

TABLE 3-2 Key Considerations in Managing Health Services the "Population Health Way": An Epidemiological Perspective *(continued)*

Epidemiological Perspective Management Issues	*Population Health Considerations*
5. **Implementing the interventions/ strategies** *"How should they be implemented?"*	■ Work with and consult stakeholders, recruit new partners if needed ■ Assess and change resource allocation as needed ■ Maintain ongoing communication with partners/stakeholders ■ Carry out an evaluation of activities and adjustment of strategies as needed
6. **Monitoring and evaluating progress** *"Is the intervention adequately addressing the issue?"*	■ Work with and consult stakeholders ■ Assess progress toward outcome objectives ■ Disseminate findings to expand the evidence base ■ As required, modify goals, outcomes, and strategies and recruit new partners

Source: Adapted from Health Canada, Population and Public Health Branch, Strategic Policy Directorate, 2001 draft, "The Population Health Template: Key Elements and Actions That Define a Population Health Approach," monograph, 17.

The American Medical Association (AMA) also produced a primer on the "how to" of population-based medicine.[53] Specifically, the AMA suggested several principles that promote a population health perspective.[54] The belief is that incorporating these principles into medical care and health services management can facilitate the process to optimize health. The principles they suggest are as follows:

■ A *holistic* view to treat the patient's unique characteristics and also the societal influences on the patient

■ A *systems approach* to coordinate and integrate the delivery of care by using multidisciplinary teams and multiorganizational arrangements for referral

■ An *epidemiological foundation* to improve objectivity in clinical and policy decision making

■ An *anthropologic view* to understand the *patient's* perspective of his/her health

■ *Distributive justice* to recognize and reduce the unequal distributions of illness, disease, disability, and death across different groups[55]

Population Health Key Elements

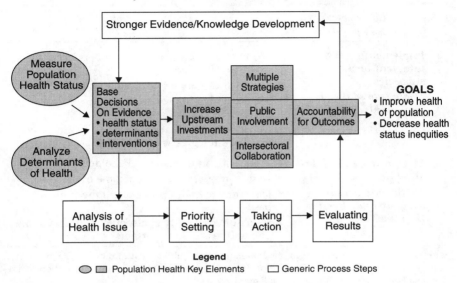

FIGURE 3-5   Population Key Elements. *Source:* Health Canada, Population and Public Health Branch, Strategic Policy Directorate, 2001 draft, "The Population Health Template: Key Elements and Actions That Define a Population Health Approach," monograph.

Health services managers who utilize these examples outlined by Health Canada and the AMA will ensure that their planning and management approach will be responsive to the populations in the communities and to the individuals in their clinics. The key elements in the population-based approach are identified in Figure 3-5.

Planning Health Services Management

Steps in the Planning Process

The planning process consists of a series of steps, as illustrated in Table 3-3. These are not in an immutable order but are followed in a more or less systematic way. The planning process is inherently cyclical and continual.

The first two steps, the identification of needs and problems and the establishment of priorities, are preliminary to program planning. This part of strategic planning allows the determination of priorities among the different problems and consequently provides justifications for the actions or programs. In other words, health program planning must take place within a larger strategic planning process.[56]

TABLE 3-3 How Population Health Planning and Health Management Functions Correspond

Population Health Planning		Health Management Functions	
Steps	Population Health Key Elements*	Function Approach	Process Approach
1. Identify needs and problems	Analysis of health issues		Technical
2. Establish priorities	Priority setting	Planning	
3. Set objectives			
4. Specify activities to attain objectives	Taking action		Administrative and political
5. Mobilize and coordinate resources		Organizing, directing, coordinating	
6. Evaluation	Evaluating results	Controlling	Technical

*Summary of steps shown in Figure 3-5

Source: G. E. A. Dever ©.

The first four steps correspond to the narrowly defined planning functions of management. The fifth, mobilization and coordination of resources, involves the organizing, directing, and coordinating of managerial functions; the sixth step, evaluation, refers to the controlling function. The first and last steps of planning constitute the technical aspect from identification of needs and evaluation. The administrative and political processes operate concurrently with the other parts.[57]

Concepts of Needs

These are central to any level of health planning and they need a target population. The process basically targets identification of population needs for health services and health planning, medical care organization, and health care sociology. Need as defined by Donabedian is "some disturbance in health and well-being."[58] Such a disturbance is always a perception and its assessment depends on who is doing the perceiving. There are at least two perspectives on need: that of the client and that of the provider. The definition of need is conditioned by value judgments and by the comprehension or framework of health within which the description is found. Regardless, information on the various approaches to needs assessment is essential to the analysis and evaluation of health problems. The various approaches are identified in Table 3-4.

TABLE 3-4 Need Assessment Approaches

Approach	Method	Information Processing Function	Measurement Expertise Needed	Time and Resources Needed
Indicator Approach				
Health Indicators	Analysis of statistics on life expectancy, morbidity, mortality, and disability	Compilation	Moderate to high	Moderate
Social Indicators	Analysis of social statistics related to health and health care utilization	Compilation	Moderate to high	Moderate
Extrapolation/ Assumption	Need extrapolations based on epidemiological data from reference population	Compilation Integration	Moderate	Minimal
Survey Approach	Analysis of service utilization or rates under treatment	Compilation	Moderate	Moderate
	Survey sample of labor and service facilities	Compilation and Development	Moderate	Moderate
	Survey sample of general population	Development	High	Extensive
	Survey sample of service or provider population	Development	High	Moderate

TABLE 3-4 Need Assessment Approaches *(continued)*

Approach	Method	Information Processing Function	Measurement Expertise Needed	Time and Resources Needed
Consensus-Reaching Approach	Community forum	Integration	Low	Moderate
	Nominal group	Development	Moderate	Minimal
	Key informants	Development	Moderate	Minimal
	Delphi technique	Development and Integration	Moderate	Moderate
	Community impressions	Development Compilation Integration	Moderate	Minimal

Source: Adapted from "Need Identification and Program Planning in the Community Context," by L. M. Siegel, C. C. Attkisson, and L. G. Carson in *Evaluation of Human Service Programs*, ed. C. C. Attkisson, with permission of Academic Press, Inc. ©1978, 226; from *Guide to Health Needs Assessment: A Critique of Available Sources of Health Care Information*, by L. W. Chambers, C. A. Woodward, and C. Dok with permission of the Canadian Public Health Association, ©1980, 32; and from *Determining Health Needs*, by Robin E. MacStravic with permission of Health Administration Press, © 1978, p. 268, as reprinted in "Program Planning in a Small Community Health Care Setting," by Carol Clemenhagen and Francois Champagne with permission of *Health Care Management Review* 7, no. 1 (Winter 1982), ©1982, 47–55.

Needs Assessment Approaches[59]

Approaches vary in complexity, cost, time necessary for completion, and relative effectiveness.[60] Three functions characterize needs assessment approaches: compilation (collecting data from already existing sources); development (producing new information); and integration (synthesizing information originating from inside and outside the system boundaries).[61]

Indicator Approaches

There are three: health, social, and extrapolation/assumption. Because needs for care are based on health status of the population, indicators used to measure those factors can measure needs as well. The health indicators are developed through analysis of morbidity, mortality, and more recently, disability data. Sources of this information include hospital admission and discharge reports; notifiable disease statistics; maternal, neonatal, and infant mortality statistics; life expectancy tables; and disability indexes for specific populations.[62]

Social indicators are relevant to health needs because they correlate with utilization of care.[63] Need is inferred from the measurement of the social conditions. The social indicators are generally used as rough pointers, since the relationship between social factors and health may be tenuous.[64] Sources of information for construction of social indicators include statistics on age, sex, education, ethnic background, housing, employment, and food consumption.

The extrapolation/assumption method implies epidemiological data on the prevalence and incidence of diseases and certain health conditions in a smaller reference population. The purpose is to estimate expected health needs associated with these same conditions in a larger population.

Survey Approaches

There are four elements here: analysis of utilization, rates under treatment, labor and service facilities, and sample surveys.

The analysis-of-utilization method of assessment examines need in terms of the demand for services. Demand is measured by the types and amount of services utilized. This method assumes that no need exists that does not result in utilization of services and that those usually totally meet the need expressed.[65] This analysis compares utilization among income, ethnic, or other groups.

The rates-under-treatment method looks specifically at instances of service utilization. For example, a survey of service encounters (e.g., clinic visits), during a specific period can be undertaken. Data such as client characteristics, services received, health status, transportation problems, and waiting times can be collected in specifically designed encounter forms or abstracted from agency records. Information is obtained through the organization that provides services.[66] This measure of need is biased toward heavy service users.

The method involving labor and services facilities is based on the assumption that individuals receiving care do in fact need it. The extent to which providers and facilities cannot cope with the existing utilization represents the degree of need.[67] This measure of need is biased toward heavy service users.

Sample surveys of the general population assess needs by collecting data on health problems, disability, and needs perception directly from respondents, often in their homes. An alternate approach consists of interviewing service users at the point of utilization. This method collects information from a group that has had at least some contact with health services. Like the rates-under-treatment, this one misses nonusers. A survey of persons involved in providing services could collect data on their perceptions of clients needs. These opinions would reflect the professional perspective.[68]

Consensus-Reaching Approaches

This segment involves five factors: community forum (focus groups), the nominal group, key informants, the Delphi technique, and community impressions.

The consensus-reaching approach focuses on means by which lay and professional views of health care needs can be assessed in participative group discussions (i.e., focus group). The community forum is an open meeting to which all members are invited to present views on their area's needs or it may be an invited list of a select few to elicit views on a specific topic. This approach is justified as a supplement to more thorough methods and is used to verify findings and build a supportive consensus.[69]

The nominal group process consists of a very structured, multiphase meeting of individuals who are closely associated with the problem area being assessed. For example, a small target group of health care consumers and facility administrators and staff members can meet to define the nature of health care needs in the community. A preset, orderly procedure is followed so that the ideas are defined individually and independently at first, then enumerated and clarified in the group through a round-robin process. The group then rates these ideas by secret ballot. The result is a rank order of needs defined by the group.[70]

In the key informant method, interviews are conducted with the community residents or local workers who have extensive firsthand experience in the area under study. The data collected is aggregated to obtain an overall picture of the community from the key informant's perspectives.[71]

The Delphi technique is defined as a method for systematic solicitation and collection of judgments on a particular topic through a set of carefully designed sequential questionnaires interspersed with feedback of opinions derived from earlier responses.[72] This technique collects and refines judgments from experts through a reiterative process. It produces a collective agreement as to the nature of existing community health care needs or a prediction of future wants. Opinions are usually submitted anonymously. Variations in the question structure, rules governing aggregation of judgments, and the interaction of respondents, among other things, determine its specific form.[73]

The community impressions method integrates information collected in interviews with small groups of key informants with an as-wide-as-possible range of existing indicator, utilization, or survey data. The scenario of needs developed in this manner then is validated through the community forum process.[74]

Health Services Management and Needs Identification

Health services management requires and even presupposes a pragmatic look at the identification of needs and problems. Health services managers must determine which services should be offered and to whom.

The first[75] steps of the planning process respond to these two basic questions. The first planning step, regardless of the different meanings of concepts of need, boils down to a description of the population surrounding the organization; description of its health problems and of its utilization in health services; analyses; and the identification of resources present in the community to address such factors (Figure 3-6).

Description of the Population

The description of the population to be served by the organization is essential to the planning and management of health care. The population should be analyzed by demographic, socioeconomic, and geographic attributes.

Description of Health Problems

Three major approaches to needs assessment are the indicator, the survey, and the consensus-reaching approaches. By using a combination of approaches, the purpose of a given needs assessment is more productive and adequate than any single method. The contribution of epidemiology to

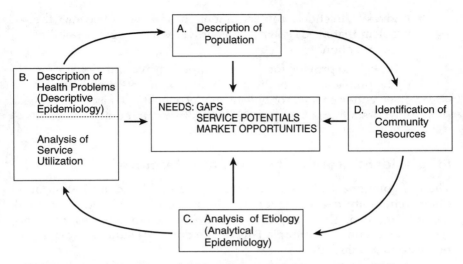

FIGURE 3-6 Identification of Health Needs and Problems. *Source:* G. E. A. Dever ©.

health services management, however, is examined here primarily as to the indicator approach, which is essentially the descriptive-epidemiologic approach. The health services managers analyze the morbidity, mortality, and risk factors using the epidemiological principle, methods, and techniques. Morbidity includes disease, discomfort, and disability—both acute and chronic. Risk factors related to elements with each of the four dimensions of the health field concept (biology, environment, lifestyle, and health care organization). Included in this category are the "health maintenance needs" or needs for "services presumed to benefit people who are well by improving or protecting their good health."[76]

Analysis of Etiology

Once problems are identified, it is useful to try to determine their source or, as Blum puts it, the "prime forces [that] causally underlie them."[77] Using data and knowledge from analytic epidemiology, the health problem, expressed in terms of mortality or morbidity, can be translated into its precursory risk factor in one or all of the four dimensions of the health field. This approach is useful for three main reasons:

■ "The immediate search and analysis of precursor risk factors to major causes of ill health reveal that certain precursors are common to many conditions."[78]

■ It gives a direction for intervention: The risk factor becomes the problem that needs solving; this provides a concrete possibility of intervention.

■ It is likely to provide for a more comprehensive and global view of the problems and of the possibilities of intervention by using an extended ecologic or holistic model of health. It also indicates the possibilities of cooperation with other community agencies.

Step 1. Identification of Community Resources

The last component of the first planning step is the identification of all other community resources that are addressing or could address the risk factors identified. These might include public health agencies, hospitals, schools, or community groups. This can be done in a summary manner or by marketing techniques.

Needs: Gaps and Market Opportunities   From the demographic evaluation of the population of the epidemiologic description and analysis of mortality, morbidity, and risk factors data there should emerge a clear picture of the health problems and their needs in the area. This constitutes the input into the second step of the planning process: the setting of priorities.

Step 2. Determination of Priorities

Once problems that the organization could address are identified, health services managers must determine which ones are the most important and therefore call for the most attention in planning and relocating resources.[79]

Many criteria, including some highly political ones, come into play in the determination of priorities. One source lists the following factors: "Time horizon, scope, and range of problems, range of interested parties, degree of uncertainty, degree of complexity, and degree of consensus."[80] Epidemiology plays an important role in decision making and rationalizing priorities. Anderson comments: "Because health needs at any time exceed the resources available, choices must be made. The community physician (epidemiologist) has the function of providing the evidence which is to guide the political and policy choices about alternatives, particularly in the second and third stages of planning."[81]

Epidemiology's contribution to the determination of priorities is based on a simple notion: The health problems that are the most important are those that cause the greatest loss and are most amenable to prevention and amelioration.[82] Two epidemiologic criteria can be used in this second planning step.

Magnitude of Loss Epidemiologic techniques can be used to estimate loss of life because of a given cause of mortality, or similarly time lost because of morbidity. The relative importance of risk factors can be assessed through the use of epidemiologic concepts such as attributable risk, absolute risk, excess risk, and relative risk.

Amenability of Loss to Prevention or Reduction[83] The second set of criteria that epidemiology can contribute to the determination of priorities is the sensitivity of the problem to a health program or the "readiness with which the disease may be prevented or its adverse effects minimized."[84] This amenability or sensitivity can be determined in any of the following ways:[85]

- Normatively, using expert's judgment and consensus
- Empirically, based on the experience of other regions, states, or countries
- Operationally, using some type of cost-benefit analysis—the lower the cost of a program in achieving a predetermined objective, the more amenable or sensitive it is to prevention or reduction

Step 3. Setting Objectives

Once priorities are determined, program planning can take place for each group of problems or risk factors. Epidemiology's contribution in this step is mostly expressing the objectives in a quantified way (using incidence or prevalence rates).

Step 4. Activities to Attain Objectives

For the objectives to be met they must be translated operationally into activities or services. This also involves the prediction, identification, and allocation of resources that will be needed to produce the services required. The fourth planning step starts with the generation of ideas for possible ways of achieving the objectives. The analysis of risk factors performed in step 1, using the four dimensions or inputs to health, can and should be of much help and creative inspiration in developing alternatives. Once alternatives are generated, they should be evaluated using cost-benefit analysis, comparing the benefits obtained from each alternative with the cost and risks of adopting it.

Step 5. Mobilization, Coordination of Resources

The activities to achieve the objectives have been chosen, and the appropriate resources have been determined and allocated. The fifth step of the planning cycle is the actual delivery of the services. The contribution of epidemiology is minimal, limited to the collection of data that can be used to monitor the program and its effects and, subsequently, to evaluate it more formally.

Situations can arise in which a "definite form of service cannot be determined from the beginning and in which epidemiology can be used to design and conduct experiments and pilot implementations to guide subsequent decisions."[86]

Step 6. Evaluation

The evaluation component contains three areas of concern: costs, activities, and outcomes. These are more commonly called fiscal, process, and outcome evaluation.

- Fiscal evaluation focuses on and determines cost accountability.
- Process evaluation determines program activity in terms of the following:
  - Population that receives the benefits by age, sex, race, or other demographic variables
  - Program organization, staffing, and funding
  - Program location and timing

  Process evaluation is a measure of program efforts or proposed activities rather than a program's effects or results.
- Outcome evaluation delineates program objectives in terms of effects to determine whether a change in health status occurred as a result of the effort.

The following observations are relevant to program evaluation:

- Most management decisions are based on intuition rather than on facts.
- The purpose of evaluation is to answer the practical questions of administrators who want to know whether to continue a program, to extend it to other sites, to modify it, or to close it down.

Evaluation is more productive when it is a continuous process with a continuous feedback loop to the administrators, supervisors, and program managers who make decisions.

Epidemiology directly contributes to health program evaluation in at least two ways.[87] First, the ideal design for evaluation remains the controlled clinical trial.[88,89] Second, the measures of outcomes are almost necessarily epidemiological measures of the health status of the population. In this regard, the contribution and use of epidemiology is essentially the same as that described in step 1, to which the cyclical nature of the planning process now returns the operation.

Summary

This chapter examined the role of epidemiology in health services management, first by looking at the different uses of epidemiology, then by analyzing the nature of management. The central theme of management is decision making. A global planning process whose aim is essentially to aid managerial decision making was described. It was noted that this planning process and the management process basically correspond. The planning process was used to examine epidemiology's contributions to health services management. Specifically, the planning process has outlined the various levels of health planning as they relate to the policies, strategies, and operations applied to a wellness model. Emerging out of this process is the population-based health planning approach that provides a blueprint for health services managers to focus on population in communities. Finally, health services managers are provided needs assessments methods for incorporation into the population-based perspective.

References

1. J. P. Fox, C. E. Hall, and L. R. Elveback, *Epidemiology: Man and Disease* (Toronto: Macmillan Company, 1970), 10.
2. K. Park, *Park's Textbook of Prevention and Social Medicine*, 14th ed. (Jabalpur, India: Barnarsidas Bhanot Publishers, 1994), XX; J. N. Morris, *Uses of Epidemiology*, 3d ed. (Edinburgh: Churchill Livingstone, 1975), 80.
3. Park, *Park's Textbook of Prevention and Social Medicine*, XX; Morris, *Uses of Epidemiology*, 80.
4. Morris, *Uses of Epidemiology*, 121.
5. International Epidemiological Association, *Epidemiology—A Guide to Teaching Methods* (Edinburgh: Churchill Livingstone, 1973), 8.
6. P. J. Fos and D. J. Fine, *Designing Health Care for Populations: Applied Epidemiology in Health Care Administration* (San Francisco: Jossey-Bass, 2000), 1–10.
7. Morris, *Uses of Epidemiology*, 121.
8. Park, *Park's Textbook of Preventive and Social Medicine*, 80.
9. Fos and Fine, *Designing Health Care for Populations*, 6–10.
10. D. Mowbray, "The Management Process," in *Epidemiology and Health*, ed. W. W. Holland and S. Gilderdale (London: Henry Kimpton Publishers, 1977), 155.
11. S. T. Fleming, F. D. Scutchfield, and T. C. Tucker, *Managerial Epidemiology* (Chicago, Ill.: Health Administration Press and Washington, D.C.: AUPHA Press, 2000), 123–145.
12. B. B. Lorgest, *Management Practices for the Health Professional*, 2d ed. (Reston, Va.: Reston Publishing Company, Inc., 1980), 39–49.
13. Fleming, Scutchfield, and Tucker, *Managerial Epidemiology*, 123–145.
14. S. A. Capper, P. M. Ginter, and L. E. Swayne, *Public Health Leadership and Management: Cases and Context* (Thousand Oaks, Calif.: Sage Publications, Inc., 2002).

15. P. H. Levin, "On Decisions and Decision Making," *Public Administration* 50, no. 19 (1972).
16. Mowbray, "Management Process," 157.
17. H. Mintzberg, "Organizational Power and Goals: A Skeletal Theory," in *Strategic Management: A New View of Business Policy and Planning*, ed. D. E. Schendel and C. W. Hofer (Boston: Little, Brown and Co., 1979), 64–80.
18. Mowbray, "Management Process," 155–156.
19. R. L. Ackoff, *A Concept of Corporate Planning* (New York: Wiley Interscience Publications, 1970), 1.
20. J. Freidmann, "A Conceptual Model for the Analysis of Planning Behavior," *Administrative Science Quarterly* 12 (1967):225.
21. J. Roeber, "Objectives, Forecasts, and Plans," *New York Times*, July 12, 1971.
22. R. Cyert and J. G. March, *A Behavioral Theory of the Firm* (Englewood Cliffs, N.J.: Prentice Hall, Inc., 1963).
23. H. A. Simon, *Administrative Behavior* (New York: Macmillan Company, 1957).
24. C. E. Lindblom, "The Science of Muddling Through," *Public Administration Review* 19 (1959):79–99.
25. D. Braybrooke and C. E. Lindblom, *A Strategy of Decision* (Glencoe, Ill.: Free Press, 1970), 268.
26. M. Q. Patton, *Utilization-Focused Evaluation* (Beverly Hills, Calif.: Sage Publications, Inc., 1978), 127–128.
27. G. E. Alan Dever, *Community Health Analysis* (Rockville, Md.: Aspen Systems, Inc. 1980), 409.
28. H. L. Blum, *Planning for Health* (New York: Human Sciences Press, Inc., 1981), 162.
29. T. T. H. Wan, "Assessing Causality: Foundations for Population-Based Health Care Managerial Decision Making," in *Epidemiology and the Delivery of Health Care Services*, 2d ed., ed. D. M. Oleske (New York: Kluwer Academic/Plenum Publishers, 2001), 75–98.
30. F. J. Jaeger, "Strategic Planning: An Essential Management Tool for Health Care Organizations and Its Epidemiological Basis," in *Epidemiology and the Delivery of Health Care Services*, 2d ed., ed. D. M. Oleske (New York: Kluwer Academic/Plenum Publishers, 2001), 99–132.
31. H. G. Hicks, *The Management of Organizations: A Systems and Human Resources Approach* (New York: McGraw-Hill Book Company, 1976), 602.
32. Fleming, Scutchfield, and Tucker, *Managerial Epidemiology*.
33. R. K. Keck, "Strategic Planning in the Health Care Industry: Concentrate on the Basic," *Health Care Issues* (September 1986).
34. Fleming, Scutchfield, and Tucker, *Managerial Epidemiology*, 139–141.
35. Blum, *Planning*, 14.
36. Fleming, Scutchfield, and Tucker, *Managerial Epidemiology*, 147–161.
37. Health Canada, Population and Public Health Branch, Strategic Policy Directorate, 2001 draft, "The Population Health Template: Key Elements and Actions That Define a Population Health Approach," monograph.
38. Health Canada, Population Health Approach—What Is the Population Health Approach, http://www.hc-sc.gc.ca/hppb/phdd/approach.html.
39. D. Coburn, et al, "Population Health in Canada: A Brief Critique," *American Journal of Public Health* 93, no. 3(2003):392–396.

40. Health Canada, "The Population Health Template," 23.
41. Health Canada, Population Health Approach.
42. Health Canada, "The Population Health Template," 1.
43. Health Canada, "The Population Health Template," 3.
44. Health Canada, "The Population Health Template," 3.
45. Health Canada, "The Population Health Template," 4.
46. Health Canada, "The Population Health Template," 4.
47. Health Canada, "The Population Health Template," 5.
48. Health Canada, "The Population Health Template," 5.
49. Health Canada, "The Population Health Template," 6.
50. Health Canada, "The Population Health Template," 6.
51. Health Canada, "The Population Health Template," 39.
52. Health Canada, Population Health Directorate, Population and Public Health, "Taking Action on Population Health," monograph (Ottawa, 1999), 38.
53. American Medical Association (AMA), *Paradigms for Clinical Practice: A Primer on Population-Based Medicine* (Atlanta: AMA, 2002).
54. AMA, *Paradigms for Clinical Practice*, 89.
55. AMA, *Paradigms for Clinical Practice*, 89.
56. R. Pineault, "La planification des services de santé: Une perspective épidémiologique," *Administration Hospitalière et Sociale* (Mars-Avril, 1979), 6.
57. C. Clemenhagen and F. Champagne, "Program Planning in a Small Community Health Care Setting," *Health Care Management Review* 7, no. 1 (Winter 1982):50.
58. A. Donabedian, *Aspects of Medical Care Administration: Specifying Requirements for Health Care* (Cambridge, Mass.: Harvard University Press, 1973), 62.
59. Clemenhagen and Champagne, "Program Planning in a Small Community Health Care Setting," 47–55.
60. R. A. Bell et al., "Service Utilization, Social Indicator, and Citizen Survey Approaches to Human Service Need Assessment," in *Evaluation of Human Service Programs*, ed. C. C. Attkisson et al. (New York: Academic Press, Inc., 1978), 256.
61. L. M. Siegel, C. C. Attkisson, and L. G. Carson, "Need Identification and Program Planning in the Community Context," in *Evaluation of Human Services Programs*, ed. C. C. Attkisson et al. (New York: Academic Press, Inc., 1978), 226–227.
62. Committee on Health Sciences, *Science for Health Services*, Science Council of Canada Report No. 22 (Ottawa: Science Council of Canada, 1974), 144.
63. Siegel, Attkisson, and Carson, "Need Identification and Program Planning in the Community Context," 227.
64. P. H. Rossi, H. E. Freeman, and S. R. Wright, *Evaluation: A Systematic Approach* (Beverly Hills, Calif.: Sage Publications, Inc., 1979), 108.
65. R. E. MacStravic, *Determining Health Needs* (Ann Arbor, Mich.: Health Administration Press, 1978), 64–66.
66. L. W. Chambers, C. A. Woodward, and C. Dok, *Guide to Health Needs Assessment: A Critique of Available Sources of Health Care Information* (Ottawa: Canadian Public Health Association, 1980), 7.
67. Chambers, Woodward, and Dok, *Guide to Health Needs Assessment*, 9–10.

68. Siegel, Attkisson, and Carson, "Need Identification and Program Planning in the Community Context," 229.
69. Rossi, Freeman, and Wright, *Evaluation*.
70. A. L. Delbecq, A. H. Van de Ven, and D. H. Gustafson, *Group Techniques for Program Planning* (Glenview, Ill.: Scott Foresman and Company, 1977), 66.
71. Siegel, Attkisson, and Carson, "Need Identification and Program Planning in the Community Context," 247.
72. Delbecq, Van de Ven, and Gustafson, *Group Techniques for Program Planning*, 10.
73. Delbecq, Van de Ven, and Gustafson, *Group Techniques for Program Planning*, 11.
74. Siegel, Attkisson, and Carson, "Need Identification and Program Planning in the Community Context," 230.
75. AMA, *Paradigms for Clinical Practice*, 89.
76. MacStravic, *Determining Health Needs*, 58.
77. H. L. Blum, "Does Health Planning Work Anywhere, and If So, Why?" *American Journal of Health Planning* 3, no. 3 (1978):43.
78. MacStravic, *Determining Health Needs*, 32.
79. Donabedian, *Aspects of Medical Care*, 164.
80. J. H. F. Brotherston et al., "Planning of Health Services and the Health Team," in *The Theory and Practice of Public Health*, ed. W. Hobson (London: Oxford University Press, 1979), 634.
81. D. O. Anderson, "Priorities and Planning," in Holland and Gilderdale, *Epidemiology and Health*, 178.
82. Donabedian, *Aspects of Medical Care*, 165.
83. Donabedian, *Aspects of Medical Care*, 164–192.
84. Donabedian, *Aspects of Medical Care*, 169.
85. Pineault, "La plantification des services de santé," 8.
86. E. G. Knox, ed., *Epidemiology in Health Care Planning* (Oxford: Oxford University Press, 1979), 124.
87. Pineault, "La plantification des services de santé," 12.
88. D. P. Byar et al., "Randomized Clinical Trials: Perspective on Some Recent Ideas," *New England Journal of Medicine* 295 (1976):74–80.
89. W. Spitzer, "What Is a Health Care Trial?" *JAMA* 233 (1975):161–163.

4

Epidemiological Measurements

Rates and Population at Risk

An important aspect of any scientific endeavor is measurement. Epidemiological measurement is an instrument that can be used to answer research questions, not be viewed as an end in itself. As seen in Chapter 3, health care managers can use epidemiology to answer questions relating to the type and amount of services they should offer to their catchment population as well as to the impact of these services. More precisely, this means using epidemiological principles, methods, and techniques to identify health problems, to determine priorities, and evaluate services. This chapter examines the epidemiological measures appropriate to these tasks.

As noted in Chapter 2, epidemiology, public health, and health services management involve the consideration of both a numerator and a denominator. The numerator is the number of cases, deaths, services, and so forth and the denominator is the population from which the numerator is taken. The denominator generally is known as the population at risk, and the individuals within the group at risk make up the numerator. A rate is simply the mathematical expression for the relation between the numerator and the denominator, together with some specification of time. For example:

$$Rate = \frac{\begin{array}{c} Number\ of\ events \\ (cases,\ deaths,\ services) \\ in\ a\ specified\ time\ period \end{array}}{\begin{array}{c} Population\ at\ risk\ of \\ experiencing\ the\ event \end{array}} \times 10^n$$

The purpose of the multiplier (10^n) is simply to produce a rate that is manageable.[1] The number of events often is so small, in relation to the denominator, that it is easier to express the numbers per 1,000 or 10,000 or other population. Rates serve another important purpose. Epidemiological measurement, like all others, depends on comparison.[2] Rates make possible a comparison of the number of events between populations and at different times. Numbers then are converted into rates to generate comparable indexes. For example, if the number of deaths for two different groups of people or for a group at two different times is compared, the number can differ only because the size of the population at risk differs. By converting to a rate, such as deaths per 100,000 persons, the size effect is removed and the rates become comparable indexes.

Guidelines for Using Rates

Rates should be used and interpreted with caution. Some comments are warranted in this regard.[3]

The Ecological Fallacy

This consists of generalizing the data collected in a particular area to all the individuals living in that area, associating an indicator with persons who were not included in its calculation, or making assertions about one unit of analysis based on the examination of another. Babbie gives several examples.[4]

- Suppose data showed that counties whose voters were relatively young gave a female candidate a greater proportion of their votes than did counties with voters of older average age. It would be tempting to conclude that young voters were more likely to vote for the female candidate than were older voters; that age affected support for the woman. Such a conclusion would run the risk of committing the ecological fallacy, because it might have been the older voters in those "young" counties who voted for the woman.

- Similarly, if the data showed that crime rates were higher in cities with large populations that are black, it might not show whether the crimes actually were committed by blacks.

- If it were found that cerebrovascular disease rates were higher in a county with a large white population than one with a smaller white population, it still could not be known that whites actually had a higher cerebrovascular death rate than blacks.

Ecological Analysis

To examine the association between a risk factor and an outcome and between geographic areas and an outcome, an ecologic analysis is performed. For example, if the smoking status of each pregnant woman, the county of residence for each pregnant woman, as well as the birth weight for each infant were known, and the state of residence and the number of well child visits for each child were known, then sample size (N) in each of the 2×2 tables to be generated for these examples would equal the total number of individuals for whom there was data.[5]

Sometimes, however, an association is to be evaluated at the aggregate level and then the N in the 2×2 table equals the total number of *groups* observed, not the individuals, and this would be an example of an ecological analysis. The groups, or units of analysis, can be geographic areas or public health facilities or clinics. For instance, the smoking and low birth weight data might look like that shown for fifty hypothetical counties in Table 4-1.

Now, the prevalence of smoking among pregnant women in a county is the risk factor and the outcome variable is the prevalence of low birth weight in a county. Consider some of the familiar statistics and measures of association and the possible interpretation in Table 4-2.[6]

Counties with a high prevalence of smoking among pregnant women have 1.7 times the risk of not meeting the Year 2010 Objective for low birth weight (≤5%). The PAR% of 29% means that the number of counties that might meet the Year 2010 Objective if smoking prevalence could be decreased to <20% in all of the counties would be $0.29 \times 35 = 10$ (rounded to nearest whole number). In other words, only 25 rather than 35 of the 50 counties would fall short of the Objective.[7]

Historically, epidemiologists have questioned the value of ecologic analysis, because the connection between the exposure and outcome is not linked at the individual level. In other words, in the preceding example, it

TABLE 4-1 Low Birth Weight and Smoking Status

	Low Birth Weight		
	>5%	≤5%	*Counties*
≥20% Smokers	25	5	30
<20% Smokers	10	10	20
TOTAL	35	15	50

Source: D. Rosenberg and A. Handler, "Measures of Association and Hypothesis Testing," in *Analytic Methods in Maternal and Child Health,* ed. A. Handler et al., 73 (Vienna, VA: Maternal and Child Health Bureau, HRSA, DHHS, 1998).

5% is the Year 2010 Objective.

TABLE 4-2 Ecological Measurement: Formulas and Interpretation

Measurement Variable	Formula	Interpretation
Prevalence	$p_1 = \dfrac{25}{30} = 0.83$	83% of the 30 counties that have greater than 20% of the mothers who smoke also have a LBW greater than 5%
Prevalence	$p_2 = \dfrac{10}{20} = 0.50$	50% of the 20 counties that have less than 20% of the mothers who smoke also have a LBW of less than 5%
Outcome Prevalence	$p_O = \dfrac{35}{50} = 0.70$	70% of the counties have a LBW of greater than 5%
"Exposure" Prevalence	$p_E = \dfrac{30}{50} = 0.60$	60% of the counties have a smoking rate of greater than 20%
Relative Risk	$\dfrac{p_1}{p_2} = \dfrac{0.83}{0.50} = 1.70$	1.7 times less likely to have ≤5% LBW, given smoking status risk or ≥20%
Population Attributable Risk %	$\dfrac{0.70 - 0.50}{0.70} \times 100 = 29\%$	% of counties that could be attributed to decreased LBW in smoking risk <20%

Source: Adapted from D. Rosenberg and A. Handler, "Measures of Association and Hypothesis Testing," in *Analytic Methods in Maternal and Child Health*, ed. A. Handler et al., 73 (Vienna, Va.: Maternal and Child Health Bureau, HRSA, DHHS, 1998).

is unknown whether the women who smoked during their pregnancies were the same ones who delivered low birth weight infants.[8]

Ratio measures and difference measures derived from a 2 × 2 table provide different types of information. The relative risk and odds ratio are used to measure the strength or the magnitude of an association between an exposure (or risk factor) and a health outcome; the attributable risk measures are used to gauge the potential public health impact of an exposure.[9]

In addition, the interpretation of the epidemiologic measures of risk must take into account the structure and type of data being used. Just as the assumption of causality did not hold when the county was the exposure variable, so too this assumption can be questioned when data is at the aggregate level or when the data is for service or systems variables. Because the traditional epidemiologic risk measures are used with many kinds of data, however, terminology and assumptions might have to be modified to accommodate a broader public health interpretation.[10]

Ecologic Designs

Whereas the association between two data elements that are not linked at the individual level is considered a cause for concern with respect to making assumptions about individuals (*ecological fallacy*), more current thinking holds that the ecologic level of analysis can be an appropriate and valid tool in its own right. Although it is usual to focus on individual risk factors and outcomes, examination of the relationship between population risk factors or exposure to a program on population level and population outcomes is also of value while developing population-based intervention strategies.[11]

In an ecologic design, the data for exposure and disease is used in aggregated form and cannot be linked at the individual level. The four cells of the table, therefore, do not contain the number of individuals with a given joint exposure-outcome status, but rather contain the number of groups (usually geographic areas or health facilities) with a given joint exposure-outcome status.[12]

In any case, the 2 × 2 table remains a very useful tool for organizing data whether or not particular risk measures will be reported. It will help the health services manager clarify the questions of interest, permit exploration of the impact of different categorization schemes, and provide a format for exploration of hypothetical changes in health status, health services, or health systems.[13]

However, if the researcher wishes to avoid these ecologic issues, then guidelines for avoiding such ecologic problems include (1) deriving indicators from a denominator that encompasses the entire population group or most of it, and (2) applying indicators with subgroup denominators only to the persons in that subgroup.

Variations in Base

These can cause some problems in comparing rates. A proportion (say 5/100) is multiplied by 100 to become a percentage (5 percent), by 1,000 to become an infant mortality rate (or 50), or perhaps by 10,000 to become a disease rate (or 500). A rate must accompany an indication of its base to be meaningful. A statement that "the rate has doubled" should be followed by the question, "What has doubled the number, rate, or ratio?" Further, a pertinent question to be asked is, "The rate per what?"

False Association

This comes about by forgetting that rates apply to aggregates and not to individuals. A neighborhood might have a high unemployment rate and a high alcoholism rate, and statistical tests would imply an association between these factors. Yet the unemployed and the imbibers might be two entirely different groups of people. Assumptions and statistical analysis must avoid inappropriate application of the statistical model and, further, should state an appropriate hypothesis with regard to the situation being investigated.

Variance of Rates with Small Denominators

Rates based on very large populations can be interpreted as fixed numbers for purposes of comparison. But as the population base becomes smaller, statistical variation becomes more prominent as an explanation of differences.

The rate has implications of a probabilistic or predictive statement. The statement that two infants died out of 75 born, for example, is simply a statement of fact. To convert this to an infant morality rate of 26—meaning 26 deaths per 1,000 live births—is by implication a statement of a long-run trend or prediction. Yet if during the following year only one infant died out of 75 born (again a statement of fact), the infant mortality rate is only 13. This so-called large decrease is a result of statistical variation, and the magnitude of the drop is exaggerated because of the use of a base of 1,000.

Yearly infant mortality rates have been used in recent years as an indicator for hospitals for their overall rating from a qualitative point of view. However, interpretations of the resulting data are questionable. Before conclusions are drawn, a time series for individual hospitals should be examined to avoid the risk of judgment based on small denominators. In addition, it is very difficult to determine the total population at risk for any one hospital.

The problem of small denominator rates arises in any statistical analysis where numbers are converted to percentages (rates per hundred). It is common practice to stratify data by age, race, morbidity, or other factors and to compare percentages of some phenomena for the different strata. The resulting data can be meaningless. Most statisticians use guidelines to determine when percentages should or should not be computed. For example, percentages might not be given for any cell with fewer than ten observations.

Rate Advantages and Disadvantages

Last year the rate of disease X in the town was 10/1,000, but this year because of an extensive effort the community managed to reduce it to 5/1,000. What impression would that statement leave? What if the rate was reduced from 100/10,000 to 50/10,000? Or from 1,000/100,000 to 500/100,000? Or from 10,000/1,000,000 to 5,000/1,000,000?

Sooner or later, reviewers would realize that they were all the same rate—and that would be correct. But how much more impressive it seems to cut 10,000 cases by half than to cut 10 cases by half.

Epidemiological Identification of Problems

The epidemiological assessment of health problems, as input to the determination of priorities and to subsequent program planning, can include three main categories of indicators: mortality, morbidity, and risk factors.

Mortality

Although mortality is far from being an ideal measure of the health of a population, it often is the most easily available and accessible—if not the only—indicator that can be used readily by health services managers (in addition to statistics on health services utilization and demographic data, discussed in Chapters 9 and 10).

Crude Rates

The simplest mortality measure is the crude death rate (CDR), stated as the number of deaths per unit of population (usually 1,000). All of these rates concern the number of deaths occurring during a specified time period, usually one year. Thus:

$$CDR = \frac{Total\ deaths}{Population\ at\ risk} \times 1,000$$

For example, the crude death rate for Georgia (2002) is derived as follows:

$$CDR = \frac{65,265\ Deaths}{8,560,310\ Population} \times 1,000$$

$$= 7.6\ deaths/1,000\ population$$

Specific Rates

A rate can be made specific for sex, age, race, cause of death, or a combination of these. These specific rates (SR) are illustrated in Table 4-3. Such specific rates usually are needed to understand the epidemiological aspects of disease and population dynamics.[14]

As the table shows, death rates vary greatly by race, sex, and age. Specific rates allow health care managers to target their programs to the appropriate population subgroups. Similarly, age/cause, sex/cause, and race/cause rates bring an even more revealing and useful picture of the mortality patterns.

As can be seen in the data for Georgia (2002), there are wide variations in the death rates for cancer and motor vehicle accidents by age groups. Without much further analysis, health services managers can have an indication that any program to reduce the impact of motor vehicle accidents should be directed toward the teen and young adult population and the elderly, although the actual number of deaths is less than half of the deaths to the 20–29 age group.

Two other specific rates of a slightly different nature also are often used by epidemiologists: the case fatality rate (CFR) and the proportionate mortality rate (PMR):

$$CFR\ (\%) = \frac{Deaths\ by\ cause}{Number\ of\ individuals\ with\ the\ specified\ disease\ (cause)} \times 100$$

This rate represents the risk of dying during a definite period of time for individuals who have this particular disease.[15] Case fatality rates also can be made specific for age, sex, race, or any other factors considered important.

The proportionate mortality rate (PMR) represents the proportion of all deaths resulting from a specific cause. It is useful because it permits the estimation of the proportion of lives to be saved by reducing or eradicating a given cause of death. The PMR can be derived as follows:

$$PMR\ (\%) = \frac{Deaths\ by\ cause}{Total\ deaths} \times 100$$

Although most authors refer to it as such, the PMR is not really a rate but a ratio, because the denominator is not the population at risk. A ratio usually compares the number of persons in a population with a specific characteristic to the number of persons in that same population without the characteristic.[16] Contrary to a rate a ratio, therefore, cannot be viewed as a

TABLE 4-3 Specific Death Rates (SR)

Definition	Georgia (2002)
$SR_{race} = \dfrac{Total\ deaths\ by\ race}{Population\ by\ race} \times 1,000$	$SR_{white} = \dfrac{47,125}{5,782,168} \times 1,000 = 8.2$
	$SR_{black} = \dfrac{17,678}{2,462,419} \times 1,000 = 7.2$
$SR_{sex} = \dfrac{Total\ deaths\ by\ sex}{Population\ by\ sex} \times 1,000$	$SR_{male} = \dfrac{32,191}{3,718,346} \times 1,000 = 8.7$
	$SR_{female} = \dfrac{33,074}{366,089} \times 1,000 = 90.3$
$SR_{age} = \dfrac{Total\ deaths\ by\ age}{Population\ by\ age} \times 1,000$	$SR_{20-29} = \dfrac{1,242}{1,255,809} \times 1,000 = 1.0$
	$SR_{>75} = \dfrac{31,926}{366,089} \times 1,000 = 87.2$
$SR_{cause} = \dfrac{Total\ deaths\ by\ cause}{Total\ population} \times 100,000$	$SR_{cancer} = \dfrac{13,937}{8,560,310} \times 100,000 = 162.8$
	$SR_{MVA} = \dfrac{1,492}{8,560,310} \times 100,000 = 17.4$

TABLE 4-3 Specific Death Rates (SR) *(continued)*

Definition	Georgia (2002)
$SR_{age/cause} = \dfrac{Total\ deaths\ by\ age/cause}{Population\ by\ age} \times 100,000$	$SR_{20-29/cancer} = \dfrac{75}{1,255,809} \times 100,000 = 5.9$
	$SR_{>75/cancer} = \dfrac{5,099}{366,089} \times 100,000 = 1,392.8$
	$SR_{20-29/MVA} = \dfrac{285}{1,255,809} \times 100,000 = 22.7$
	$SR_{>75/MVA} = \dfrac{122}{366,089} \times 100,000 = 33.3$

Source: G. E. A. Dever.

probability statement. A hospital manager might calculate the proportion of deaths and/or operations for heart patients. This statistic compared with other such data would provide the manager with essential planning data. Mortality measures traditionally used as health status indicators are shown in Table 4-4.

Adjusted or Standardized Rates

As stated previously, one of the purposes of epidemiological measurement is the comparison between groups and time. Crude and specific death rates do not, however, lend themselves to such comparisons because they ignore the fact that different populations have different compositions, mostly in terms of age structure. Similarly, the age composition of a population varies in time, making the use of crude and specific rates more hazardous for comparison purposes.

The adjustment or standardization of rates is a statistical procedure that removes the effect of differences in composition.[17] Because of its marked effect on mortality (and morbidity), age is the variable used most commonly for adjustment. Sometimes other variables need to be adjusted, instead of or in addition to age, such as sex and race if the composition of the populations to be compared is known or suspected to be dissimilar with regard to these variables. The age structure of a population is a potent marker for a number of social, economic, and political developments for various population segments. Age structure is also strongly linked to the morbidity and mortality profiles of any given population.

The following age ranges are commonly used to produce an age-standardization (adjusted) mortality rate: <1, 1–4, 5–14, 15–24, 25–44, 45–64, 65–84, and 85 and over.

Other age groupings can also be used appropriately. Most chronic diseases are positively associated with chronological age and, because populations have different age structures, age is a potent confounder and needs to be standardized (adjusted) when these populations are to be compared for morbidity and mortality rates.

Two basic methods of rate adjustment or standardization are the direct and the indirect. Although the following discussion deals with birth weights and neonatal mortality rates in two different hospital groups, other variables such as age, sex, and racial distribution in the populations of interest can be adjusted by the same methods.

Direct Method—Birth Weight and Infant Mortality   The direct method of birth weight adjustment involves the application of birth weight–specific rates observed in each of the populations (in this case hospital groups A and B) compared to an arbitrarily chosen structure (in this case all live births in the hypothetical state population) called the standard population. A standard

TABLE 4-4 Mortality Measures Most Used as Health Status Indicators

No.	Indicator	Numerator	Denominator	Usually Expressed per Number at Risk
1.	**Crude Death Rate** Crude; specific for age, sex, socioeconomic area, etc.	Number of deaths during a given time interval	Estimated mid-interval population	1,000
2.	**Cause-Specific Death Rate** Crude by cause; specific for age, race, sex, socioeconomic area, etc.	Number of deaths assigned to a specific cause during a given time interval	Estimated mid-interval population	100,000
3.	**Proportional Mortality Ratio** Crude by cause; specific for age, race, sex, socioeconomic area, etc.	Number of deaths assigned to a given disease during a given time interval	Number of deaths from all causes reported during the same time interval	100(%)
4.	**Case Fatality Rate** Crude; specific for age, race, sex, socioeconomic area, etc.	Number of deaths assigned to a specific cause during a given time interval	Number of new cases of that disease reported during the same time interval	100(%)
5a.	**Fetal Death Rate I** Crude; specific for age of mother, race, socioeconomic area, etc.	Number of fetal deaths of 28 weeks or more gestation reported during a given time interval	Number of fetal deaths of 28 weeks or more gestation reported during the same interval plus number of live births during same interval	1,000
5b.	**Fetal Death Rate II** Crude; specific for age of mother, race, socioeconomic area, etc.	Number of fetal deaths of 20 weeks or more gestation reported during a given time interval	Number of fetal deaths of 20 weeks or more gestation reported during the same interval plus the number of live births during the same interval	1,000

TABLE 4-4 Mortality Measures Most Used as Health Status Indicators *(continued)*

No.	Indicator	Numerator	Denominator	Usually Expressed per Number at Risk
6a.	**Fetal Death Ratio I** Crude; specific for age of mother, race, socioeconomic area, etc.	Number of fetal deaths of 28 weeks or more gestation during a given time interval	Total number of live births during the same time interval	1,000
6b.	**Fetal Death Ratio II** Crude; specific for age of mother, race, socioeconomic area, etc.	Number of fetal deaths of 20 weeks or more gestation recorded during a given time interval	Number of live births recorded during the same time interval	1,000
7a.	**Perinatal Mortality Rate I** Crude; specific for age of mother, race, socioeconomic area, etc.	Number of fetal deaths of 28 weeks or more gestation reported during a given time interval plus the reported number of infant deaths under seven days of life during the same time interval	Number of fetal deaths of 20 weeks or more gestation reported during the same time interval plus the number of live births during the same time interval	1,000
7b.	**Perinatal Mortality Rate II** Crude; specific for age of mother, sex, socioeconomic area, etc.	Number of fetal deaths of 20 weeks or more gestation reported during a given time interval plus the reported number of infant deaths under 28 days of life during the same time interval	Number of fetal deaths of 20 weeks or more gestation reported during the same time interval plus the number of live births reported during the same time interval	1,000

TABLE 4-4 Mortality Measures Most Used as Health Status Indicators (*continued*)

No.	Indicator	Numerator	Denominator	Usually Expressed per Number at Risk
8.	**Infant Mortality Rate** Crude; specific for race, sex, socioeconomic area, birth weight, cause of death, etc.	Number of child deaths under one year of age reported during a given time interval	Number of live births reported during the same time interval	1,000
9.	**Neonatal Mortality Rate** Crude; specific for race, sex, socioeconomic area, birth weight, cause of death, etc.	Number of deaths under 28 days of age reported during a given time interval	Number of live births reported during the same time interval	1,000
10.	**Postneonatal Mortality Rate** Crude; specific for race, sex, socioeconomic area, cause of death, etc.	Number of infant deaths from 28 days of age up to, but not including, one year reported during a given time interval	Number of live births reported during the same time interval	1,000
11.	**Maternal Mortality Rate** Crude; specific for age of mother, race, socioeconomic area, etc.	Number of deaths assigned to causes related to pregnancy during a given time interval	Number of live births reported during the same time interval	10,000

Source: Adapted from *Descriptive Statistics, Rates, Ratios, Proportions and Indices,* U.S. Department of Health, Education, and Welfare, Public Health Service (Atlanta: Centers for Disease Control, 1977), 3–8.

population can be that of the United States, a given state, or any other known population structure, including one or a combination of those being compared. Common standardization of rates is distinguished from other stratification methods in controlling for confounding by its use of external standard population in addition to populations being compared.

For example, a "U.S. Standard Million" sometimes is used, representing the composition of a hypothetical population of one million people having the same proportion in each age or other variable group as the United States has as a whole. Thus, in essence, the death rates in the populations to be compared are being recalculated by assuming that they have the same age or other variable distribution (or structure) as that of the standard population. As an illustration, neonatal mortality rates in two hypothetical hospital groups are compared as follows.

Hospital Group A: Composed of community hospitals without neonatal intensive care units that transfer most of their high-risk pregnant women to the tertiary care center for safe delivery

Hospital Group B: Composed of tertiary care hospitals with neonatal intensive care units (NICUs)

The confounder in the two hospital groups is the birth weight distribution because the tertiary hospital group serves more high-risk pregnant women than the community hospital group and the birth weight is an important predictor of neonatal mortality. Data stratifications for the two groups are shown in Table 4-5.

The crude relative risk of infant death (if birth weight distribution is disregarded) when the two hospital groups are compared is 1 (6.2/6.2). Standardizing mortality by birth weight will help determine if the relationship is a fair reflection of the mortality experience in the two hospital groups (Table 4-6).[18]

A directly standardized relative risk is calculated using data from the standard population and the preceding rates from the two hospital groups. The direct standardization is calculated as follows:

Adjusted Rate for the Community Hospitals (Hospital Group A) =

$$\frac{(5,000 \times 353.3) + (35,000 \times 16.0) + (460,000 \times 2.0)}{500,000} = 6.5$$

Adjusted Rate for Tertiary Care Hospitals (Hospital Group B) =

$$\frac{(5,000 \times 216.7) + (35,000 \times 11.7) + (460,000 \times 1.0)}{500,000} = 3.9$$

$$\text{Crude Relative Risk} = \frac{6.2}{6.2} = 1.0$$

$$\text{Standardized Relative Risk} = \frac{6.5}{3.9} = 1.7$$

TABLE 4-5 Data Adjustment—Infant Mortality by Birth Weight for Hospital Groups A and B

Birth Weight (Grams)	Deaths	Births	Percentage of Total Births	Birth Weight–Specific Death Rate per 1,000 Live Births	Crude Infant Mortality Rate per 1,000
1. Hospital Group A (Community Hospitals without NICUs)					
<1,500	53	150	1	353.3	
1,500–2,499	12	750	5	16.0	
≥2,500	28	14,100	94	2.0	
TOTAL	93	15,000	100		6.2
2. Hospital Group B (Hospitals with NICUs)					
<1,500	65	300	2	216.7	
1,500–2,499	14	1,200	8	11.7	
≥2,500	14	13,500	90	1.0	
TOTAL	93	15,000	100		6.2

Source: Adapted from *Analytic Methods in Maternal and Child Health* by A. Handler et al. (Vienna, Va.: MCH Bureau, HRSA, DHHS, 1998), 93–94.

While calculating an adjusted relative risk, it is necessary to calculate what appears to be the adjusted rates for each population. These recalculated rates reflect what would be expected in the standard population if it had the morbidity and mortality experience of the populations being compared. Note that the adjusted rates of 6.5 and 3.9 do not reflect the real mortality risks in the two hospital groups. They are by-products of the standardization procedure and cannot be used as helpful measures in decision-making situations. They can lead to misleading conclusions.[19]

The adjusted relative risk of 1.7 shows that the community hospitals have elevated neonatal mortality compared to the tertiary care centers (even though the unadjusted crude relative risk was 1). Without adjustment, the better survival of neonates born in the tertiary care centers would have been masked or overlooked due to the disparity in the birth weight distribution of the infants served by the two hospital groups. Even though the tertiary hospital group has a higher incidence of low birth weight births than the community hospitals (10% vs. 6%), they have a lower infant mor-

TABLE 4-6   All Live births And deaths in the State (External Standard = All Live Births)

Birth Weight (Grams)	Deaths	Births	Percentage of Total Births	Birth Weight– Specific Death Rate per 1,000	Crude Infant Mortality Rate per 1,000
<1,500	1,375	5,000	1	275.0	
1,500–2,499	490	35,000	7	14.0	
≥2,500	460	460,000	92	1.0	
TOTAL	2,325	500,000	100		4.7

Source: Adapted from *Analytic Methods in Maternal and Child Health* by A. Handler et al. (Vienna, Va.: MCH Bureau, HRSA, DHHS, 1998), 94.

tality rate within each birth weight stratum (216.7 vs. 353.3, 11.7 vs. 16.0, and 1.0 vs. 2.0).[20]

Direct Method—Mortality Rates   The direct method of age adjustment involves the application of the age-specific rates observed in each of the populations being compared to an arbitrarily chosen structure called the standard population. A standard population can be that of the United States, of a given state, or any other known population structure, including one or a combination of those being compared.[21]

For example, a "U.S. Standard Million" sometimes is used, representing the composition of a hypothetical population of one million people that has the same proportion in each age group as the United States as a whole.[22] Thus, in essence, the death rates in the populations to be compared are recalculated by assuming that they have the same age distribution as that of the standard population. To illustrate, suppose that the populations to be compared have expected x and y numbers of deaths if they both have a "standard" age structure; that is, the same age distribution as the standard population selected. For instance, between 1991 and 2000, County A had a death rate from acute myocardial infarction of 203 per 100,000 population. For the same period, the state rate was 152.7 per 100,000. This difference can result from a different age structure. To take away the effects of the age distribution, it is appropriate to age-adjust the county rate to the standard (state) age distribution. The direct method of age adjustment is shown in Table 4-7. This table

TABLE 4-7 Direct Age Adjustment of Rates

Age Group	Age-Specific County Rate per 100,000	State Population (1991–2000)	Proportion of State Population	County Rates Times Proportion*
20–29	2.6	8,354,955	0.1716	0.45
30–44	45.1	9,015,340	0.1851	8.35
45–59	312.0	7,080,165	0.1454	45.36
60–74	832.5	4,715,510	0.0968	80.61
>74	1,514.0	1,526,865	0.0314	47.47
Total State Population		48,696,875		182.24

Source: G. E. A. Dever.

*The age-adjusted rate is the summation of this column

shows that the age-adjusted death rate from acute myocardial infarction is 182.24 per 100,000 in the county. This still is higher than the state rate but much less so than before age adjustment. Consequently, some of the difference between the state and county rates can be attributed to a different age distribution. There are several issues in the choice of the standard population.

An age-adjusted death rate is a hypothetical index, designed to facilitate comparisons among populations, rather than a true measure of risk. And age-adjusted death rate (by the direct method) answers the question: What would the death rate in a study population be *if* that population had the same age distribution as the standard population? So in theory any population distribution can be used as the standard; it is only a set of weights applied to the age-specific death rates. The choice of the standard population will not usually have a great effect on the relative levels of the age-adjusted rates that are being compared. But it is important to remember that age-adjusted death rates can be compared to each other only if they are adjusted to the same standard.[23]

For many years the National Center for Health Statistics has used the 1940 U.S. population as the standard for age-adjusting death rates. Converted to a population of one million with the same proportions at each age as in the 1940 population, this standard is sometimes referred to as the "standard million." An advantage of consistently using this same standard population is that it promotes comparisons of age-adjusted death rates, especially when examining trends over time from 1940 to the present. A disadvantage of using this standard is that the size of the adjusted rate is often very different from the size of the crude rate in the study population.[24]

Take the example of heart disease mortality in North Carolina. In 1993, the crude heart disease death rate was 277.0 per 100,000 population. Age-adjusted to the 1940 United States population standard, the 1993 heart disease death rate for North Carolina was 151.4. The 1993 U.S. heart disease death rate, age-adjusted to the 1940 United States standard, was 145.3. This shows that the 1993 heart disease death rate in North Carolina was slightly higher than that in the United States, after adjustment for differences in age distribution. However, the North Carolina adjusted rate of 151.4 is much lower than the crude rate in 1993 of 277.0 (i.e., it is not an accurate measure of the risk of death from heart disease in 1993). This is primarily due to (1) the 1940 United States population is much younger than the 1993 North Carolina population, and (2) heart disease death rates are much higher in the older age groups. So standardizing to a much younger population results in a much lower age-adjusted death rate. In recognition of this problem, the National Center for Health Statistics has proposed that the year 2000 U.S. population be used as the recommended standard population. This will mean that the age-adjusted death rates will generally be much more similar in size to contemporary crude death rates. However, it will also mean that time-series comparisons of age-adjusted death rates will have to be re-computed using the new standard and that rates adjusted to the 1940 standard cannot be compared to rates adjusted to the new standard.[25]

One should be especially careful when assessing trends over time using age-adjusted death rates. It is essential that rates for different years be adjusted to the same population before making comparisons. Also, if the standard population is very different from the populations of the years being compared (as is often the case when using the 1940 U.S. standard), changes in the adjusted rates over time might not be an accurate reflection of the actual changes in the risk of death.[26]

Indirect Method The direct method of rate adjustment requires a knowledge of the age-specific death rates in all populations to be compared. If these age-specific rates are not known for the populations in which age adjustments are sought, or if the numbers are too small to produce stable rates, the indirect method of standardization (or adjustment) can be used.[27]

This indirect method is, in a sense, the reverse process: Where the direct method applies the rates from the populations to be compared to a standard population structure, the indirect method applies the rates from the standard population (that is, a standard set of rates) to the distributions of the different populations to be compared. In applying these standard rates to the populations being studied, it is possible to estimate the number of deaths (once again, the expected deaths) that would have occurred in these groups if the people who make them up had been dying at the same (age-specific) rate as those in the standard population. Addition of the age-specific expected deaths produces a total of expected deaths in each population that can be compared to the total observed deaths. This comparison usually is done by calculating the standardized mortality ratio (SMR) as follows:

$$SMR = \frac{Observed\ deaths}{Expected\ deaths} \times 100$$

If the SMR is greater than 100, it means more deaths occurred in the observed population than would be expected, based on the rates in the standard population. Similarly, a ratio less than 100 indicates fewer deaths than expected. For example, an SMR of 140 indicates 40 percent excess deaths as compared to the standard population, whereas an SMR of 85 indicates 15 percent fewer deaths. Using the same example as before, the indirect age adjustment method of the rates in County A is shown in Table 4-8.

The indirect age-adjusted rate in the county is 170.54 per 100,000. To calculate the SMR, it is necessary to use the actual number of deaths in the state (instead of the death rate). The product of those actual deaths times the ratio of the county population to the state population in each age group gives the expected number of deaths in the county in each age group, as in Table 4-9.

TABLE 4-8   Indirect Age Adjustment Method

Age Group	Age-Specific State Rate per 100,000	County Population (1991–2000)	Proportion of County Population	State Rates Times Proportion*
20–29	1.5	230,890	0.1609	0.24
30–44	27.2	246,305	0.1716	4.67
45–59	217.4	230,460	0.1606	34.91
60–74	680.9	156,880	0.1093	74.44
>74	1,588.1	50,860	0.0354	56.28
Total State Population		1,435,035		170.54

Source: G. E. A. Dever.

*The age-adjusted rate is the summation of this column

TABLE 4-9   Application of SMR Calculations

Age Group	Deaths in State (D)	County Population (A)	State Population (B)	Expected Deaths (D × A/B)
20–29	125	230,890	8,354,955	3.45
30–44	2,451	246,305	9,015,340	66.96
45–59	15,390	230,460	7,080,165	500.95
60–74	32,110	156,880	4,715,510	1,068.27
>74	24,429	50,860	1,526,865	813.73
Total				2,453.36

Source: G. E. A. Dever.

This means that if the county had the same age distribution as the state, 2,453 deaths from acute myocardial infarction could have been expected. The actual number of deaths was 2,912. Thus, the age-adjusted SMR is derived as follows:

$$SMR = \frac{2,912}{2,453} \times 100 = 118.7$$

The age-adjusted SMR indicates that, even in controlling for the age structure, there were proportionately 18.7 percent more deaths from acute myocardial infarction in the county than in the state.

The SMR has at least two distinct advantages over the direct method of rate adjustment.

First, knowledge of the age distribution of deaths in the population of interest is not required. Only the number of persons in each age group in this population and the age-specific death rate in the standard population are necessary. Because it is often much easier to obtain the data from the standard population (for example, the United States as whole, or an individual state) than from a smaller population, this could be a major advantage.

Second, the SMR makes comparison among diseases much easier, because it is a ratio whose value is directly comparable across diseases. On the other hand, the results of direct standardization are adjusted rates with comparisons that have direct meaning only for a given cause of death or disease.

Comparison of the Direct and Indirect Methods   The direct method of adjustment is generally preferred where the numbers of deaths in the study population are large enough to produce stable age-specific death rates. A big advantage of the direct method is that the adjusted rates of a number of different study populations can be directly compared to each other if they are all adjusted to the same standard population. This allows mortality comparisons assuming a constant age distribution across all of the study populations. The indirect method is often used if mortality rates by age cannot be calculated for the study population, or if the numbers of deaths in the study population are too small to produce stable age-specific death rates. A problem with the indirect method is that the adjusted rate for the study population can be compared only with the rate of the standard population. Different study populations cannot be compared to each other because the adjusted rates are not based on a common age distribution. In other words, differences in the rates can still be due to differences in age distribution, because the rates are adjusted to the age distribution of each particular study population rather than to a common standard.[28]

When used as health status indicators, crude, specific, and adjusted rates have advantages and disadvantages depending on the special circumstances in which each is being applied. Table 4-10 lists some of the advantages and disadvantages of the application of each of these rates.

TABLE 4-10 Advantages and Disadvantages of Indirect Standardization Methods

Rate	Advantages	Disadvantages
Crude	They are summary rates, easy to generate from minimal data, and allow comparison between countries or regions of the world.	Present limited information and ignore necessary information on population subgroups such as age, race, gender, and other important variables. They fail to identify differences among these population subgroups.
Adjusted	Allow populations and population subgroups to be compared even with differences in population subgroups. Also allow appreciation of the magnitude of the problems being analyzed even when population data is relatively small compared to the standard.	Adjusted rates can mask the true rates. They are usually a reflection of the standard population instead of the populations of interest.
Specific	Provide detailed information about population subgroups such as age, race, gender, and other variables. They are also good for epidemiologists and public health managers in decision-making processes.	Can be more complex and cumbersome to generate when different population subgroups are being considered.

Source: Adapted from *Epidemiology: An Introductory Text*, by J. S. Mausner and A. K. Bahn (Philadelphia: W. B. Saunders Company, 1974), 138.

Morbidity and Risk Factors

Although mortality statistics are the most used and easily available health indicators, there can be no doubt they offer only an incomplete picture of the health problems of a population. For this reason, data on morbidity, showing the spread of disease, discomfort, and disability—both acute and chronic—is also necessary.

Incidence Rate

Morbidity data usually is presented through incidence and prevalence rates. An incidence rate (IR) indicates the rate at which people without a particular disease develop it during a specified period of time (e.g., the number of new cases of a disease over a period of time), usually one year.[29] To illustrate:

$$IR = \frac{\text{Number of new cases of a disease over a period of time}}{\text{Population at risk}} \times 100$$

Prevalence Rate

A prevalence rate (PR) measures the number of people in a population who have a particular disease. The point prevalence rate indicates the number of people who have a disease at a given point in time, whereas the period prevalence rate (less commonly used) measures the number who had the disease over a period of time. These rates can be calculated as follows.

$$\text{Point } PR = \frac{\text{Number of existing cases of a disease at a point in time}}{\text{A disease at a point in time}}$$

$$\text{Period } PR = \frac{\text{Number of existing cases of a disease during a period}}{\text{Total population}}$$

Period prevalence is constructed at a specific time plus new cases (incidence) and recurrences during a succeeding time period.[30] Both incidence and prevalence rates should be made specific for age, sex, race, or other important factors. They also can be adjusted by the same methods as for mortality rates. Incidence and prevalence rates obviously are closely related. Prevalence is a function of incidence and of duration of a disease (D), thus:

$$PR = IR \times D$$

Similarly, mortality (crude death rate) is a function of the incidence and the case fatality rate:

$$CDR = IR \times CFR$$

Both incidence and prevalence rates are important and fundamental tools to assess health problems of a population. The incidence rate is an indicator of risk: a high incidence rate indicates a high risk of disease. The prevalence rate can be used by health services managers as an indicator of workload or need for personnel and facilities. A high prevalence can be the result of increased survival because of improved medical care or behavioral or environmental changes. Similarly, a low prevalence can reflect either a rapid fatal process or rapid and effective care.

Health services managers also need to look at risk factors, or phenomena, within each of the four dimensions of the health field: biology, lifestyle, environment, and health care organization (Chapters 8 and 9, on health services utilization and demography, respectively, deal more specifically with factors of biology and health care organization). Lifestyle and environmental factors can be described in a way similar to diseases—for example, an incidence rate for cigarette smoking or drug consumption or the prevalence rates of pests that present disease risks.

Data on morbidity and risk factors should be used as often as possible. The main problem, however, lies in obtaining the figures. Contrary to mortality data, specifics on morbidity often are not routinely reported and collected. Ways to obtain information on morbidity and risk factors include using data collected by insurance plans, hospitals, employers, schools, or any other providers or third-party organizations; using data from special surveys such as the United States National Health Survey, the Canadian Health Survey, the World Health Organization, those conducted by universities, health planning agencies, or others; and by conducting a special survey. That last alternative, of course, is complex and costly. Data concerning infectious diseases is available from the U.S. Public Health Service Centers for Disease Control and Prevention as well as from state and county health departments.

Hospital Morbidity Data   Morbidity data that indicate various diagnostic categories is available in hospital records and should provide a particularly useful source of information to detect changes in disease patterns. This source of information can be of major importance to the health services manager or administrator in a hospital or other health care facility.

The problem of time lag related to a discharge diagnosis is important to this aspect of morbidity data from hospital records. In certain situations, the admission diagnosis could be used by the health services manager for the investigation of the disease patterns. In this situation, however, the critical component is the lack of an appropriate denominator for determining population-at-risk. The numerator would be the number of cases categorized by diagnostic group. The difficulty comes when trying to compute rates without really knowing the true population-at-risk. If the market area for a hospital is well defined, then it is possible to utilize the population within that market area for the population-at-risk. At no time should a health care manager calculate at-risk rates using the denominator of the in-hospital population. A more likely statistic at that point would be a proportionate mortality rate (PMR).

Various problems can be expected when estimating the incidence and prevalence of various diseases in the hospital setting. Basing estimates on hospital admissions will be less valid for chronic diseases than for those characterized as acute illnesses. Using in-hospital data will result in losing many cases of acute and minor illnesses that are diagnosed and treated in physicians' offices, outpatient departments, or ambulatory care settings. Thus, the concept of denominators is much more critical in the case of acute and minor illnesses than in the chronic case.

Because of these concerns, hospital records have been underutilized as a valuable source of information. To overcome some of these concerns, hospitals in a metropolis or other common market area could join together in a common computer service. It would then be possible to have a systematic collection of admission and discharge diagnostic data. There are national systems and some state hospital associations that are currently utilizing this approach. The result of these endeavors is an epidemiological surveillance system, which provides many opportunities for the hospitals to do effective health services planning and management.

Mortality and morbidity data can be referred to as health status indicators. A health status indicator is a single, unidimensional measure obtained from a single component (variable). Two or more variables also can be combined into a health status index: a composite measure summarizing data from two or more components (variables). Because an index allows the inclusion and weighting of the many dimensions of health (physical, mental, social), theoretically it is preferable to single indicators. The construction of an index, however, requires elaborate statistical techniques and methodologies. Although this is an intense and burgeoning field of research, results that could be applied on a small scale by health services managers have yet to be described.[31,32,33,34,35]

The Significance of Rates

The epidemiological approach to the determination of health problems rests on the comparison of mortality and morbidity rates in the population of concern to the health services manager with some other standard or target rate. The identification of a problem has meaning only in relation to some standard. A standard then refers to the value associated with a particular indicator (criterion) that is acceptable to the decision makers.

For example, an infant mortality rate of 20 per 1,000 has marginal meaning by itself. It is necessary to know something about the variability or stability of this rate. This rate then must be compared with an infant mortality rate in another geographical area or another time period or with some arbitrarily or preordained set standard or target value.

When comparing rates, the issue arises as to how much of a difference or deviation from the standard is significant. This involves three factors: the variability of rates, the significance of the difference between two rates, and the significance of excess deaths.

The Variability of Rates

An observed mortality or morbidity rate cannot be taken as a true rate for an area. An observed rate is an estimate of the true rate and, as is the case with any estimate, is subject to chance variation. As Kleinman points out, the rationale is that the number of deaths in an area, for example, varies by chance depending on the size of the population and the probability of death—the true mortality rate.[36] As the size of the population increases, the chance component becomes less important and the observed mortality rate becomes a better estimate of the true rate. For example, if an area has few deaths, the observed death rate can be very different from the true rate. Consequently, the variability of rates must be assessed. This can be done easily through basic statistical measures.

Standard Deviation   This is the most important measure of dispersion about the mean value of a distribution and forms the basis for most statistical analysis. It consists of the square root of the sum of the squared deviations of each value from the mean, divided by the number of observations, or:

$$S = \frac{\sqrt{\left[\sum_{i=1}^{n}\left(X_i - \overline{X}\right)^2\right]}}{n}$$

where:

S = standard deviation

$(X_i - \overline{X})^2$ = the mean value $\overline{X}$ from the value of X_i, then squared

n = number of observations

One unique property of the standard deviation in the normal distribution is that 68 percent of the observed values will fall within one standard deviation on either side of the mean; 95 percent within about two standard deviations; and 99 percent within three standard deviations. As shown later, this property has important consequences in the statistical analyses of testing hypotheses and significance levels.

When measuring a population factor such as an infant mortality rate, it is helpful to estimate the true rate for the population. Because every value in the population cannot be measured, however, some smaller number of measurements is used and from these the true mean is estimated. Thus, when a population mean or some other population parameter is to be determined, a small sample of the total population is taken and the true population mean estimated from the sample. If all possible samples of a given size were taken from the same population, the result would be a distribution of sample means with the shape of a normal distribution.

Regardless of the shape of the population distribution, however, the distribution of the sample means will be about normal. This is expressed in the central limit theorem, which states that for almost all populations the sampling distribution of the means will be distributed about normally, given a sufficient sample size. Sufficient sample size generally is considered to be thirty or more elements. This theorem allows inferences to be drawn about population means and mortality rates from information extracted from samples in time or space.

Like a population distribution, a distribution of sample means also involves a variance. The variance of the sample mean is equal to the variance calculated from a sample divided by the size of the sample used to calculate the variance:

$$S_{\bar{x}}^2 = \frac{S^2}{n}$$

The square root of the variance of the sample mean is called the standard error of the mean, denoted:

$$S_{\bar{x}} = \sqrt{\frac{S^2}{n}} = \frac{S}{\sqrt{n}}$$

where:

$S_{\bar{x}}$ = standard error of the mean

S = standard deviation

n = number of observations

The standard error of the mean is the statistic that permits statements to be made regarding population estimates of the true mean with specified levels of confidence.

Similarly, the standard error of a rate is the standard deviation of the (theoretical) sampling distribution of the rate. The standard error is used to estimate the range within which the true population lies. This range is called the confidence interval, and the probability with which it is asserted that the true population rate is contained within that interval is called the degree of confidence.

The value most commonly used for the degree of confidence is .95, or 95 percent. This means users can be 95 percent confident that the true rate lies within the calculated confidence interval. To look at it another way, there is 95 percent probability that the confidence interval includes the true rate and 5 percent probability that it does not. When chance of error equals 5 percent and is not acceptable, then the 99 percent confidence interval is commonly used.

Confidence Intervals   The calculation of the confidence interval is based on the assumption that the distribution of the observed rates can be approximated by the standard normal curve. Elementary texts on statistics discuss the theoretical aspects of the construction of confidence intervals and of inferential statistics.[37,38,39,40,41,42] This analysis is limited to three methods for the construction of confidence intervals. A more in-depth discussion is presented in Chapter 10, "Small Area Analysis—Epidemiological Assessment."

Method 1   If a rate for a population at a given time has been computed, it can be considered a sample estimate of the true rate or a sample in time or space, thereby allowing confidence interval estimations to be used. An estimate of the true rate reflects the true rate plus random error. To construct a confidence interval for the rate, the following formula is used.[43]

95 percent confidence limits:

$$Upper\ limit = \frac{1,000}{n}\left[d + 1.96\sqrt{d}\right]$$

$$Lower\ limit = \frac{1,000}{n}\left[d - 1.96\sqrt{d}\right]$$

where:

d = number of deaths upon which rate is based

n = denominator of rate (i.e., the target population)

Similarly, the 99 percent confidence limits are as follows:

$$CI = \frac{1,000}{n}\left[d \pm 2.58\sqrt{d}\right]$$

FIGURE 4-1   Calculating a Confidence Interval for a Population Rate

1. Find the square root of d	$\sqrt{d}$
2. Multiply the square root of d by 1.96	$1.96 \times \sqrt{d}$
3.a. For the upper limit, add d to $1.96\sqrt{d}$	$d + 1.96\sqrt{d}$
3.b. For the lower limit, subtract $1.96\sqrt{d}$ from d	$d - 1.96\sqrt{d}$
4. Divide 1,000 by n	$1,000/n$
5.a. Multiply the quotient in step 4 ($1,000/n$) by the sum in 3.a ($d + 1.96\sqrt{d}$) to get the upper limit	
5.b. Multiply the quotient in step 4 ($1,000/n$) by the difference in step 3.b to get the lower limit	

The step-by-step procedure for calculating the 95 percent confidence interval is shown in Figure 4-1. For the 99 percent confidence interval, 1.96 is replaced with 2.58. If the death rate is greater than 100 per 1,000, $\sqrt{d}$ is replaced with $\sqrt{d[\,1 - (\,d\,/\,n\,)\,]}$. If the rate is of some base other than 1,000 (10,000 or 100,000), this base is exchanged for 1,000 (as previously shown).

The procedure for calculating 95 percent confidence intervals using Method 1 is illustrated in Figure 4-2. The confidence interval calculated there shows that it is possible to be 95 percent confident that the true death rate lies between 5.20 and 6.85 deaths per 1,000.

Method 2   A 95 percent confidence interval for more than thirty observations also can be derived from the following formula:

$$CI = p \pm 1.96 \sqrt{\left[\frac{p \times q}{n}\right]}$$

where:

   CI = confidence interval

   p = the rate

   $q = (1 - p)$

   n = the population for the rate

To calculate the confidence interval:

   1. Divide the rate (p) by 1,000 to put it on a per-person basis.
   2. Multiply the rate (p) by 1 minus the rate (q): $p \times q$.

FIGURE 4-2 Method 1 Procedure for Calculating 95 Percent Confidence Interval for a Population Rate

In DeKalb County, Georgia, in 1998, there were 205 deaths of white males aged 45 to 64 years. A total of 34,006 white males lived in the county. The death rate was 6.03 per 1,000:

$$\left(\frac{205}{34,006} \times 1,000\right) = 6.03$$

The 95 percent confidence interval is:

$$CI = \frac{1,000}{n}\left[d \pm 1.96\sqrt{d}\right]$$

1. $\sqrt{205} = 14.32$
2. $14.32 \times 1.96 = 28.07$
3.a. $205 + 28.07 = 233.07$ (+ for high limit)
3.b. $205 - 28.07 = 176.93$ (– for low limit)
4. $1,000/34,006 = 0.0294$
5.a. $0.0294 \times 233.07 = 6.85$
5.b. $0.0294 \times 176.93 = 5.20$

$$CI = 5.2 \text{ to } 6.85 \ (95\%)$$

3. Divide the product of $p \times q$ by the population for the rate (n):
$$\frac{p \times q}{n}.$$

4. Find the square root for the preceding quotient: $\sqrt{\left[\dfrac{p \times q}{n}\right]}$.

5. Multiply the preceding square root by 1.96. That is: $1.96 \times \sqrt{\left[\dfrac{p \times q}{n}\right]}$ (multiply the product by the number used to get the rate to a per-person basis).

6. To find the two specified confidence limits, add the preceding product to the rate for the high limit and subtract the product

from the rate for the low limit. Thus, the confidence interval =

$$\text{rate} \pm 1.96 \sqrt{\left[\frac{p \times q}{n}\right]}.$$

The procedure for calculating 95 percent confidence intervals using Method 2 is illustrated in Figure 4-3.

Method 3   The third and simplest method to calculate the confidence interval approximates the standard error of the rate. The standard error (SE) of a rate can be calculated easily.

$$SE = \frac{r}{\sqrt{d}}$$

where:

    r = the rate

    d = observed number of deaths (upon which the rate is based)

The 95 percent confidence interval is constructed using the following formula.

    $CI_{(95\%)} = \text{rate} \pm (1.96 \times SE)$

FIGURE 4-3   Method 2 Procedure for Calculating 95 Percent Confidence Interval for a Population Rate

---

Using the data for DeKalb County (Figure 4-2), the 95 percent confidence interval for the 1998 death rate among white males ages 45 to 64 (mortality rate is 6.03) is:

$$CI = \frac{1,000}{n}\left[d \pm 1.96\sqrt{d}\right]$$

1. $6.03/1,000 = 0.00603$
2. $0.00603 \times 0.99397 = 0.00599$ (0.99397 is obtained by subtracting 0.00603 from 1.0, as defined for q)
3. $0.005999/34.006 = 0.0000001$
4. $\sqrt{0.0000001} = 0.0003162$
5. $1.96 \times 0.0003162 = 0.0006197 \times 1,000 = 0.6197$ (multiplying by 1,000 returns the rate to a per 1,000 population basis)
6. $6.03 + 0.6197 = 6.65$ (high limit)
7. $6.03 - 0.6197 = 5.41$ (low limit)

        CI = 5.41 to 6.65 (close to the first method)

The 99 percent confidence interval would simply be:

$$CI_{(99\%)} = \text{rate} \pm (2.58 \times SE)$$

A step-by-step procedure to calculate the 95 percent confidence interval is as follows:

1. Find the square rood of d: $\sqrt{d}$.
2. Calculate the standard error (SE): divide the rate (r) by the square root of d ($\sqrt{d}$).
3. Multiply the SE by 1.96.
4. Add the preceding product to the rate for the high limit and subtract it for the low limit.

This procedure is illustrated in Figure 4-4.

The three methods described can be used to assess the variability of any rate, including the standardized mortality rate (SMR) and birth rates. Method 3 uses an approximation of the SE of a rate but is the simplest and easiest to calculate and is more than adequate for use in health services management. Using Method 3, the SE of an SMR is as follows:

$$SE = \frac{SMR}{\sqrt{d}}$$

where:

d = number of observed deaths

FIGURE 4-4 Method 3 Procedure for Calculating 95 Percent Confidence Interval for a Population Rate

Using the data from Figure 4-2:

1. $\sqrt{205} = 14.32$
2. $SE = 6.03 / 14.32 = 0.421$
3. $1.96 \times 0.421 = 0.825$
4. $6.03 + 0.825 = 6.855$ (high limit)
5. $6.03 - 0.825 = 5.205$ (low limit)

   CI = 5.205 to 6.855 (close to the other two methods)

And the *SE* of a birth rate (*r*) is as follows:

$$SE = \frac{r}{\sqrt{b}}$$

where:

  b = number of births

Significance of Difference between Two Rates

When comparing a rate with an arbitrarily set standard, goal, or target value, the confidence interval for the observed rate (the rate to be compared with the standard) provides the significance of the difference: If the standard is included in the confidence interval of the observed rate, there is no significant difference at the level of confidence chosen.

The situation is somewhat more complex, however, when comparing rates of two different areas or of two different times for the same area. This requires a direct extension of the concept of a confidence interval. The objective is to determine whether a significant difference exists between the rates or whether the difference is caused solely by random effects. Different methods must be used depending on whether or not the rates are independent.

When Rates Are Independent Two rates are said to be independent when they do not include any of the same observations or events (births, deaths, and so on) in their numerator. A death included in one death rate should not be included in a second rate. Thus, rates from overlapping time periods (e.g., from 1980 to 1990 and from 1985 to 1995) or from geographical hierarchy (e.g., comparing a county rate to the one for the district or state it is part of) are not independent. For example, independent rates are those from two different counties.

To determine whether there is a significant difference between two independent rates, the confidence interval for the ratio between the two rates, or the difference between the two independent rates, is used.[44] The ratio between two rates is defined as follows:

$$R = \frac{r_1}{r_2}$$

where:

  R = ratio
  r_1 = rate for area 1 or period 1
  r_2 = rate for area 2 or period 2

The 95 percent confidence interval for the ratio (R) is defined as follows:

$$R \pm 1.96R\sqrt{\left(\frac{1}{d_1}\right)+\left(\frac{1}{d_2}\right)}$$

where:

d_1 = number of events (deaths, etc.) for area 1 or period 1 (i.e., the rate numerator)

d_2 = number of events for area 2 or period 2

To establish a significant difference, it must be determined whether the confidence interval contains 1. If not, it can be stated that the two rates are significantly different. If the interval does contain 1, it cannot be concluded that a significant difference exists. As an example, suppose a typical Georgia county has the following infant mortality data for 1991–1995 and 1996–2000 (Table 4-11). The 95 percent confidence interval is as follows:

$$1.96R\sqrt{\left(\frac{1}{d_1}\right)+\left(\frac{1}{d_2}\right)}=1.96(1.5)\sqrt{\left(\frac{1}{120}\right)+\left(\frac{1}{60}\right)}$$

$$=1.96(1.5)(0.1577)=0.463$$

$$1.5+0.463=1.963 \; (Upper \; limit)$$

$$1.5-0.463=1.036 \; (Lower \; limit)$$

$$CI(95\%)=1.036 \; to \; 1.963$$

Thus, the rate for 1991 to 1995 can be said, with 95 percent confidence, to be from 1.036 to 1.963 times the 1996 to 2000 rate. Because the interval does not

TABLE 4-11   Infant Mortality, 1991–1995 and 1986–2000, Georgia

Year	Number of Infant Deaths	Number of Live Births	Infant Mortality Rate (per 1,000)
1991–1995	120	4,000	30
1996–2000	60	3,000	20
			$R = 30/20 = 1.5$

Source: G. E. A. Dever.

contain 1, there is a statistically significant difference in the county's infant mortality rates at different times. On the other hand, if the interval did contain 1, there would not be a statistically significant difference.

An alternate form of computing the 95 percent confidence interval for the ratio between two rates is to use the confidence intervals for each rate. If the confidence limit is defined as the value that is added to and subtracted from the rate to give the confidence interval, the formula is as follows:

$$CL = 1.96 \times SE = 1.96 \times \left(\frac{1}{\sqrt{d}} \right)$$

where:

SE = standard error (see Method 3 for calculating confidence
        interval)

The confidence interval for the ratio R then is this:

$$CL = R \pm R \sqrt{ \left(\frac{CL_1}{r_1} \right)^2 + \left(\frac{CL_2}{r_2} \right)^2 }$$

where:

CL_1 = confidence level for rate 1
CL_2 = confidence level for rate 2
r_1, r_2 = rates for county periods 1 and 2, respectively

Using this method for the previous example, the confidence level would be this:

$$CL_1 = 1.96 \times \left(\frac{30}{\sqrt{120}} \right) = 1.96 \times 10.74 = 5.37$$

$$CL_2 = 1.96 \times \left(\frac{20}{\sqrt{60}} \right) = 1.96 \times 2.582 = 5.06$$

and:

$$CL = R \pm R \sqrt{\left(\frac{CL_1}{r_1}\right)^2 + \left(\frac{CL_2}{r_2}\right)^2}$$

$$= 1.5 \pm 1.5 \sqrt{\left(\frac{5.37}{30}\right)^2 + \left(\frac{5.06}{20}\right)^2}$$

$$= 1.5 \pm 1.5(0.31) = 1.5 \pm 0.465$$

$$Upper\ limit = 1.5 + 0.465 = 1.965$$

$$Lower\ limit = 1.5 - 0.465 = 1.035$$

$$CL = 1.035\ to\ 1.965$$

The confidence interval does not include 1, which indicates that the two rates are significantly different at the 95 percent level. On the other hand, if the interval did contain 1, there would not be a statistically significant difference. The confidence interval (shown here) is similar to what was obtained using the previous formula. In some instances there could be slight differences in the outcome (CI) due to approximation of the standard error used in calculating the confidence limit in this last method.

These two formulas for the construction of the confidence interval for the ratio between two independent rates are valid only when the denominator (r_2) is based on 100 or more events (e.g., deaths). An alternate way to test the difference between two independent rates is to construct a confidence interval directly for the difference (and not for the ratio). The confidence interval for the difference between two independent rates ($D = r_1 - r_2$) is given by the following expression:

$$D \pm \sqrt{CL_1^2 + CL_2^2}$$

where:

$$D = \text{difference between the two rates}$$
$$CL_1, CL_2 = \text{confidence limits for rates 1 and 2}$$

The confidence limit (CL) then is the value that is added to and subtracted from the rate to construct the confidence interval of the rate:

$$CL = 1.96 \times SE = 1.96\left(\frac{r}{\sqrt{d}}\right)$$

where:

$$d = \text{number of deaths (for a death rate)}$$

In this case, if the interval includes zero, it cannot be concluded that the difference between the two rates is significant. In the previous example:

$$D = r_1 - r2 = 30 - 20 = 10$$
$$CL_1 = 5.37 \qquad CL_2 = 5.06$$
$$CL = D \pm \sqrt{CL_1{}^2 + CL_2{}^2}$$
$$= 10 \pm \sqrt{(5.37)^2 + (5.06)^2}$$
$$= 10 \pm 7.34$$
$$Upper\ limit = 10 + 7.34 = 17.34$$
$$Lower\ limit = 10 - 7.34 = 2.62$$
$$CL = 2.62\ to\ 17.34$$

The 95 percent confidence interval for the difference between the two rates ranges from 2.62 to 17.34. Because this interval does not include zero, there is 95 percent confidence that the difference between the two rates is significant.

A typical example is the difference in infant mortality rates between two counties, A and B. An illustration of the preceding method is shown in Table 4-12.

The confidence limits (95 percent) are as follows:

$$Tift\ County:\ CL_1 = 1.96 \times \left(\frac{16.2}{\sqrt{141}} \right) = \pm 2.67$$

$$Camden\ County:\ CL_2 = 1.96 \times \left(\frac{13.0}{\sqrt{74}} \right) = \pm 2.96$$

The confidence interval for the difference between the rates is as follows:

$$Difference\ D = 16.2 - 13.0 = 3.2$$
$$Confidence\ Interval = D \pm \sqrt{CL_1{}^2 + CL_2{}^2}$$
$$= 3.2 \pm \sqrt{(2.67)^2 + (2.96)^2}$$
$$= 3.2 \pm 3.98$$
$$= -0.78\ to\ 7.18$$

TABLE 4-12 Infant Mortality Rates for Counties A and B

County	Infant Deaths	Births	Infant Mortality Rate (per 1,000)
Tift	141	8,717	16.2
Camden	74	5,672	13.0

Source: G. E. A. Dever.

Thus, the 95 percent confidence interval would be (−0.78 to 7.18). Since the interval does include zero, it can be concluded that the rates for the two counties are not significantly different.

When Rates Are Not Independent When comparing a rate to a standard rate (that is, when rates may not be independent), a slightly more complex formula is needed:

$$\mu = (r - s)\sqrt{\frac{n}{s - s^2}}$$

where:

> r = the observed rate or rate to be compared
> s = the standard rate (state, region, nation, etc.)
> n = the denominator (population on which the rate is based)

The formula is calculated as follows:

1. Square (multiply by itself) the standard rate s: ($s \times s = s^2$). Change all rates to a per-person basis (divide by the rate's denominator).
2. Subtract the square of s from s: $s - s^2$.
3. Divide the denominator on which the rate is based n by the difference of $s - s^2$: $\dfrac{n}{(s-s^2)}$

4. Find the square root of the quotient from the last step: $\sqrt{\dfrac{n}{s-s^2}}$
5. Subtract the standard rate s from the observed rate r: $r - s$
6. Multiply the square root in the fourth step by the difference in the fifth step: $\mu = (r - s)\sqrt{\dfrac{n}{s - s^2}}$

If μ exceeds 1.96, it can be concluded that the rate differs significantly at the 95 percent confidence level from the standard rate to which it is compared. If it exceeds 2.33, it is significantly different at the 98 percent level; and if it exceeds 2.58, it is significantly different at the 99 percent level. For example, a county has a population of 16,400 persons and a death rate of 20.9 per 1,000. The objective is to find out whether this is significantly different from the state rate of 16.8 per 1,000.

> Observed rate r = 20.9 per 1,000
> Standard rate s = 16.8 per 1,000

Population (denominator n on which the rate is based) = 16,400

1. $(0.0168) = 0.0168 \times 0.0168 = 0.000282$
2. $0.0618 - 0.000282 = 0.016518$
3. $16,400/0.016518 = 992,856.27$
4. $\sqrt{992,856.27} = 996.42173$
5. $0.0209 - 0.0168 = 0.0041$
6. $0.0041 \times 996.42173 = 4.09$ (μ)

Because the value of 4.09 (μ) is greater than 2.58, it can be concluded that the difference between the rates is significant at the 99 percent confidence level—in other words, there is 99 percent confidence that the death rate in the county is higher than in the state.

When rates are based on a very few number of events (e.g., births, deaths, cases), the actual number of events is used instead of the rate.

$$\mu = \frac{(o - e)}{e}$$

where:

o = the observed number(s) to be compared

e = the standard number (state, region, nation, etc.)

To calculate this formula:

1. Find the square root of the standard number e: $\sqrt{e}$
2. Subtract the standard number e from the observed number o: $o - e$
3. Divide the difference between the observed and standard numbers (step 2) by the square root of $\frac{(o-e)}{e}$

Thus, the significance of a higher infant mortality rate for a county as compared to the state can be determined by the following:

$$\mu = \frac{(o - e)}{e}$$

Observed rate o = 20.2 per 1,000 (65 deaths)

Standard rate e = 17.5 per 1,000 (117 deaths)

1. $\sqrt{117} = 10.81$
2. $65 - 117 = -52$
3. $-52/10.81 = -4.81$

Because the value −4.81 in absolute terms (that is, without considering the sign) is greater than 2.58, it can be concluded that the two rates are significantly different at the 99 percent confidence level.

The Significance of "Excess Deaths"

As noted, the epidemiological approach to the identification of health problems rests on comparisons. A problem is defined by an excess of morbidity or mortality. Although this discussion is limited to excess deaths, the same concepts and techniques can be applied to excess morbidity when the data is available.

The analysis of excess deaths requires two major steps. Initially, it must be determined whether or not there is a difference between the number of deaths expected and the number actually occurring. Once this difference is determined, the second step is to test it to ascertain whether it merely results from chance or actually is significant statistically. To conduct this analysis, the following data inputs are required.

1. Data on the population being investigated:
   - Population (demographic data categorized by age, sex, race, occupation, or other specifics)
   - Mortality data by cause of death, either in actual number observed or in death rates
2. Data on the standard population

The standard population is the basis for comparing the group being investigated. The standard population can be the state's, the nation's, a county's, or some other geographical area larger than the group being analyzed. Data regarding the standard population must be identical, however, to those available for the group being studied.

If death rates are the desired area of investigation, then they must be available for the selected standard population. Similarly, if age breakdowns are used, they also must be available for the standard population. The standard, however, should resemble the population being investigated as closely as possible.

For example, if counties within a state are under scrutiny, the state should be used as the standard population. With this data, the expected number of deaths can be derived for the population being investigated. The next section provides two methodologies for testing the significance of differences between observed and expected deaths, using numbers and rates of deaths.

Determining the Number of Expected Deaths

Each of the methodologies in this section is statistically valid for health problem analysis and should produce the same results. The selection of one methodology over the other, therefore, depends solely upon the availability of data—and personal preference.

Utilizing the Actual Number of Deaths   The expected number of deaths can be calculated using the following formula:

$$E = \frac{P_1}{P_2} \times D$$

where:

E = expected deaths
P_1 = population being investigated
P_2 = standard population
D = actual deaths in standard population

The ratio $\frac{P_1}{P_2}$ should be age-sex-race specific: If the subject is deaths among white males 55 to 64, both P_1 and P_2 should refer to the number of white males of these ages; on the other hand, if deaths among the overall population are being looked at, P_1 and P_2 should refer to the total population.

For example, in Georgia between 1994 and 1998 there were 1,004 deaths from liver cirrhosis among males ages 45 to 64 years. The state population for this age group during this period was 3,547,396. Bibb County (the county being investigated) had a total population of 70,978 for the age group during the same period. Assuming that the risk of dying from liver cirrhosis was the same in Bibb County as the state as a whole, the expected number of deaths in Bibb County would be calculated as follows.

$$E = \frac{P_1}{P_2} \times D$$

$$= \frac{70,978}{3,547,396} \times 1,004$$

$$= 0.02 \times 1,004$$

$$= 20.1$$

Thus, 20.1 (rounded to 20) is the expected number of deaths of males ages 45 to 64 due to liver cirrhosis during the period under consideration in Bibb

County. Comparing this expected number to the actual number of deaths (30 in Bibb County being investigated), a difference of 10 deaths is identified. To determine whether these deaths represent excess, however, a test of significance must be performed.

Utilizing Death Rates   If death rates instead of actual number of deaths are available from the standard population, the expected number of deaths is given by the following equation:

$$E = P_1 \times M_2$$

where:

P_1 = population being investigated

M_2 = specific death rate in the standard population

Since $M_2 = \dfrac{D}{P_2}$, it can be seen this is algebraically equivalent to the previous method.

Testing the Significance of Results

In the previous example, Georgia had a death rate from liver cirrhosis of 2.83/10,000 population among males ages 45 to 64, or 1,004 deaths.

$$E = 70,978 \times \frac{2.83}{10,000} = 20.086 \ (expected\ deaths)$$

Once the difference between the expected and the observed (actual) deaths is determined, a statistical test must be applied to determine whether it has significance, at least statistically. If the difference shows a statistical significance, then an elevated number of expected deaths is not likely to be a result of chance alone. Associated with significance level, however, there always is a certain possibility that X events in 100 could have occurred solely on the basis of chance.

Two approaches for testing this significance are presented in this section. In the first method, standard mortality ratios (SMRs) are developed and tested utilizing the standard error (SE) and confidence intervals (CI). The second method illustrates the chi-square "goodness of fit" test.

Although each of these methods is sound for this purpose, the SMR can be used more easily by a wide range of health services managers with limited statistical backgrounds. It requires fewer restrictions than the chi-square test, and it is equally sound statistically. The SMR requires more subjective judgment to interpret the results, but the chi-square test is bound by more statistical parameters and, thus, is more rigorous. Although no subjective judgments are to be made, the chi-square test is more complex and can require some statistical expertise to perform.

Standardized Mortality Ratio (SMR)   The SMR has already been described in the indirect method of rate adjustment. It is calculated as follows:

$$SMR = \frac{Observed\ deaths}{Expected\ deaths} \times 100$$

An SMR of 100 indicates that the observed number of deaths equals the expected number of deaths. An SMR of 130 indicates 30 percent excess deaths; one of 90, 10 percent fewer deaths than expected. The next step is to calculate the confidence interval of the SMR. Using Method 3 for calculation of a 95 percent confidence interval (see Figure 4-4), the 95 percent confidence interval of an SMR is obtained by the following equation:

$$CI = SMR \pm (1.96 \times SE)$$

where:

$$SE = \frac{SMR}{\sqrt{d}}$$

$d =$ number of observed deaths

Data on observed and expected deaths in a county, as compared to a state, is presented in Table 4-13.

TABLE 4-13   Observed and Expected Deaths from Heart Disease for County A, by Age Group, Georgia, 1999–2002

Age Group	Expected Deaths	Observed Deaths
20–29	16	16
30–39	18	20
40–49	22	18
50–59	51	56
60–69	55	72
70–79	62	64
80–89	22	28
90+	14	15
Total	260	289

Source: G. E. A. Dever.

$$SMR = \frac{Observed}{Expected} \times 100$$

$$SMR = \frac{260}{289} \times 100 = 89.97$$

$$SE = \frac{SMR}{\sqrt{d}} = \frac{89.97}{\sqrt{260}} = 5.58$$

$$CI\ (95\%) = 89.97 \pm (1.96 \times 5.58)$$

$$Upper\ limit = 89.97 + 10.94 = 100.91$$

$$Lower\ limit = 89.97 - 10.94 = 79.03$$

$$CI = 79 \text{ to } 101$$

The interpretation of the confidence interval of an SMR is as follows:

1. If the lower and upper confidence limits are distributed above and below 100 (i.e., if the lower limit is below 100 and the upper limit is above 100), then there is no significant difference between the observed and the expected deaths.

2. If the lower confidence limit is above 100, then the observed deaths are significantly higher than expected (i.e., it is unlikely that the excess is merely a chance occurrence).

3. If the upper confidence limit is below 100, then the observed deaths are significantly fewer than expected.

4. If a confidence interval is quite wide, regardless of whether both limits are above or below 100, then more years of data is required, or the data should be grouped, before any conclusions can be reached. Although no clear-cut rules specify what constitutes a "wide" range, it is fair to say that a range of 50 or more would be excessive.

In the preceding example, the decision is difficult to make because the upper limit is barely over 100. It can only be concluded that the SMR seems modestly, although not significantly, low at the 95 percent confidence level (it would be significant, however, at the 90 percent level).

Chi-square (χ^2) Test   The chi-square or "goodness of fit" test provides a way to compare an observed frequency with an expected frequency distribution. The formula for chi-square is as follows:

$$\chi^2 = \sum \frac{(O-E)^2}{E}$$

where:

χ^2 = chi-square

Σ = sum across all groups

O = observed deaths

E = expected deaths

Table 4-14 presents the calculation of chi-square for the data presented in Table 4-13. The computed chi-square of 6.97 is compared with a tabular value of χ^2 with $(k - r)$ degrees of freedom, where k equals the number of categories that can be calculated $(O - E)^2 / E$ (i.e., the number of age groups in this example), and r equals the number of restrictions (quantities) that were determined from observed data and used in calculating the expected frequencies.[45]

In most cases, where the expected frequencies are determined by using one of the two methods just described, the only observed quantity involved in calculating the expected frequencies is the population (P_1). When this is the case, the degrees of freedom are $(k - 1)$. In the example in Table 4-14, there are no restrictions because the expected frequencies were not calculated from observed data.

There are, then, eight degrees of freedom (eight age groups). The value of the χ^2 for eight degrees of freedom at the 95 percent level is 15.5. If the calculated value (6.97) is less than the tabular value, then it can be said that there is no significant difference between the observed and the expected

TABLE 4-14 Calculation of Chi-Square (χ^2) for Observed and Expected Deaths from Hearth Disease for County A, 1994–1998

Age Group	Observed Deaths	Expected Deaths	$\frac{(O - E)^2}{E}$
20–29	16	16	0.00
30–39	18	20	0.20
40–49	22	18	0.89
50–59	51	56	0.45
60–69	55	72	4.01
70–79	62	64	0.06
80–89	22	28	1.29
90+	14	15	0.07
Total	260	289	6.97

$\chi^2 = 0.0 + 0.20 + 0.89 + 0.45 + 4.01 + 0.06 + 1.29 + 0.07$
$\chi^2 = 6.97$

Source: G. E. A. Dever.

deaths. If it is greater than the tabular value, then the difference is statistically significant.

The results of both approaches (SMR and χ^2) provide a statistically significant level that allows the health services manager to determine whether or not any excess deaths were indeed representative of a morbidity/mortality problem.

Evidence, Not Proof

Statistical significance provides evidence of differences, characteristics, or associations but does not provide proof. This is because statistical significance is based on several underlying assumptions, including those involving the properties of the distribution and the sample results.

In statistical significance testing, the concern is with the probability of making an error (or of being correct), given the results obtained. Thus, if there is a given confidence level (or a 5 percent error level), what really is being said is that 95 times out of 100 the resulting value exceeds two standard errors.

Further, if the value exceeds the established critical level and falls outside the range of likely values, two things are possible. Either the true mean is different from the one hypothesized (rejection of the false null hypothesis), or the true mean is not different from the one hypothesized; that is, the sample value selected falls in the 5 percent region only by chance (rejection of a true null hypothesis).

Of similar importance, statistical significance deals with probabilities based on repeated sampling from a given population. For any one sample, the true probability is either .0 or 1.0: either the sample statistic is a reliable estimate of the true population parameter or it is not.

Although the confidence level (often referred to as α) indicates the probability of having a value that exceeds the critical region by chance, it does not indicate the probability that the true statistic is actually different from the hypothesized one. The latter is the β probability, or the power of the test, dealing with the ability to detect a false null hypothesis. Although the computation of the β probability is much more difficult than it is for α, it is important to realize that once the desired level and the sample size are set, the β level is fixed.

Because this β level value is usually not known and often is very small, it cannot be concluded that it is true, even when a null hypothesis is not rejected. Rather, it is said that the results are inconclusive or, more commonly, that the null hypothesis was not rejected. Thus, depending on the results from a test of significance, there is a greater likelihood of making an error—either rejecting a true null hypothesis or failing to reject a false null hypothesis. Any test for significance should consider these probabilities of error, and the decision maker should weigh the consequences carefully.

Practical Significance and Decision Making

When statistical significance is commonly reported in testing hypotheses or making inferences—based on the theory of sampling distribution and mathematics—serious concern also should be shown for its practical significance: the real impact or cost of difference. Practical significance can be assessed only by someone familiar with the hypothesis being tested or with the program being evaluated.

It is possible that a difference can be statistically significant though so small as to be meaningless in terms of pragmatic impact. This is especially true when dealing with large samples or rates based on large populations. Because statistical significance is a function of both sample size and population variation, it is quite possible that in a large sample any differences will be significant. Thus, consideration must be given to the real impact of a statistically significant difference on the program or population being tested.

A problem for the health care administrator, then, is the difference between statistical and practical significance. In health services, where data on large populations is available, indexes such as mean or rates can always be significantly different in a statistical sense. The health professional must decide whether the differences are of a magnitude significant enough to justify action, such as revising a program.

A common problem in evaluation testing arises when a key index has increased significantly, according to a statistical expert, but the administrator senses that the size of the increase has no programmatic importance. Survey reports on population often cite differences that are described as "significantly greater" and "significantly longer," but that even to an untrained analyst do not seem to matter much.

A final warning about repeated testing for significance: Tests are designed so that the error probability in any one test is small. Yet, if several tests are made, it is quite likely that true null hypotheses based on chance occurrences can be rejected. Such repeated testing of a number of related factors often is done when searching for relationships rather than testing specific hypotheses. When statistical significance is found in such cases, the probability is quite high that chance occurrence caused rejection.

Summary

Health services managers can use many of the techniques and measurements presented here. The concept of a rate and population at risk are central to the analysis of problems related to the management of health services. This chapter provided the tools and methods for epidemiological investigation into the effective delivery of health services.

The epidemiological measures of rates and their significance allow administrators to determine the magnitude of a problem and whether it warrants further analysis. Much more practical uses for these statistical and epidemiological methods are to monitor current conditions and establish future needs. Finally, determining the significance of the results obtained can be more of a practical decision than a statistical one—the possibility of which health care managers need to consider.

References

1. P. E. Sortwell and J. M. Last, "Epidemiology," in *Maxcy-Rosenau Public Health and Preventive Medicine,* 11th edition, ed. J. M. Last (New York: Appleton-Century-Crofts, Inc., 1980), 14.
2. Sortwell and Last, "Epidemiology," 14.
3. P. A. Buescher, "Problems with Rates Based on Small Numbers," *Statistical Primer,* no. 12 (1997):1–6.
4. E. R. Babbie, *The Practice of Social Research* (Belmont, Calif.: Wadsworth Publishing Co., 1979), 91.
5. D. Rosenberg and A. Handler, "Measures of Association and Hypothesis Testing," in *Analytic Methods in Maternal and Child Health,* ed. A. Handler et al., 73 (Vienna, Va.: Maternal and Child Health Bureau, HRSA, DHHS, 1998).
6. Rosenberg and Handler, "Measures of Association and Hypothesis Testing," 73.
7. Rosenberg and Handler, "Measures of Association and Hypothesis Testing," 74.
8. Rosenberg and Handler, "Measures of Association and Hypothesis Testing," 74.
9. Rosenberg and Handler, "Measures of Association and Hypothesis Testing," 74.
10. Rosenberg and Handler, "Measures of Association and Hypothesis Testing," 74–75.
11. Rosenberg and Handler, "Measures of Association and Hypothesis Testing," 80.
12. Rosenberg and Handler, "Measures of Association and Hypothesis Testing," 80.
13. Rosenberg and Handler, "Measures of Association and Hypothesis Testing," 75.
14. L. Gordis, *Epidemiology,* 2d ed. (Philadelphia: W. B. Saunders Company, 2000), 31–62.
15. Gordis, *Epidemiology,* 31–62.
16. Gordis, *Epidemiology,* 31–62.
17. T. C. Timmreck, *An Introduction to Epidemiology,* 3d ed. (Boston: Jones and Bartlett Publishers, 2002), 121–122.
18. Handler et al., Analytic Methods in Maternal and Child Health, 94.
19. Handler et al., Analytic Methods in Maternal and Child Health, 95.
20. Handler et al., Analytic Methods in Maternal and Child Health, 95.
21. R. N. Anderson and E. Arias, "The Effect of Revised Populations on Mortality Statistics for the United States, 2000," *National Vital Statistics Reports* 51, no. 9 (2003):1–24.
22. Anderson and Arias, "The Effect of Revised Populations on Mortality Statistics for the United States, 2000," 1–24.

23. P. A. Buescher, "Age-Adjusted Death Rates," *Statistical Primer*, no. 13 (1998):1–9.
24. P. A. Buescher, "Age-Adjusted Death Rates," *Statistical Primer*, no. 13 (1998):1–9.
25. P. A. Buescher, "Age-Adjusted Death Rates," *Statistical Primer*, no. 13 (1998):1–9.
26. Buescher, "Age-Adjusted Death Rates," 1–9.
27. Sortwell and Last, "Epidemiology," 25.
28. Buescher, "Age-Adjusted Death Rates," 1–9.
29. Timmreck, *An Introduction to Epidemiology*, 133–140.
30. Timmreck, *An Introduction to Epidemiology*, 153–154.
31. G. E. A. Dever, *Community Health Analysis: A Holistic Approach* (Rockville, Md.: Aspen Systems, Inc., 1980), 80–85.
32. J. Elinson and A. E. Siegmann, eds., *Socio-Medical Health Indicators* (Farmingdale, N.Y.: Baywood Publishing Company, Inc., 1979).
33. "1976 Health Status Indexes Conference—An Annotated Guide to the Papers," *Health Services Research* 4 (Winter 1976):335.
34. A. C. Michalos, ed., *Social Indicators Research* 64, no. 3 (2003):209–224.
35. R. D. Crosby, R. L. Kolotkin, and G. R. Williams, "Defining Clinical Meaningful Change in Health-Related Quality of Life," *Journal of Clinical Epidemiology* 56 (2003):395–407.
36. J. E. Kleinman, "Infant Mortality," *Statistical Notes for Health Planners* 2 (July 1976):4.
37. R. W. Broyles and E. M. Lay, *Statistics in Health Administration*, (Rockville, Md.: Aspen Systems, Inc., 1979), 1:570.
38. Rimm et al., *Basic Biostatistics in Medicine and Epidemiology*, (NY, Appleton-Century Crofts, 1980):37–42.
39. D. G. Altman et al., eds., *Statistics with Confidence*, 2d ed. (London: BMJ Books, 2000).
40. H. Motulsky, *Intuitive Biostatistics* (New York: Oxford University Press, 1995).
41. D. G. Altman, *Practical Statistics for Medical Research* (London: Chapman and Hall, 1991).
42. L. E. Daly and G. J. Bourke, *Interpretation and Uses of Medical Statistics*, 5th ed. (Oxford: Blackwell Science Ltd., 2000).
43. J. E. Kleinman, "Mortality," *Statistical Notes for Health Planners* 3 (February 1977):6.
44. Kleinman, "Mortality," 6.
45. D. E. Drew and E. Keeler, "Algorithms for Health Planners," *Hypertension* 6 (August 1977):63.

5

Identifying Problems, Determining Priorities

Manager's Use of Mortality Indicators

Several epidemiological measurements, techniques, and concepts were described in Chapter 4 that are useful in identifying health problems. Based on some of those methods, this chapter presents a concrete, overall epidemiological approach that can be used easily by health services managers to identify problems in their populations. However, when appropriate, any of the alternatives discussed can be used.

This approach is centered on the standardized mortality ratio (SMR) as an initial screening device. The age-sex-race rates then are used within each diagnostic (cause-of-death) grouping. Table 5-1 presents the data for Georgia County A and the state of Georgia. Data for five years is used because, when dealing with small areas, there is too much variability to make annual rates significant.[1] Similarly, cause-of-death diagnoses are grouped into larger diagnosis-related groups. Only actual numbers of deaths are used. In some instances, especially in counties with fewer deaths and less population, it would be appropriate to expand the time from the five years, as presented here, to ten years. This would further decrease the variability in the rates, making comparisons more valid. Calculations of the SMRs are shown in Table 5-2 and the construction of the 95 percent confidence intervals and the corresponding significance in Table 5-3. Population data is available for each year between 1998 and 2002. To construct the five-year population, therefore, the 1998 to 2002 populations for each year are summed.

Identifying the Problems

Table 5-3 shows definite problems in County A. Heart diseases in general and acute myocardial infarction in particular are significantly higher in the county than in the state. A substantially higher number of homicides also

TABLE 5-1 Leading Causes of Death in County A and Georgia; All Ages, Sexes, and Races, 1998–2002

Year	Heart Diseases*	Cerebro-vascular Disease	Lung Cancer	Motor Vehicle Accidents	All Other Accidents	Pneumonia	Homicides
				County A			
1998	1,007 (235)	240	227	102	83	131	85
1999	935 (226)	273	232	98	76	118	86
2000	954 (224)	276	200	95	96	144	84
2001	923 (207)	276	223	80	103	131	77
2002	928 (220)	242	235	107	96	158	84
Total	4,748 (1,112)	1,307	1,117	482	454	682	416
				Georgia			
1998	16,571 (5,201)	3,889	3,723	1,478	1,311	2,048	801
1999	16,775 (5,190)	4,040	3,886	1,535	1,418	1,991	728
2000	16,903 (4,833)	4,243	3,686	1,586	1,389	2,099	723

TABLE 5-1 Leading Causes of Death in County A and Georgia; All Ages, Sexes, and Races, 1998–2002 (continued)

Year	Heart Diseases*	Cerebro-vascular Disease	Lung Cancer	Motor Vehicle Accidents	All Other Accidents	Pneumonia	Homicides
			Georgia				
2001	16,949 (4,683)	4,269	3,911	1,594	1,457	2,152	640
2002	17,274 (4,820)	4,153	3,969	1,616	1,473	2,258	663
Total	84,472 (24,727)	20,594	19,175	7,809	7,048	10,548	3,555

Source: Representative of data from OASIS, Office of Health Information and Policy, Division of Public Health, Georgia Department of Human Resources, *http://oasis.state.ga.us.*

*Includes acute myocardial infarction, other ischemic heart disease, other heart diseases, and diseases of the arteries. Numbers in parentheses indicate deaths from acute myocardial infarction

	Population	
Year	County A	Georgia
1998	577,108	7,048,990
1999	583,172	7,192,305
2000	586,603	7,334,274
2001	587,730	7,486,242
2002	593,850	7,642,207
Total	2,928,463	36,704,018

TABLE 5-2 SMRs for Selected Causes of Death in County A, 1998–2002, Georgia; All Ages, Sexes, and Races

| | Calculation of Expected Deaths[1] | | | | Observed Deaths | SMR[2] |
| | A | B | C | D | E | F |
Cause of Death	Local Population[3] (P[1])	State Population[4] (P[2])	Actual Deaths in the State (d)	Expected Deaths $\frac{Col\ A}{Col\ B} \times Col\ C$	Observed Deaths in Area	$\frac{Col\ E}{Col\ D} \times 100$
Heart Disease*	2,928,463	3,670,418	84,472 (24,727)	6,740 (1,973)	4,748 (1,112)	70.4 (56.4)
Cerebrovascular Disease	2,928,463	3,670,418	20,594	1,643	1,307	79.5
Lung Cancer	2,928,463	3,670,418	19,175	1,530	1,117	73.0
Motor Vehicle Accidents	2,928,463	3,670,418	7,809	632	482	76.3
All Other Accidents	2,928,463	3,670,418	7,048	562	454	80.8

TABLE 5-2 SMRs for Selected Causes of Death in County A, 1998–2002, Georgia; All Ages, Sexes, and Races (continued)

Cause of Death	Calculation of Expected Deaths[1]				Observed Deaths	SMR[2]
	A	B	C	D	E	F
	Local Population[3] (P_1)	State Population[4] (P_2)	Actual Deaths in the State (d)	Expected Deaths $\frac{Col\ A}{Col\ B} \times Col\ C$	Observed Deaths in Area	$\frac{Col\ E}{Col\ D} \times 100$
Pneumonia	2,928,463	3,670,418	10,548	842	682	81.0
Homicide	2,928,463	3,670,418	3,555	284	416	146.5

Source: Representative of data from OASIS, Office of Health Information and Policy, Division of Public Health, Georgia Department of Human Resources, *http://oasis.state.ga.us.*

1. Expected deaths $= \dfrac{P_1}{P_2} \times d$

   where: P_1 = Local population
   P_2 = State population
   d = Number of actual deaths in state (standard)

2. $SMR = \dfrac{Observed\ deaths}{Expected\ deaths} \times 100$

3. 1998–2000 Local population = (sum of the five-year populations from Table 5-1). Because we have five years of mortality data, we need five years of population data. One must match the numerator and denominator.

4. 1998–2002 State population = (sum of the five-year populations from Table 5-1).

   *Numbers in parentheses indicate deaths from acute myocardial infarction

TABLE 5-3 Confidence Interval and Significance, County A, 1998–2002, Georgia; All Ages, Sexes, and Races

Cause of Death	A. SMR (from Column F, Table 5-2)	Standard Error[1]				Confidence Limits (Interval, 95%)		Significance + If Lower Limit > 100 − If Upper Limit < 100 0 if UL > 100, LL < 100
		B. Number of Observed Deaths	C. Square Root of Observed Deaths	D. SE = Col A / Col B	E. SE × 1.96	F. Col A − Col E Lower Limit	Col A + Col E Lower Limit	
Heart Disease*	70.4 (56.4)	4,748 (1,112)	68.91 (33.35)	1.02 (1.69)	2.0 (3.3)	68.4–72.4 (53.1)–(59.7)		− −
Cerebrovascular Disease	79.5	1,307	36.15	2.20	4.3	75.2–83.8		−
Lung Cancer	73.0	1,117	33.42	2.18	4.3	68.7–77.3		−
Motor Vehicle Accidents	76.3	482	21.95	3.47	6.8	69.5–83.1		−
All Other Accidents	80.8	454	21.31	3.79	7.4	73.4–88.2		−
Pneumonia	81.0	682	26.12	3.10	6.1	74.9–87.1		−
Homicide	146.5	416	20.39	7.18	14.1	131.9–160.6		+

Source: Representative of data from OASIS, Office of Health Information and Policy, Division of Public Health, Georgia Department of Human Resources, *http://oasis.state.ga.us.*

1. Standard Error (SE) $= \dfrac{SMR}{\sqrt{d}}$

   where: d = Number of observed deaths in area being investigated

*Numbers in parentheses indicate deaths from acute myocardial infarction.

occur in the county as compared to the state. Cancer of the lung, motor vehicle accidents, and other accidents are not higher (or significantly lower) than in the state. Pneumonia seems to be borderline—somewhat higher in the county but barely significant.

It should be noted that county and state mortality are compared, so identification of problems is based on the state average. It might be desirable to apply another standard: for example, even though lung cancer is not higher in the county than in the state it could still be considered a problem if the state incidence were regarded as too high. Furthermore, the analysis encompasses all ages, sexes, and races; although an SMR might not be significant for the overall population, it might still be important in a specific age, sex, or race group.

The next step, then, is to look at the specific rates. Although this analysis is limited to age-specific rates, it also is advisable to look at age-sex-race rates. Table 5-4 presents these age (life stage) rates (a blank space does not represent zero deaths but unavailable data due to information that was limited to the top ten leading causes of death in each age group).

Table 5-4 serves several purposes. It shows the age at which each cause of death is most prevalent. For example, motor vehicle accidents are the leading cause of death in adolescence and early adulthood, whereas pneumonia is most prevalent in infants and older adults. There is also a preponderance of other accidents in infancy and late adulthood. Health services managers can use this data to target a program specifically to the most appropriate group. It is also interesting to note that the data for heart diseases, including acute myocardial infarction, and cerebrovascular disease is higher in the state than in the county from early to late adulthood, including older adulthood.

The table also shows whether there is a problem in a specific age (or race) group that does not show up in the overall SMR. In the example, this does not seem to be the case. If it were, however, the solution would be to calculate the specific SMR, to use the formula for testing the significance of the difference between two rates (not independent), or to calculate the confidence interval of the county rate if it is to be compared with an arbitrary standard (a goal or target).

Infant Mortality—An Example

Another important cause of death is infant mortality. Between 1998 and 2002, there were 49,017 births in County A, as compared to 577,753 in the state.[2] In the county 456 infant deaths occurred (rate = 9.3/1,000 births), while in the state there were 5,287 (rate = 92/1,000 births). The significance can be estimated using either the SMR or the direct comparison of the rates.

TABLE 5-4 Cause-Specific Mortality Rates* by Life State; County A and Georgia, 1998–2002

Area	Heart Diseases**	Cerebro- vascular Disease	Lung Cancer	Motor Vehicle Accidents	All Other Accidents	Pneumonia	Homicides
INFANCY (Under 1 Year)							
County	24.5 (—)	—	—	—	—	12.3	—
State	28.5 (—)	7.9	—	7.4	20.5	16.9	10.2
CHILDHOOD							
Early (1–9 years)							
County	1.7 (—)	—	—	5.6	5.9	—	1.4
State	2.0 (—)	0.4	—	7.1	7.3	0.8	1.2
Later and Adolescence (10–19 years)							
County	3.1 (—)	—	—	13.3	3.4	—	19.5
State	2.7 (—)	0.4	—	21.6	6.7	0.6	8.9
ADULTHOOD							
Young (20–44 years)							
County	24.6 (1.7)	5.3	—	20.1	8.9	3.4	20.8
State	36.9 (5.0)	4.8	—	24.4	12.2	3.1	15.1

TABLE 5-4 Cause-Specific Mortality Rates* by Life State; County A and Georgia, 1998–2002 (continued)

Area	Heart Diseases**	Cerebro- vascular Disease	Lung Cancer	Motor Vehicle Accidents	All Other Accidents	Pneumonia	Homicides
ADULTHOOD							
Middle (45–64 years)							
County	216.9 (29.1)	34.5	64.5	14.6	12.7	11.0	7.5
State	280.4 (76.7)	40.4	86.0	19.6	18.2	14.0	7.4
Late (65+ years)							
County	2,166.7 (380.7)	427.4	297.3	24.4	92.9	232.1	4.5
State	2,481.7 (502.4)	461.0	338.5	32.8	83.6	243.7	4.8

Source: Representative of data from OASIS, Office of Health Information and Policy, Division of Public Health, Georgia Department of Human Resources, *http://oasis.state.ga.us.*

— Denotes the number is below a set standard to be given; therefore, it is suppressed

*Rates expressed as deaths per 100,000 population

**Numbers in parentheses refer deaths from acute myocardial infarction

$$SMR = \frac{Observed\ deaths}{Expected\ deaths} \times 100$$

$$Expected\ deaths = \frac{P_1}{P_2} \times Deaths\ in\ state$$

$$Expected\ deaths = \frac{49,017}{577,753} \times 5,287 = 448.6$$

$$SMR = \frac{456}{448.6} \times 100 = 101.6$$

The standard error (SE) is:

$$SE = \frac{SMR}{\sqrt{d}} = \frac{101.6}{\sqrt{456}} = 4.8$$

The confidence interval (CI) is:

$$CI = \pm SE \times 1.96 \ (using\ 95\%\ confidence\ limit)$$

$$= \pm 4.8 \times 1.96 = \pm 9.4$$

$$Upper\ limit = 101.6 + 9.4 = 111$$

$$Lower\ limit = 101.6 - 9.4 = 92.2$$

$$CI = 92.2\ to\ 111$$

Because the confidence interval includes 100, it can be concluded that there is no significant difference in infant mortality between County A and the state rate. The same conclusion can be reached using the following formula (see also Chapter 4):

$$\mu = (r - s)\sqrt{n\,/\,s - s^2}$$

where:

r = County rate = $9.3\,/\,1,000 = 0.0093$

s = State rate = $9.2\,/\,1,000 = 0.0092$

n = Denominator of county rate = $577,753$ (births)

$$= (0.0093 - 0.0092) \times \sqrt{\frac{577,753}{(0.0092 - 0.000085)}} = 0.797$$

Because μ is smaller than 1.96, it can be concluded that the two rates are not significantly different at the 95 percent confidence level. It is also interesting to calculate the confidence interval of rates, allowing the comparison with an arbitrarily set standard or goal. For example, is the county rate significantly higher than a goal of 7 deaths per 1,000 births? The 2000 or 2010 objective for the nation is usually the set point for comparing a local geography or program to the nation. The confidence interval is given by the following equation:

$$CI = Rate \pm 1.96 \times SE$$

where:

$$SE = \frac{Rate}{\sqrt{Deaths}}$$

$$SE = \frac{9.3}{\sqrt{456}} = 0.436 \ or \ 0.44$$

$$CI = 9.3 \pm (1.96 \times 0.44) = 9.3 \pm 0.86$$

$$Upper \ limit = 9.3 + 0.86 = 10.16$$

$$Lower \ limit = 9.3 - 0.86 = 8.44$$

This means that, just by chance, the county rate can vary between 8.44 and 10.16 (95 percent of the time). Thus, it is significantly higher than a target value of 7.0.

In summary, health services managers can identify the specific health problems of their area by the following steps.

1. Calculate the SMRs across all ages, sexes, and races to determine the causes of death that are excessive as compared to a standard (state, national, or other).
2. Look at the specific age-sex-race rates to determine further specific problems.
3. Calculate the significance of any difference found in step 2.

Determination of Priorities

Once problems are identified, questions remain as to which should be addressed, which are the most important. Epidemiology can contribute to the determination of priorities.

Proportionate Mortality Ratio

The simplest and perhaps the preliminary epidemiological measure for determining priorities is the proportionate mortality ratio (PMR). As dis-

TABLE 5-5   Age-Specific PMRs

	Deaths by Cause		
Age Group	All Causes	Accidents	PMR for Accidents (%)
1–4	125	42	33.6
65–74	4,291	118	2.8

cussed earlier, the PMR represents the percentage of all deaths that result from a specific cause.

$$PMR = \frac{Death\ by\ cause}{Total\ deaths} \times 100$$

The PMR indicates the relative importance of causes of death and consequently provides an estimate of the number and population of lives saved by reducing or eradicating a specific cause. On the other hand, the PMR can be misleading because its magnitude depends on the number of deaths from causes other than the one under consideration.[3] An example is displayed in Table 5-5. Even though death rates from accidents are higher among the elderly, the proportion of deaths from that cause is greater for young children. This of course is because total deaths from all other causes are much higher in the elderly. Care must be exercised, therefore, when comparing PMRs across age groups.

In addition to the PMR, epidemiology provides two main sets of criteria for determining priorities: magnitude of the loss and amenability to prevention or reduction.

Magnitude of Loss, Years of Life Lost

The development of priorities can be based on losses from death, from morbidity, or from both.[4] Losses can be expressed in terms of time, productive time, or income foregone. Added losses can be added to each because of the cost of care. The years-of-life-lost (or YLL) indicator can be used to calculate the estimated number lost for each cause of death. The resulting rank or prioritization of causes of deaths will be quite different from that obtained using the PMR, with only the erode number of deaths.

This is because most deaths occur at an older age, but many more life years are lost when death occurs at a younger age than expected. Mortality in older age groups probably is least amenable to health services, so the

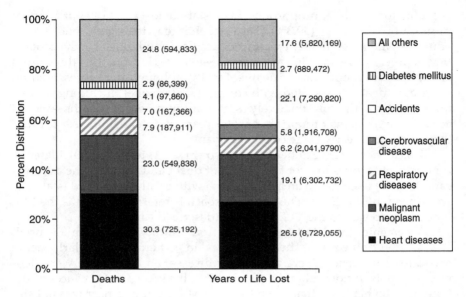

FIGURE 5-1 Number and Percent Distribution of Selected Causes of Death and Potential Years of Life Lost. *Source:* Data derived from *National Vital Statistics Report* 49, no. 11 (Atlanta: Centers for Disease Control and Prevention, National Center for Health Statistics, 2001).

opposite might be true for morbidity or disability. The YLL, thus, might be a useful indicator in the prioritization of problems for purposes of health service management.[5] Figure 5-1 illustrates the ranking of causes of death in the United States, using both the erode number of deaths and the estimated years of life lost.[6]

As shown in the left-hand bar, the six leading causes of death in 1999 were heart diseases, malignant neoplasms (cancer), respiratory diseases, cerebrovascular disease (stroke), accidents, and diabetes. Together they accounted for 75.0 percent of all deaths; of these, heart disease represents 30.3 percent, cancer 23.0 percent, and accidents only 4 percent. Respiratory diseases represent approximately 8 percent of all deaths, while diabetes is about 3 percent.

The right-hand bar shows the impact of the six leading categories on years of life lost, based on life expectancy rates at each age. Heart disease and accidents dominate the YLL category with 26 percent and 22 percent, respectively. Heart disease impacts older age groups more frequently, so it accounts for a smaller proportion of years of life lost (26.46%) but a higher proportion of deaths (30.3%). Because children, teenagers, and young adults are the most frequent victims of accidents and violence, the proportion of potential years of life lost from those causes is more than three times as high as the proportion of deaths. Finally, although not represented on the graph, deaths associated with congenital anomalies, including perinatal mortality—though relatively small in number of deaths—would account for a sizable proportion of total years of potential life lost because they occur at an early stage of the life span.

Basically, the YLL can be used in two ways: (1) to simply calculate the number of life years lost for each cause of death and compare the different causes, or (2) to compare an area (county) with another standard (state), as was done with the SMR. The latter approach is referred to here as the YLL index, as opposed to the YLL indicator (described earlier).

Once again, the data for 1998–2002 from County A in Georgia is used. It was determined that heart diseases in general (particularly acute myocardial infarction), cerebrovascular disease, and homicide were definite problems. It now might be decided that the state rate for cancer of the lung was too high and that, even though SMR for lung cancer was not significantly higher in the county than in the state, it still had to be considered a problem.

For purposes of this example, the priority analysis is limited to cerebrovascular disease, homicide, and lung cancer. Table 5-6 illustrates the calculation of the YLL indicator. Age 74.5 years was chosen arbitrarily as the life expectancy, that is, the age to which the population normally could aspire. All deaths are assumed to occur at midpoints of the age groups so the expected number of years lost is calculated as 65 minus the midpoint of the age group. The table shows the cause of death costing the most years of life is homicide, followed by cerebrovascular disease, even though the latter accounts for almost seven times as many deaths as homicide does. Lung cancer is second in number of deaths but third in YLL.

To compare the county with the state in terms of YLL using the YLL index, it is necessary to adjust for differing age distributions by calculating the expected number of deaths for each age group. The expected YLL can then be computed; the YLL index is the ratio of observed to expected YLL.

$$YLL\ index = \frac{Observed\ years\ of\ life\ lost}{Expected\ years\ of\ life\ lost} \times 100$$

TABLE 5-6 Estimated YLL Indicators; County A, Georgia, 1998–2002

Indicators	Age Group	Deaths		Average YLL		Estimated YLL
A. Cerebrovascular	Under 1	3	×	74.5	=	223.5
Disease	1–9	1	×	70.0	=	70.0
	10–19	0	×	59.5	=	0.0
	20–44	70	×	42.5	=	2,975.0
	45–64	198	×	21.0	=	4,158.0
	65 and over	1,035	×	5.0	=	5,175.0
	Total	**1,307**				**12,601.5**
B. Homicide	Under 1	4	×	74.5	=	298.0
	1–9	5	×	70.0	=	350.0
	10–19	75	×	59.5	=	4,462.5
	20–44	277	×	42.5	=	11,772.5
	45–64	43	×	21.0	=	903.0
	65 and over	11	×	5.0	=	55.0
	Total	**415**				**17,841.0**
C. Cancer of	Under 1	0	×	74.5	=	0.0
the Lung	1–9	0	×	70.0	=	0.0
	10–19	0	×	59.5	=	0.0
	20–44	27	×	42.5	=	1,147.5
	45–64	370	×	21.0	=	7,770.0
	65 and over	720	×	5.0	=	3,600.0
	Total	**1,117**				**12,517.5**

Source: Representative of data from OASIS, Office of Health Information and Policy, Division of Public Health, Georgia Department of Human Resources, *http://oasis.state.ga.us.*

Interpretation and calculation of the significance of the YLL index are identical to that of the SMR. Table 5-7 presents the calculation of the expected YLL.

$$Expected\ deaths = \frac{P_1}{P_2} \times d$$

where:

P_1 = County population

P_2 = State population

d = Deaths in the state

TABLE 5-7 Estimated YLL Index; County A, Georgia, 1998–2002

Indicators	Age Group	County Population (P_1)	State Population (P_2)	Deaths in State (d)	Expected Deaths $\left(\dfrac{P_1}{P_2} \times d\right)$	Average YLL	Expected YLL
A. Cerebro-vascular Disease	Under 1	40,748	557,311	44	3.2	74.5	238.4
	1–9	356,198	4,952,875	22	1.6	70.0	112.0
	10–19	384,273	5,305,425	19	1.4	59.5	83.3
	20–44	1,331,085	14,887,225	715	63.9	42.5	2,715.8
	45–64	574,000	7,352,501	2,971	231.9	21.0	4,869.9
	65 and over	242,164	3,648,681	16,821	1,116.4	5.0	5,582.0
	Total						**13,601.4**
B. Homicide	Under 1	40,748	557,311	57	4.2	74.5	312.9
	1–9	356,198	4,952,875	59	4.2	70.0	294.0
	10–19	384,273	5,305,425	474	34.3	59.5	2,040.9
	20–44	1,331,085	14,887,225	2,243	200.5	42.5	8,521.3
	45–64	574,000	7,352,501	547	42.7	21.0	896.7
	65 and over	242,164	3,648,681	174	11.5	5.0	57.5
	Total						**12.123.2**

TABLE 5-7 Estimated YLL Index; County A, Georgia, 1998–2002 (continued)

Indicators	Age Group	County Population (P_1)	State Population (P_2)	Deaths in State (d)	Expected Deaths $\left(\dfrac{P_1}{P_2} \times d\right)$	Average YLL	Expected YLL
C. Cancer	Under 1	40,748	557,311	0	0.0	74.5	0.0
of the	1–9	356,198	4,952,875	0	0.0	70.0	0.0
Lung	10–19	384,273	5,305,425	1	0.1	59.5	6.0
	20–44	1,331,085	14,887,225	502	44.9	42.5	1,908.3
	45–64	574,000	7,352,501	6,321	493.5	21.0	10,363.5
	65 and over	242,164	3,648,681	12,351	819.7	5.0	4,098.5
	Total						**16,376.2**

Source: Representative of data from OASIS, Office of Health Information and Policy, Division of Public Health, Georgia Department of Human Resources, *http://oasis.state.ga.us.*

The YLL indexes (age-adjusted) are as follows:

$$Cerebrovascular\ disease = \frac{12,601.5}{13,601.4} \times 100 = 93$$

$$Homicide = \frac{17,841.0}{12,123.2} \times 100 = 147$$

$$Cancer\ of\ the\ lung = \frac{12,517.5}{16,376.2} \times 100 = 76$$

The confidence interval (CI) for the YLL index is calculated as described previously:

$$95\%\ CI = YLL \pm 1.96 \times SE$$

where:

$$SE = \frac{YLL}{\sqrt{d}}$$

Thus, for:

Cerebrovascular disease:

$$CI = 93 \pm 1.96 \times \frac{93}{\sqrt{1,307}} = 93 \pm 5.0$$

$$CI = 88.0\ to\ 98.0$$

Homicide:

$$CI = 147 \pm 1.96 \times \frac{147}{\sqrt{415}} = 147 \pm 14.1$$

$$CI = 132.9\ to\ 161.1$$

Cancer of the lung:

$$CI = 76.0 \pm 1.96 \times \frac{76.0}{\sqrt{1,117}} = 76.0 \pm 4.5$$

$$CI = 71.5\ to\ 80.5$$

This means it is possible to be 95 percent confident that from about 2 to 12 more years of life are lost in the state than in the county because of cerebrovascular disease, from about 33 to 61 percent more years of life lost (YLL) in the county than in the state are due to homicide, and significantly less—19 to 28 percent less—in the county than in the state are from cancer of the lung.

It is interesting to note that the results of the YLL index are somewhat different from those of the SMR. The SMR for homicide indicates about 61 percent difference between the state and the county, but the YLL index shows a deficit of 47 percent when compared to that of the state. This is because of two factors.

1. The YLL index, unlike the SMR, emphasizes the differences in age-specific mortality in younger ages.
2. The YLL index is age-adjusted, whereas the SMRs were not age-adjusted. This can be done in calculating the expected deaths for each age group, as for the YLL, instead of directly determining the overall expected deaths across all ages. This age adjustment removes any variations in mortality that can occur because of a different age distribution in the county and in the state.

When data is available, the magnitude of loss for morbid conditions can also be calculated. Obviously, this is valuable information because it is a direct indicator of the burden of diseases in the population. Such loss is often expressed in terms of disability days.

Risk Factors and Priorities

Another epidemiological strategy in the determination of priorities is to calculate losses because of risk factors. As should be clear by now, risk factors are the cornerstone of epidemiology. It was shown earlier how the concept of causality is expanded in epidemiology by the concept of risk. It was also shown how health can be conceived of as resulting from the interaction of multiple risk factors grouped in four health-field dimensions. In that sense, risk factors are the key to an effective and efficient health strategy, mostly through preventive action.

In the planning and management of health programs, therefore, it is important to be able to estimate the impact of each risk factor on the population. This gives an estimate of the potential impact of a program directed toward some risk factors in reducing mortality and morbidity. Such estimates consequently help managers to determine the relative importance—prioritization—of each risk factor for which a program could be developed.

Absolute and Relative Risk

The incidence rate of a disease is a measurement of risk. The incidence rate in a group of people exposed to a risk factor can be called the absolute risk of the disease. An even more meaningful action is to compare this risk with that of people who are not exposed to that factor. The ratio of the incidence rate in the exposed to the incidence rate in the nonexposed is called the relative risk (RR).

$$RR = \frac{Incidence\ rate\ among\ exposed}{Incidence\ rate\ among\ nonexposed}$$

Using the concept of relative risk, a 2×2 data table illustrating the long-term relationship between cigarette smoking and development of lung cancer can be used to explain the relationship of smoking and lung cancer, where in Table 5-8:

A = Population of smokers with lung cancer
B = Population of smokers without lung cancer
C = Population of nonsmokers with lung cancer
D = Population of nonsmokers without lung cancer

Relative risk (RR) is the ratio of the incidence of lung cancer among smokers divided by the incidence of lung cancer among nonsmokers, assuming

TABLE 5-8 Data Illustrating Lung Cancer and Smoking Status

	Lung Cancer		
	Yes	No	
Smokers	A (150)	B (4,850)	5,000 (N_1)
Nonsmokers	C (60)	D (4,940)	5,000 (N_2)
Total	210	9,790	10,000

Source: G. E. A. Dever.

that a prospective study where incidence of the diseases can be calculated. Therefore:

$$RR = \frac{A}{A+B} \div \frac{C}{C+D}$$

$$RR = \frac{A}{N_1} \div \frac{C}{N_2}$$

$$RR = \frac{A}{N_1} \times \frac{N_2}{C}$$

Therefore, using the data from Table 5-8:

$$RR = \frac{150}{5,000} \times \frac{5,000}{60} = 2.5$$

This means the risk of lung cancer among this population of 10,000 is 2.5 times higher among the smokers than the nonsmokers when the two groups are matched by age, sex, race, geographical location, and other confounding variables.

In another example, Doll and Hill studied death rates among British male physicians who smoked.[7] Among heavy smokers, they found death rates of 1.66 per 1,000 for lung cancer, 2.63 for other cancers, and 1.41 for other respiratory diseases. This compared with 0.07 (lung cancer), 2.01 (other cancers), and 0.81 (other respiratory diseases) among nonsmokers. Using the formula, the relative risk of lung cancer among heavy smokers in this survey is 23.7 (1.66 ÷ 0.07 = 23.7), for other cancers 1.3 (2.63 ÷ 2.01 = 1.3), and for other respiratory diseases, 1.7.

Doll and Hill also found death rates of 5.99 versus 422 (heavy smokers vs. nonsmokers) for coronary thrombosis (a RR of 1.4), and for other causes, rates of 7.19 vs. 6.11 (RR = 12). The rate for all causes of death in the survey is 18.84 for heavy smokers contrasted with 13.25 for nonsmokers, giving a RR for all causes of 1.4.

In this particular example, relative risk is a measurement that illustrates the association between nonsmokers and heavy smokers for certain causes of death in the physician population. In general, for all causes, the risk of death is 1.4 times as great for heavy smokers as nonsmokers, and in particular for lung cancer, the risk of death for heavy smokers is almost 24 times as great as that of nonsmokers.[8]

As described in Chapter 2, the three main types of epidemiological study are prospective, retrospective, and cross-sectional. Only prospective studies can provide an incidence rate by following a group of people (usually two groups, exposed and nonexposed) forward in time and observing the development of disease. With data from prospective studies, relative risk can be calculated with few problems. Cross-sectional studies provide a measure of the prevalence of disease at one point in time. An estimate of the relative risks can be calculated from such studies by obtaining the ratio of the prevalence rates between the exposed and the nonexposed.

Much more frequently, however, epidemiological data are derived from retrospective studies. In these, data is collected from two groups of people, one having a specific disease or condition and the other not having it, to determine whether they were or were not exposed to the same risk factors. For example, data can be collected from people who have lung cancer and from others, comparable in terms of age, sex, race, and other variables, who do not to determine their smoking habits. From such studies four categories are obtained.

	With the Disease (Cases)	Without the Disease (Controls)
Exposed	A	B
Nonexposed	C	D

It is known that a given number (A) of people with the disease were exposed to the factor, a given number (B) without the disease also were exposed, and so on. However, the population at risk is not known, so the incidence rates cannot be calculated. These four groups do not represent the total populations exposed and not exposed. However, the relative risk can be estimated by using the odds ratio, also known as the risk ratio or the cross-ratio. The estimate of relative risk is obtained by the following:

$$RR = \frac{A \times D}{B \times C}$$

where A, B, C, and D are defined as above.

For example, a retrospective study to determine the smoking habits of a group of lung cancer patients and of a matched group of patients with other diseases was conducted. The following (smokers were defined as those who averaged at least one cigarette a day over the ten years preceding the onset of the present illness) was determined from the focus groups:

	Patients with Lung Cancer	Patients with Other Conditions	
Smokers	1,350	1,296	2,646
Nonsmokers	7	61	68
Total	1,357	1,357	

The relative risk can be estimated as follows:

$$RR = \frac{1{,}350 \times 61}{7 \times 1{,}296} = 9.08$$

This estimate represents a risk (odds ratio) of lung cancer nine times greater among smokers than nonsmokers.

Attributable Risk   The proportion of cases of a disease or a cause of death attributable to a risk factor also can be calculated. The attributable risk can be defined as the difference between exposed and nonexposed groups in the incidence rate of a disease or condition. The data shows that the incidence of lung cancer attributable to heavy smoking is 1.59 per 1,000 (1.66 − 0.07). The rate of 1.59 per 1,000 is referred to as the excess risk.[9]

A proportion (ratio) is another way of expressing the attributable risk, known as the attributable risk percent (AR%). This represents the percentage of risk that can be attributed to the risk factor. The ratio can be calculated either for the exposed population (AR% in the exposed) or for the total population (AR% in the population).

$$\text{AR in the exposed} = \frac{IR_e - IR_{ne}}{IR_e} \times 100$$

$$\text{Population AR} = \frac{IR_e - IR_{ne}}{IR_e + IR_{ne}} \times 100$$

where:

IR_e = Incidence rate among exposed

IR_{ne} = Incidence rate among nonexposed

Using data from Doll and Hill's study of lung cancer produces this result:

$$\text{AR in heavy smokers} = \frac{1.66 \times 0.07}{1.66} \times 100 = 95.8\%$$

Thus, 95.8 percent of deaths from lung cancer can be attributable to heavy smoking. The population AR% in this example cannot be calculated because the incidence rate of nonheavy smokers is lacking (only the incidence rate among nonsmokers is available). If the death rate from lung cancer among all smokers is 0.85/1,000 and among nonsmokers is 0.07/1,000, then:

$$AR\% \text{ in smokers} = \frac{0.88 - 0.07}{0.88} \times 100 = 92\%$$

$$\text{Population } AR\% = \frac{0.88 - 0.07}{0.88 + 0.07} \times 100 = 85\%$$

This means that 92 percent of deaths from lung cancer among smokers can be attributed to smoking and that 85 percent of lung cancer deaths among the total population can also be attributed to smoking. The latter figure (population attributable risk) represents the maximum proportion of lung cancer that can be assigned to cigarette smoking.

As for relative risk, the population AR% can be calculated even when incidence rates are not available (in retrospective studies).

$$\text{Population } AR\% = \frac{B(RR - 1)}{1 + B(RR - 1)} \times 100$$

where:

RR = Relative risk

B = Proportion of those exposed in the population

For example, if the relative risk of lung cancer among smokers is 9.08, and it is known that 50 percent of the general population are smokers, then:

$$\text{Population } AR\% = \frac{0.50(9.08 - 1)}{1 + 0.50(9.08 - 1)} \times 100 = 80\%$$

Both attributable and relative risks can be helpful in determining priorities. Table 5-9 illustrates the relationship and complementary components of these epidemiological measures. In this example, smokers are at 12 times greater risk of dying from lung cancer than nonsmokers and at 1.4 times greater risk from cerebrovascular disease. It can be said that smoking influences the death rates from lung cancer much more than those from cerebrovascular disease. The attributable (excess) risks indicate, however, that 78 lung cancer deaths and 177 cerebrovascular deaths per 100,000 are attributable to smoking. This means that smoking influences a greater number of deaths from cerebrovascular disease than from lung cancer.[10]

Relative risk, thus, is a better measurement of the causal association between a risk factor and a disease (or cause of death), whereas the attributable risk gives an estimate of the possible reduction in morbidity and mortality from the elimination of the risk factor.

TABLE 5-9 Comparison of Relative and Attributable Risks

	Death Rates per 100,000	
	Lung Cancer	*Cerebrovascular Disease*
Smokers	85	599
Nonsmokers	7	422
Relative risk $= $	$\dfrac{85}{7} = 12.1$	$\dfrac{599}{422} = 1.4$
Attributable risk $=$ (excess risk)	$85 - 7 = \dfrac{78}{100,000}$	$599 - 422 = \dfrac{177}{100,000}$

Source: Adapted from *Epidemiology: An Introductory Text* by J. S. Mausner and A. K. Bahn (Philadelphia: W. B. Saunders Company, 1974), 322.

Amenability to Prevention or Reduction

The second set of epidemiological criteria that can be used in determining priorities is the amenability of the disease, problem, or risk factor for prevention or reduction or its sensitivity to a health program. Consequently, it is not of much use to consider a problem to be a priority if there is nothing that can be done about it.

Amenability can be conceived of as a relationship between inputs and outputs.[11] Inputs are often stated in terms of costs or expenditures; outputs in terms of the effects of the program on the problem or the money value of such effects. This is known as a cost-benefit analysis.

Although cost-benefit analysis is popular, its regular use in health services management is far away. It is relatively easy to keep track of such costs, but the measurement and valuation of benefits present several problems. However, health services managers can still consider the amenability of a health problem by relying on the judgment of experts or the experience of others. For example, several estimates of the effectiveness of smoking cessation programs have been published. Similarly, the work of Rutstein and colleagues,[12] the Canadian Task Force on the Periodic Health Examination,[13] and the U.S. Department of Health and Human services[14] (as described in Chapter 2) can be used to determine the problems that are most amenable to prevention.

Magnitude of loss and amenability, thus, are two essentially independent properties jointly constituting guides for the determination of priorities.[15] Donabedian has outlined possible decision rules or bases for magnitude of loss and amenability to prevention or reduction by comparing magnitude of loss with accountability and the decisions on priority level for delivery of services or for research. If the magnitude of loss and amenability to prevention is high, then there is a high priority for service delivery; on the other hand, if both of these characteristics are low, then a low priority of service delivery emerges, as well as a second priority for research. Finally, when magnitude of loss and amenability of prevention alternate (i.e., high/low and low/high), there is a high priority for research and a second priority for service delivery, respectively.[16]

Problems of Measurement

This chapter and the previous one presented several epidemiological measures to be used in health services management and analyzed their statistical and practical significance. A last issue remains: the quality of these measures. For purposes here, distinctions are drawn among three components of quality of a measure: its validity, its reliability, and its sensitivity.

Validity of a Measure

Validity refers to the extent a measurement can measure what it purports to measure. Is it really measuring what was intended to be measured? The validity of epidemiological measures for identifying health problems is, of course, a big issue: Do they really measure "health problems"? The answer is even more difficult because it is not really known what "health" is.

The validity of a measure has four dimensions: face, and the three Cs, content, criterion, and construct.

Face validity refers to apparent, commonsense validity: Does the measurement appear to do what it is supposed to be doing? For example, if the number of parking tickets is used as an indicator of the health of community, that poses a big problem with face validity even though it really might be right (by some as yet unexplainable phenomenon). Face validity is important mostly in terms of the acceptability of results to outsiders.

Content validity refers to the extent of measuring all aspects, dimensions, or components of what is intended to be measured. This is, of course, the major drawback to health indicators or single measures of health. For example, an infant mortality rate unquestionably is not a content-valid measure of health, even though infant mortality often is used as the single indicator. There is no way to assess the content validity of a measurement mathematically. The only guideline is to break down what is to be measured into as main components as possible. For example. if the subjects are physiological, psychological, and social health, indicators can be found for each. These indicators can be used either separately or combined into a health index.

Criterion validity refers to the extent to which it is possible to explain or predict what is wanted to be measured (a distinction can be made between predictive and concurrent criterion validity). This can be assessed by looking at the correlation of the measurement with some other criteria, either retrospectively or futuristically (when those criteria become available). For example, the predictive criterion validity of smoking can be assessed as a health problem indicator by looking at the association between smoking and death. In this case, the relative and attributable risks associated with smoking demonstrate that smoking is a good predictor of health problems.

Finally, construct validity refers to the general definition of validity: that is, the extent to which managers are really measuring what they say they are. Several methods have been proposed to assess construct validity. These all are complex, however, and are described well in other excellent sources.[17,18,19] In general, all of these methods aim to correlate the measure to be construct-validated with other measures that are known to be construct-valid.

An oversimplified example would be if an attempt were made to devise a new aptitude scale, perhaps a shorter version. It is known that several such scales have been construct-validated. If the new scale correlates highly with the others, then there could be relative confidence in its construct validity.

Reliability of a Measure

Reliability refers to the reproducibility or constancy of the measurement. If a measure is used several times, how close will be the different results? This is not directly related to validity, however. A classic example is a weight scale: Suppose a person is weighed five times in quick succession and the measurement is always the same. It could be said that the scale was reliable. However, it might be maladjusted and add twenty pounds to the real weight—five times in quick succession. Even though reliable in its consistency, the scale does not give a valid measure. Assessment of the reliability of a single indicator is quite straightforward: Repeated applications of the indicator must correlate together closely. For multidimensional indexes, some statistical techniques are available.[20,21,22]

Sensitivity of a Measure

The sensitivity of a measure refers to its ability to include a great proportion of what it is measuring. This is the opposite of its specificity, or its ability to exclude as much false information as possible. Infant mortality rates, for example, are sensitive indicators because they include most of the routinely reported infant deaths and omit many "false" deaths (i.e., deaths that could not be allocated to another group).

Sensitivity and specificity most often relate to screening measures. A screening measurement (or test) can be either sensitive or specific. A sensitive screening measure should be wide enough to include as many real cases of the disease as possible; in doing so, however, it also will include a high number of false cases (it will not be specific).

Summary

Two of the major problems facing all decision makers, including health services managers, are the identification of a problem and the resulting difficulty of determining priorities. This chapter shows how the SMR—the standardized mortality rate—is a simple but reliable method and can be used to identify various problems from an epidemiological perspective. The determination of priorities can be accomplished by several methods, of which the PMR, years of life lost, risk factors, and amenability to prevention are discussed.

Each is useful and valid for setting priorities in health management. Certainly all techniques and methods are subject to variability and errors, so for this reason the concepts of validity, reliability, and sensitivity are discussed. It is contended here that health services managers using these epidemiological measures will be more sophisticated in the analysis of health care utilization.

References

1. T. Lofton et al., *Planning Information Reports (PIR), 1994–1998* (Atlanta: Georgia Department of Human Resources, Division of Public Health, Office of Health Information and Policy, 2000).
2. Lofton et al., *Planning Information Reports (PIR)*.
3. T. C. Timmreck, *An Introduction to Epidemiology*, 3d ed. (Sudbury, Mass.: Jones and Bartlett Publishers, 2002), 124–125.
4. A. Donabedian, *Aspects of Medical Care Administration: Specifying Requirements for Health Care* (Cambridge, Mass.: Harvard University Press, 1973), 165.
5. J. C. Kleinman, "Infant Mortality," *Statistical Notes for Health Planners* 2 (July 1976):12.
6. Centers for Disease Control and Prevention, National Center for Health Statistics, *National Vital Statistics Report* 49, no. 11 (2001).
7. R. Doll and A. B. Hill, "A Study of the Aetiology of Carcinoma of the Lung," *British Medical Journal* (1952): 2(4877):1271–1286.
8. R. Doll and A. B. Hill, "Lung Cancer and Other Causes of Death in Relation to Smoking. A Second Report on the Mortality of British Doctors," *British Medical Journal* (1956): 12(5001):1071–1081.
9. Timmreck, *An Introduction to Epidemiology*, 145.
10. Doll and Hill, "A Study of the Aetiology of Carcinoma of the Lung," 1271–1286.
11. Donabedian, *Aspects of Medical Care*, 170.
12. D. D. Rutstein et al., "Measuring the Quality of Medical Care—A Clinical Method," *New England Journal of Medicine* 294 (1976):582–588.

13. Minister of Supply and Services, Health and Welfare, Canada, *The Periodic Health Examination Monograph—Report of a Task Force to the Conference of Deputy Ministers of Health* (Ottawa, 1980) 194.
14. U.S. Department of Health and Human Services, Public Health Service, Office of Public Health and Science, Office of Disease Prevention and Health Promotion, *Clinician's Handbook of Preventive Services*, 2d ed. (McLean, Va.: International Medical Publishing, Inc., 1998).
15. Donabedian, *Aspects of Medical Care*, 169.
16. Donabedian, *Aspects of Medical Care*, 169.
17. M. S. Litwin, *How to Measure Survey Reliability and Validity*, The Survey Kit TSK 7 (Thousand Oaks, Calif.: Sage Publications, Inc., 1995).
18. J. C. Nunnally and R. L. Durham, "Validity, Reliability, and Special Problems of Measurement in Evaluation Research," in *Handbook of Evaluation Research*, ed. E. L. Struemling and M. Guttertag (Beverly Hills, CA: Sage Publications, Inc., 1979):305–311.
19. E. G. Carmines and R. A. Zeller, *Reliability and Validity Assessment* (Beverly Hills, Calif.: Sage Publications, Inc., 1979), 76.
20. Carmines and Zeller, *Reliability and Validity Assessment*, 76.
21. G. W. Bohrnstedt, "A Quick Method for Determining the Reliability and Validity of Multiple-Item Scales," *American Sociological Review* 34 (August 1969):39.
22. L. S. Cronbach, "Coefficient Alpha and the Internal Structure of Tests," *Psychometrika* 16 (1951):297.

6

Descriptive Epidemiology: Person

The Patterns of Disease and Health

Descriptive epidemiology is concerned with the observation and description of the occurrence, distribution, size, and progression of health and causes of disease and death in populations. Chapter 5 showed how health services managers can use epidemiological measures to determine the occurrence and size of health problems in a population of interest. The basic premise of epidemiology, however, is that disease and health do not occur randomly but in patterns reflecting the operation of the underlying causes.[1]

These patterns of occurrence can be described by answering three broad questions: Who is affected? Where does the problem occur? When does the problem occur? The answers give managers a more detailed understanding of health problems in their communities and serve in the development of programs (program planning) to meet these needs.

Knowledge of the distribution and progression of health and disease in the population increases the effectiveness of programs by allowing, among other things, the identification of specific target groups.

This chapter examines the distribution of disease by person (who); Chapter 7 deals with place (where) and time (when) of occurrence. The use of the term "disease" is broadened here to encompass such other problems as motor vehicle and all other accidents, homicide, and suicide—all of which are included in epidemiological statistics as causual factors in deaths and other conditions that impact health.

Demographic Variables

Age, sex, and racial or ethnic origin are the three main demographic variables that characterize the distribution of health and disease in a population.

The Role of Age

Age is the personal attribute most strongly related to disease occurrence. In fact, age association is so strong that it almost always is necessary to control (eliminate) the effect of differences in age distribution when comparing disease occurrences in the two populations, or at two points in time, through age adjustment of rates—unless, of course, there is confidence that the age distributions are quite similar. Some diseases can occur almost exclusively in a particular age group; others over a wider age span but tending to be more prevalent at certain levels than at others.

The relationship between age and disease occurrence can be examined in several ways. Age-specific rates can (1) measure the risk of disease in each group, (2) examine the leading diseases in each group, and (3) trace the age progression of a particular disease.

Life Stage Disease Patterns   Table 6-1 lists the leading age-specific (life stage pattern) health problems in the state of Georgia (1999–2001), whereas Tables 6-2, 6-3, 6-4, and 6-5 rank the life stage (age)-specific leading causes of mortality for males and females, white and black and others for the United States (1999–2001). Definite patterns are peculiar to each age group (the influence of race and sex is discussed in later sections). The problems of infancy are primarily congenital and are related to immaturity. During childhood, accidents (motor vehicle and other), infectious diseases, and homicide and other forms of violence and abuse are the most prevalent problems. The major killers in adolescence are motor vehicle accidents, other accidents, suicide, and homicide. Alcohol and drug abuse, as well as unwanted pregnancies, also are characteristic problems. As individuals grow older, accidents, homicide, and suicide slowly are replaced as major killers by chronic diseases, mostly heart disease, stroke, and cancer.

Age-Specific Rates   Age-specific rates can also be used to trace the progression of a particular disease through the life stages. Figure 6-1 shows death rates per 100,000 for males and females, by age. The identification of trends by age-specific death rates gives information on the evaluation of death rates over time. It demonstrates that death rates in both groups are high for infancy but declined quite significantly from 1955 to 2000. All age groups show a decline or have remained relatively flat, as in the 15–24 and 25–34 age groups.

The distribution of health and disease in a population is a function of many attributes and characteristics of its members. These factors can be grouped into three sets of variables: demographic, social, and lifestyle.

TABLE 6-1 Leading Age-Specific Life Style Health Problems, Georgia, 1999–2001 •

Life Stage and Age	Health Problems	Life Stage and Age	Health Problems
Infancy (birth through first year)	Anoxia and hypoxia	**Adolescence** (13–19 years)	Adolescent pregnancy
	Low birth weight		Alcohol
	Congenital anomalies		Drug abuse
	Pneumonia		Motor vehicle accidents
	Accidents		All other accidents
	Sudden infant death syndrome		Suicide
	Down's syndrome		Homicide
	Hyaline membrane disease		Venereal diseases
	Phenylketonuria (PKU)		Dental disease
			Mental/emotional problems
			Sports injuries
Early Childhood (1–4 years)	Accidents	**Early Adulthood** (20–29 years)	Homicide
	Infectious diseases		Suicide
	Child abuse		Anxiety
	Lead poisoning		Depression
	Development attrition		Mental illness
			Motor vehicle/other accidents
Childhood (5–12 years)	Accidents		Cancers
	Cancers		Ischemic heart disease
	Influenza and pneumonia		Complications of pregnancy
	Homicide		Cirrhosis of the liver
	Leukemia		Nervous conditions
	Morbidity (infection of ear, nose, throat, other)		Back, limb, and hip injuries
	Malnutrition		Gallbladder disease
	Dental disease		

TABLE 6-1 Leading Age-Specific Life Style Health Problems, Georgia, 1999–2001• (continued)

Life Stage and Age	Health Problems	Life Stage and Age	Health Problems
Young adulthood (30–44 years)	Ischemic heart disease	**Late Adulthood** (60–74 years)	Ulcer
	Motor vehicle accidents		Frequent constipation
	Cancers		Hypertension
	Stroke		Hernia
	Heart attack		Upper gastrointestinal disorders
	Homicide		Gallbladder conditions
	Suicide		Respiratory conditions
	Mental illness		Ischemic heart disease
	Depression		Stroke
			Heart attack
			Diabetes
			Cancers
			Influenza and pneumonia
			Chronic obstructive pulmonary disease (COPD)
Middle Adulthood (45–59 years)	Ischemic heart disease		
	Heart attack		
	Cancers		
	Stroke		
	Cirrhosis of the liver		
	Diabetes		
	Motor vehicle accidents		
	Suicide		
	Respiratory conditions		
	Hypertension		

TABLE 6-1 Leading Age-Specific Life Style Health Problems, Georgia, 1999–2001 • (continued)

Life Stage and Age	Health Problems
Older Adulthood (75 + years)	Hernia Dependency Frequent constipation Gallbladder conditions Senility Arthritis Rheumatism Heart conditions

Source: G. E. Alan Dever, "Passages: Predictability of Mortality through the Life Stages," Georgia Department of Human Resources, Division of Public Health, 1980, 399. And C.D.C.—National Vital Statistics Report, *Deaths: Preliminary Data for 2002*, Kochanek, K. D. and B. L. Smith, Division of Vital Statistics Vol. 52 No. 13 Feb 11, 2004, pp 27–29.

TABLE 6-2   Ten Leading Causes of Death by Life Stages; U.S. 1999–2001, White Males

	Infancy (First Year)		Childhood (Ages 1–4)			Late Childhood (5–12)	
Rank	Cause of Death	Number	Rank	Cause of Death	Number	Cause of Death	Number
1	Congenital Anomalies	6,857	1	Unintentional Injury	2,434	Unintentional Injury	2,888
2	Short Gestation	3,940	2	Congenital Anomalies	593	Malignant Neoplasms	1,008
3	SIDS	2,821	3	Malignant Neoplasms	573	Congenital Anomalies	360
4	Maternal Pregnancy Comp.	1,493	4	Homicide	354	Homicide	266
5	Respiratory Distress	1,170	5	Heart Disease	228	Heart Disease	214
6	Placenta Cord Membranes	1,107	6	Septicemia	113	Suicide	146
7	Unintentional Injury	1,020	7	Influenza and Pneumonia	104	Influenza and Pneumonia	90
8	Bacterial Sepsis	780	8	Perinatal Period	88	Benign Neoplasms	89
9	Circulatory System Disease	709	9	Benign Neoplasms	71	Chronic Lower Respiratory Disease	75
10	Atelectasis	694	10	Cerebrovascular	48	Septicemia	75

Exercise: Calculate rate based on number by life stage. To complete this task, determine the appropriate numerator and denominator. Compare rates across life stages by disease category. Note the variations.

TABLE 6-2 Ten Leading Causes of Death by Life Stages; U.S. 1999–2001, White Males (continued)

	Adolescence (Ages 13–19)		Early Adulthood (Ages 20–29)			Young Adulthood (30–44)	
Rank	Cause of Death	Number	Rank	Cause of Death	Number	Cause of Death	Number
1	Unintentional Injury	13,008	1	Unintentional Injury	25,613	Unintentional Injury	39,478
2	Suicide	3,794	2	Suicide	10,053	Heart Disease	24,007
3	Homicide	2,164	3	Homicide	5,538	Malignant Neoplasms	20,296
4	Malignant Neoplasms	1,319	4	Malignant Neoplasms	3,081	Suicide	19,383
5	Heart Disease	607	5	Heart Disease	2,031	HIV	8,800
6	Congenital Anomalies	423	6	HIV	616	Homicide	6,666
7	Chronic Lower Respiratory Disease	112	7	Congenital Anomalies	598	Liver Disease	6,182
8	Cerebrovascular	107	8	Cerebrovascular	378	Diabetes Mellitus	3,065
9	Influenza and Pneumonia	102	9	Diabetes Mellitus	323	Cerebrovascular	2,960
10	Benign Neoplasms	74	10	Influenza and Pneumonia	284	Influenza and Pneumonia	1,485

TABLE 6-2 Ten Leading Causes of Death by Life Stages; U.S. 1999–2001, White Males (continued)

| | Middle Adulthood (Ages 45–49) | | Late Adulthood (Ages 60–74) | | | Older Adulthood (Ages ≥75) | |
Rank	Cause of Death	Number	Cause of Death	Number	Rank	Cause of Death	Number
1	Malignant Neoplasms	110,504	Malignant Neoplasms	286,975	1	Heart Disease	516,570
2	Heart Disease	108,206	Heart Disease	252,205	2	Malignant Neoplasms	319,077
3	Unintentional Injury	29,054	Chronic Lower Respiratory Disease	54,878	3	Cerebrovascular	112,551
4	Liver Disease	17,971	Cerebrovascular	36,038	4	Chronic Lower Respiratory Disease	100,507
5	Suicide	15,484	Diabetes Mellitus	26,936	5	Influenza and Pneumonia	54,931
6	Diabetes Mellitus	11,503	Unintentional Injury	18,108	6	Diabetes Mellitus	36,537
7	Cerebrovascular	10,956	Liver Disease	14,098	7	Alzheimer's Disease	36,015
8	Chronic Lower Respiratory Disease	9,512	Influenza and Pneumonia	11,881	8	Unintentional Injury	29,870
9	HIV	5,631	Nephritis	10,366	9	Nephritis	28,676
10	Viral Hepatitis	4,055	Aortic Aneurysm	8,979	10	Parkinson's Disease	20,814

Source: Office of Statistics and Programming, National Center for Injury Prevention and Control, CDC, *http://webapp.cdc.gov/sasweb/ncipc/leadcaus10.html*, produced with data from the National Center for Health Statistics (NCHS) Vital Statistics System.

TABLE 6-3 Ten Leading Causes of Death by Life Stages; U.S. 1999–2001, Black Males

	Infancy (First Year)			*Childhood (Ages 1–4)*			*Late Childhood (5–12)*	
Rank	*Cause of Death*	*Number*	*Rank*	*Cause of Death*	*Number*	*Rank*	*Cause of Death*	*Number*
1	Short Gestation	3,114	1	Unintentional Injury	699	1	Unintentional Injury	1,057
2	Congenital Anomalies	1,635	2	Homicide	251	2	Malignant Neoplasms	219
3	SIDS	1,381	3	Congenital Anomalies	218	3	Homicide	117
4	Maternal Pregnancy Comp.	864	4	Heart Disease	92	4	Congenital Anomalies	111
5	Respiratory Distress	651	5	Malignant Neoplasms	90	5	Chronic Lower Respiratory Disease	95
6	Placenta Cord Membranes	512	6	Influenza and Pneumonia	60	6	Heart Disease	89
7	Unintentional Injury	452	7	Perinatal Period	51	7	HIV	42
8	Bacterial Sepsis	435	8	Chronic Lower Respiratory Disease	44	8	Suicide	38
9	Circulatory System Disease	287	9	Septicemia	36	9	Anemias	33
10	Necrotizing Enterocolitis	280	10	Anemias	26	10	Benign Neoplasms	28

TABLE 6-3 Ten Leading Causes of Death by Life Stages; U.S. 1999–2001, Black Males (continued)

	Adolescence (Ages 13–19)			Early Adulthood (Ages 20–29)			Young Adulthood (30–44)	
Rank	Cause of Death	Number	Rank	Cause of Death	Number	Rank	Cause of Death	Number
1	Homicide	2,919	1	Homicide	8,190	1	HIV	8,203
2	Unintentional Injury	1,963	2	Unintentional Injury	4,139	2	Heart Disease	7,379
3	Suicide	472	3	Suicide	1,481	3	Unintentional Injury	6,906
4	Malignant Neoplasms	303	4	Heart Disease	975	4	Homicide	5,385
5	Heart Disease	269	5	HIV	841	5	Malignant Neoplasms	4,307
6	Congenital Anomalies	137	6	Malignant Neoplasms	594	6	Suicide	1,633
7	Chronic Lower Respiratory Disease	104	7	Diabetes Mellitus	167	7	Cerebrovascular	1,296
8	Anemias	48	8	Chronic Lower Respiratory Disease	166	8	Diabetes Mellitus	1,007
9	HIV	45	9	Anemias	164	9	Liver Disease	908
10	Diabetes Mellitus	29	10	Congenital Anomalies	124	10	Nephritis	590

TABLE 6-3 Ten Leading Causes of Death by Life Stages; U.S. 1999–2001, Black Males (continued)

	Middle Adulthood (Ages 45–49)		Late Adulthood (Ages 60–74)		Older Adulthood (Ages ≥75)	
Rank	Cause of Death	Number	Cause of Death	Number	Cause of Death	Number
1	Heart Disease	24,364	Malignant Neoplasms	39,086	Heart Disease	40,540
2	Malignant Neoplasms	21,997	Heart Disease	37,390	Malignant Neoplasms	31,734
3	HIV	5,910	Cerebrovascular	7,635	Cerebrovascular	10,069
4	Unintentional Injury	5,820	Diabetes Mellitus	5,439	Chronic Lower Respiratory Disease	5,722
5	Cerebrovascular	4,588	Chronic Lower Respiratory Disease	4,679	Diabetes Mellitus	4,520
6	Diabetes Mellitus	3,406	Nephritis	2,995	Influenza and Pneumonia	4,262
7	Liver Disease	2,789	Unintentional Injury	2,652	Nephritis	3,696
8	Homicide	1,811	Septicemia	2,401	Septicemia	3,135
9	Nephritis	1,792	Influenza and Pneumonia	2,069	Unintentional Injury	2,122
10	Chronic Lower Respiratory Disease	1,588	Hypertension	1,531	Alzheimer's Disease	1,985

Source: Office of Statistics and Programming, National Center for Injury Prevention and Control, CDC, *http://webapp.cdc.gov/sasweb/ncipc/leadcaus10.html*, produced with data from the National Center for Health Statistics (NCHS) Vital Statistics System.

TABLE 6-4   Ten Leading Causes of Death by Life Stages; U.S. 1999–2001, White Females

	Infancy (First Year)			Childhood (Ages 1–4)			Late Childhood (5–12)	
Rank	Cause of Death	Number	Rank	Cause of Death	Number	Rank	Cause of Death	Number
1	Congenital Anomalies	5,972	1	Unintentional Injury	1,584	1	Unintentional Injury	1,795
2	Short Gestation	3,259	2	Congenital Anomalies	526	2	Malignant Neoplasms	877
3	SIDS	1,904	3	Malignant Neoplasms	463	3	Congenital Anomalies	331
4	Maternal Pregnancy Comp.	1,120	4	Homicide	281	4	Homicide	214
5	Placenta Cord Membranes	943	5	Heart Disease	163	5	Heart Disease	175
6	Respiratory Distress	789	6	Influenza and Pneumonia	118	6	Benign Neoplasms	101
7	Unintentional Injury	758	7	Septicemia	93	7	Influenza and Pneumonia	74
8	Circulatory System Disease	597	8	Benign Neoplasms	69	8	Cerebrovascular	59
9	Intrauterine Hypoxia	574	9	Perinatal Period	61	9	Septicemia	57
10	Bacterial Sepsis	550	10	Cerebrovascular	55	10	Chronic Lower Respiratory Disease	55

TABLE 6-4 Ten Leading Causes of Death by Life Stages; U.S. 1999–2001, White Females (continued)

	Adolescence (Ages 13–19)			Early Adulthood (Ages 20–29)			Young Adulthood (30–44)	
Rank	Cause of Death	Number	Rank	Cause of Death	Number	Rank	Cause of Death	Number
1	Unintentional Injury	5,799	1	Unintentional Injury	7,074	1	Malignant Neoplasms	8,203
2	Malignant Neoplasms	905	2	Malignant Neoplasms	2,499	2	Unintentional Injury	7,379
3	Suicide	788	3	Suicide	1,687	3	Heart Disease	6,906
4	Homicide	591	4	Homicide	1,535	4	Suicide	5,385
5	Heart Disease	378	5	Heart Disease	1,100	5	Liver Disease	4,307
6	Congenital Anomalies	279	6	Congenital Anomalies	441	6	Cerebrovascular	1,633
7	Influenza and Pneumonia	91	7	Cerebrovascular	331	7	Homicide	1,296
8	Chronic Lower Respiratory Disease	88	8	Complicated Pregnancy	267	8	Diabetes Mellitus	1,007
9	Cerebrovascular	78	9	Diabetes Mellitus	262	9	HIV	908
10	Benign Neoplasms	72	10	HIV	261	10	Chronic Lower Respiratory Disease	590

TABLE 6-4 Ten Leading Causes of Death by Life Stages; U.S. 1999–2001, White Females (continued)

Rank	Middle Adulthood (Ages 45–49)		Rank	Late Adulthood (Ages 60–74)		Rank	Older Adulthood (Ages ≥75)	
	Cause of Death	Number		Cause of Death	Number		Cause of Death	Number
1	Malignant Neoplasms	102,723	1	Malignant Neoplasms	231,058	1	Heart Disease	768,485
2	Heart Disease	38,292	2	Heart Disease	144,418	2	Malignant Neoplasms	330,834
3	Unintentional Injury	11,086	3	Chronic Lower Respiratory Disease	51,147	3	Cerebrovascular	221,133
4	Cerebrovascular	9,079	4	Cerebrovascular	33,087	4	Chronic Lower Respiratory Disease	113,252
5	Chronic Lower Respiratory Disease	9,064	5	Diabetes Mellitus	24,248	5	Alzheimer's Disease	91,912
6	Diabetes Mellitus	7,995	6	Unintentional Injury	10,872	6	Influenza and Pneumonia	82,491
7	Liver Disease	6,111	7	Influenza and Pneumonia	9,325	7	Diabetes Mellitus	54,327
8	Suicide	4,841	8	Nephritis	8,888	8	Unintentional Injury	36,757
9	Septicemia	2,939	9	Septicemia	8,315	9	Nephritis	33,693
10	Influenza and Pneumonia	2,690	10	Liver Disease	8,123	10	Septicemia	29,670

Source: Office of Statistics and Programming, National Center for Injury Prevention and Control, CDC, *http://webapp.cdc.gov/sasweb/ncipc/leadcaus10.html*, produced with data from the National Center for Health Statistics (NCHS) Vital Statistics System.

TABLE 6-5 Ten Leading Causes of Death by Life Stages; U.S. 1999–2001, Black Females

| | *Infancy (First Year)* | | | *Childhood (Ages 1–4)* | | | *Late Childhood (5–12)* | |
Rank	Cause of Death	Number	Rank	Cause of Death	Number	Rank	Cause of Death	Number
1	Short Gestation	2,489	1	Unintentional Injury	486	1	Unintentional Injury	554
2	Congenital Anomalies	1,524	2	Homicide	215	2	Malignant Neoplasms	175
3	SIDS	1,029	3	Congenital Anomalies	177	3	Congenital Anomalies	95
4	Maternal Pregnancy Comp.	686	4	Heart Disease	81	4	Homicide	92
5	Placenta Cord Membranes	443	5	Malignant Neoplasms	77	5	Heart Disease	73
6	Respiratory Distress	424	6	Influenza and Pneumonia	39	6	Chronic Lower Respiratory Disease	45
7	Unintentional Injury	355	7	Septicemia	29	7	Anemias	32
8	Bacterial Sepsis	316	8	Perinatal Period	28	8	Benign Neoplasms	30
9	Circulatory System Disease	261	9	Anemias	25	9	HIV	29
10	Necrotizing Enterocolitis	194	10	Cerebrovascular	24	10	Cerebrovascular	18

TABLE 6-5 Ten Leading Causes of Death by Life Stages; U.S. 1999–2001, Black Females (continued)

	Adolescence (Ages 13–19)			Early Adulthood (Ages 20–29)			Young Adulthood (30–44)	
Rank	Cause of Death	Number	Rank	Cause of Death	Number	Rank	Cause of Death	Number
1	Unintentional Injury	694	1	Unintentional Injury	1,284	1	Malignant Neoplasms	6,189
2	Homicide	423	2	Homicide	1,065	2	Heart Disease	4,737
3	Malignant Neoplasms	200	3	HIV	748	3	HIV	4,144
4	Heart Disease	155	4	Heart Disease	671	4	Unintentional Injury	2,607
5	Congenital Anomalies	89	5	Malignant Neoplasms	589	5	Homicide	1,547
6	Suicide	80	6	Complicated Pregnancy	197	6	Cerebrovascular	1,439
7	Chronic Lower Respiratory Disease	58	7	Suicide	196	7	Diabetes Mellitus	816
8	HIV	51	8	Diabetes Mellitus	157	8	Chronic Lower Respiratory Disease	537
9	Anemias	44	9	Anemias	141	9	Nephritis	529
10	Complicated Pregnancy	37	10	Chronic Lower Respiratory Disease	126	10	Liver Disease	526

TABLE 6-5 Ten Leading Causes of Death by Life Stages; U.S. 1999–2001, Black Females (continued)

	Middle Adulthood (Ages 45–49)		Late Adulthood (Ages 60–74)			Older Adulthood (Ages ≥75)	
Rank	Cause of Death	Number	Cause of Death	Number	Rank	Cause of Death	Number
1	Malignant Neoplasms	19,100	Heart Disease	31,134	1	Heart Disease	70,844
2	Heart Disease	14,519	Malignant Neoplasms	30,861	2	Malignant Neoplasms	30,509
3	Cerebrovascular	3,910	Diabetes Mellitus	7,445	3	Cerebrovascular	20,279
4	Diabetes Mellitus	3,264	Cerebrovascular	7,404	4	Diabetes Mellitus	9,947
5	HIV	1,974	Nephritis	3,591	5	Influenza and Pneumonia	6,135
6	Unintentional Injury	1,951	Chronic Lower Respiratory Disease	3,261	6	Nephritis	5,829
7	Chronic Lower Respiratory Disease	1,496	Septicemia	2,467	7	Alzheimer's Disease	5,332
8	Nephritis	1,479	Hypertension	1,743	8	Septicemia	5,230
9	Septicemia	1,278	Influenza and Pneumonia	1,466	9	Chronic Lower Respiratory Disease	4,621
10	Liver Disease	1,193	Unintentional Injury	1,435	10	Hypertension	3,895

Source: Office of Statistics and Programming, National Center for Injury Prevention and Control, CDC, *http://webapp.cdc.gov/sasweb/ncipc/leadcaus10.html*, produced with data from the National Center for Health Statistics (NCHS) Vital Statistics System.

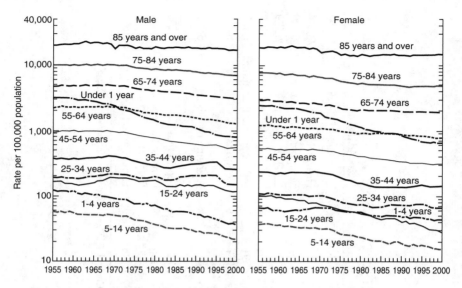

FIGURE 6-1   Death Rates by Age and Sex: U.S. 1955–2000. *Source:* Centers for Disease Control and Prevention, *National Vital Statistics Report* 50, no. 15 (2002):4.

Disease Pyramids   The disease pyramid is an alternate method of examining diseases by age as well as by sex and race (Figure 6-2). Constructed in the same manner as a population pyramid, the disease pyramid shows which age groups are affected by diseases. It provides an immediate visual analysis of disease mortality by age, sex, and race. It can illustrate the dominance of a specific age, sex, or race for the selected disease (Figure 6-3). Specific target groups can be identified, depending on the specificity of the age groups involved.

For example, an inverted pyramid indicates a disease that is concentrated in the older ages, whereas one that bulges to the left of the central axis at midpoint indicates that a disease such as cirrhosis of the liver occurs predominantly in males of middle age. The pyramid, however, does not give the absolute risk of dying by age, sex, and race because its values are not weighted according to distribution of the population for each of those groupings.

Cohort Analysis   Both age-specific rates and disease pyramids thus trace the progression of a particular disease through the age groups by showing the relationship between age and disease rates as they occur simultaneously in time.[2] The process is known as current or cross-sectional analysis. Different people therefore are involved in each age group.

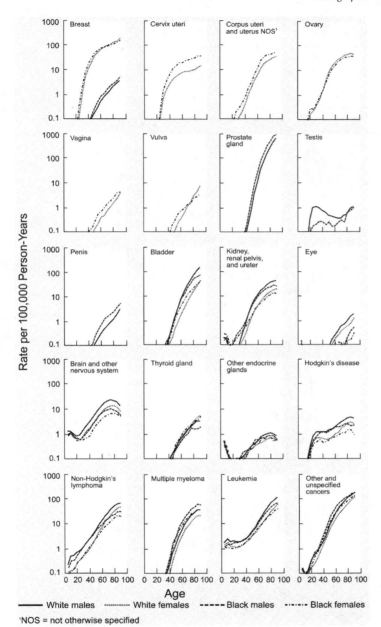

Rate per 100,000 Person-Years

Age

——— White males ·········· White females ----- Black males -··-··- Black females

¹NOS = not otherwise specified

FIGURE 6-2 Annual Age-Specific Mortality Rates for Specific Cancers by Race and Sex, U.S. 1970–1994. *Source:* S. S. Devesa et al., *Atlas of Cancer Mortality in the United States, 1950–94* (Rockville, Md.: National Institutes of Health, National Cancer Institute, 1999), 53.

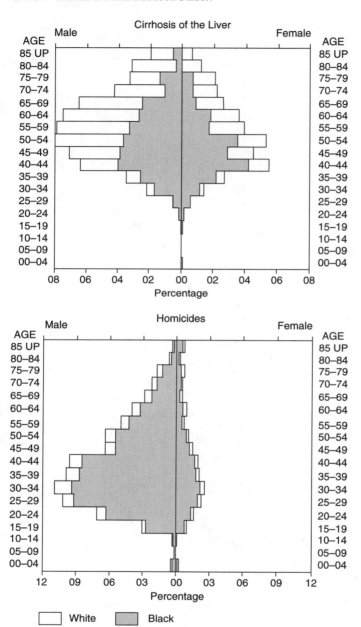

FIGURE 6-3 Disease Pyramids, Georgia, 1970–1974. *Source:* Reprinted from "Disease Patterns of the 70s," *Health Services Research and Statistics*, Georgia Department of Human Resources, Division of Physical Health (August 1976):116, 121, 137.

By contrast cohort analysis, although showing disease progression through the different age groups, follows a specific bloc of people (a cohort) through time. Several cohorts are usually identified and followed as they pass through different ages during part, or all, of their life span. Both current and cohort analysis should produce the same results except when the frequency of the disease under consideration has been changing over time.[3] Then a cohort analysis will show a truer picture of the relationship of age, or aging, on the progression of disease.

The now-classic example of this is Frost's study of tuberculosis in Massachusetts for the years 1880 to 1930.[4] Figure 6-4 shows the results of three cross-sectional analyses of the mortality rates of tuberculosis in 1880, 1910, and 1930. As for the relationship between age and tuberculosis, the three curves produce quite different results. Although all three show a high

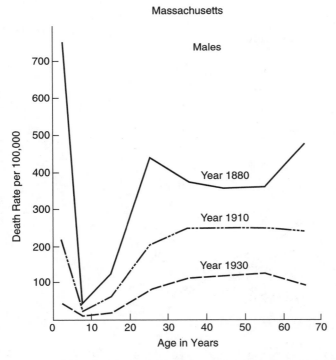

FIGURE 6-4 Cross-Sectional Analysis of Tuberculosis Death Rates. *Source:* Reprinted from "The Age Selection of Mortality from Tuberculosis in Successive Decades," by W. H. Frost with permission of the *American Journal of Hygiene,* ©1939, vol. 30, 91–96.

incidence in childhood, the current (cross-sectional) analysis of 1880 death rates shows a peak between ages 20 and 30 and another after about age 55. In contrast, the 1910 analysis shows a quite steady incidence in adulthood, whereas the 1930 curve shows a small but steady increase through adulthood, peaking between 50 and 60. How can these seemingly contradictory relationships between age and death rates from tuberculosis be explained?

A cohort analysis provides the answer. In Figure 6-5, each curve represents the death rates from tuberculosis experienced by the cohort of persons born between 1861–1870 ("cohort 1870"); 1871–1880 ("1880"); 1881–1890 ("1890"); 1891–1900 ("1900"); and 1901–1910 ("1910"). All curves show the same basic relationship between age and tuberculosis: In addition to a high incidence in early childhood, all cohorts experienced their highest death rates between ages 20 and 30, with a steady decrease thereafter. No increase is evident in older adulthood, nor is there a steady rate through adulthood.

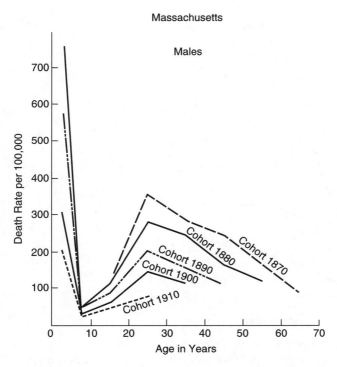

FIGURE 6-5   Cohort Analysis of Tuberculosis Death Rates. *Source:* Reprinted from "The Age Selection of Mortality from Tuberculosis in Successive Decades," by W. H. Frost with permission of the *American Journal of Hygiene,* ©1939, vol. 30, 91–96.

Frost concludes that adults and older adults have a higher rate in the cross-sectional analysis than they should have had, as shown from the results of the cohort analysis, because they belong to an older cohort with overall (through all ages) higher death rates. For example, persons in the 50 to 60 age group in the 1930 analysis (Figure 6-4) belong to the 1880 cohort (i.e., born between 1871 and 1880), which had a greater exposure to tuberculosis than any other succeeding groups.

This study supports the hypothesis that mortality from tuberculosis in adult life is predominantly endogenous (i.e., resulting from activation of latent foci) and determined largely by the degree of infection received in early life.[5]

The Role of Sex

Males and females have different mortality and morbidity patterns. The simplest way to examine these different patterns is to use the sex ratio: the ratio of male to female cases. Table 6-6 illustrates the sex and race ratios for selected causes of death by utilizing age-adjusted death rates.

Tables 6-7 through 6-10 illustrate the importance of classifying male/female ratios. These ratios range from 10-plus for cancer of the lip to a ratio of <.01 for breast cancer. An interesting classification would be to categorize the rate into 3, 2–2.99, 1–1.99, and less than 1, which would aid in the identification of a specific problem by sex. Today death rates are almost always higher among males than females, except for a few chronic conditions such as diabetes, hypertension, and a few types of cancers (Figure 6-6). In utero and neonatal death rates also are higher for males. These rates are true for both whites and blacks. Life expectancy also is greater in females and the difference is widening. A female born in 2000 can expect to live 5.4 years longer than a male born in the same year, although a female born in 1930 enjoyed only a 3.5-year advantage.[6]

The sex ratio assumes that the population is divided equally by sex. This of course is not the case. Although more males are born alive than females (106 males to 100 females), from age 20 on females exceed males in each age group and the relative difference increases with advancing age.[7] Consequently, age-specific and sex-specific rates are more useful than sex ratios in comparing health problems of males and females.

An interesting aspect of the influence of sex on disease is that, although mortality rates are higher in males, morbidity rates usually are higher in females. For females, both reported morbidity and physician visits are higher in all age groups. These sex differences can be caused by many factors. Some diseases, such as hemophilia, are genetically sex linked. Hormonal and reproductive factors also can play a role in either predisposing a given sex toward a particular disease or providing protection against it.

TABLE 6-6   Ratio of Age-Adjusted Death Rates by Sex, Race, and Hispanic Origin for the 15 Leading Causes of Death for the Total Population in 2000: United States, Percentage of Total Deaths, Death Rates, Age-Adjusted Rates for 2000, Percentage Change in Age-Adjusted Death Rates from 1999 to 2000

| | | 2000 | | | Age-Adjusted Death Rate | | | | |
| | | | | | | | Ratio | | |
Rank[1]	Cause of Death[*]	Number Deaths	Percentage of Total Deaths	Crude Death Rate	2000	Percent Change 1999 to 2000	Male to Female	Black to White	Hispanic to White Non-Hispanic
. . .	All causes	2,403,351	100.0	873.1	872.0	−1.1	1.4	1.3	0.7
1	Heart diseases	710,760	29.6	258.2	257.9	−3.7	1.5	1.3	0.6
2	Malignant neoplasms	553,091	23.0	200.9	201.0	−0.8	1.5	1.3	0.6
3	Cerebrovascular diseases	167,661	7.0	60.9	60.8	−1.6	1.0	1.4	0.7
4	Chronic lower respiratory diseases	122,009	5.1	44.3	44.3	−3.3	1.4	0.7	0.4
5	Accidents (unintentional injuries)	97,900	4.1	35.6	35.5	−1.1	2.2	1.1	0.9
6	Diabetes mellitus	69,301	2.9	25.2	25.2	—	1.2	2.2	1.5
7	Influenza and pneumonia	65,313	2.7	23.7	23.7	0.4	1.3	1.1	0.7
8	Alzheimer's disease	49,558	2.1	18.0	18.0	9.1	0.8	0.7	0.4
9	Nephritis, nephritic syndrome, and nephrosis	37,251	1.5	13.5	13.5	3.1	1.4	2.4	0.8
10	Septicemia	31,224	1.3	11.3	11.4	0.9	1.2	2.4	0.7
11	Intentional self-harm (suicide)	29,350	1.2	10.7	10.6	−0.9	4.5	0.5	0.5

TABLE 6-6 Ratio of Age-Adjusted Death Rates by Sex, Race, and Hispanic Origin for the 15 Leading Causes of Death for the Total Population in 2000: United States, Percentage of Total Deaths, Death Rates, Age-Adjusted Rates for 2000, Percentage Change in Age-Adjusted Death Rates from 1999 to 2000 (continued)

| | | | | | Age-Adjusted Death Rate | | | | |
| | | | | | | Percent Change | Ratio | | |
Rank[1]	Cause of Death[*]	Number	Percentage of Total Deaths	2000 Crude Death Rate	2000	1999 to 2000	Male to Female	Black to White	Hispanic to White Non-Hispanic
12	Chronic liver disease and cirrhosis	26,552	1.1	9.6	9.6	–1.0	2.2	1.0	1.7
13	Essential (primary) hypertension and hypertensive renal disease	18,073	0.8	6.6	6.6	4.8	1.0	2.9	0.9
14	Assault (homicide)	16,765	0.7	6.1	6.1	–1.6	3.3	5.7	3.0
15	Pneumonitis due to solids and liquids	16,636	0.7	6.0	6.0	7.1	1.8	1.1	0.5
...	All other causes	391,904	16.3	142.4	...	...	...	...	...

– Quantity zero

... Category not applicable

[1]Rank based on number of deaths

[*]Based on the *Tenth Revision International Classification of Diseases*, 1992

Source: Centers for Disease Control and Prevention, *National Vital Statistics Report* 50, no. 15 (2002): 8.

Death rates on an annual basis per 100,000 population: age-adjusted rates per 100,000 U.S. standard population based on year 2000 standard

TABLE 6-7   Cancer Mortality Rate, Male/Female Ratios;* Whites, 1970–1994

Primary Site	Male/Female Ratios
	Ratios 3 or More
Lip	11.00
Larynx	5.93
Esophagus	3.87
Bladder	3.51
	Ratios 2–2.99
Lung, trachea, bronchus, and pleura	2.90
Other oral cavity and pharynx	2.83
Other skin	2.72
Nasopharynx	2.50
Salivary glands	2.25
Kidney, renal pelvis, and ureter	2.19
Stomach	2.15
	Ratios 1–1.99
Nose, nasal cavity, and sinuses	1.93
Melanoma of skin	1.84
Rectum	1.73
Leukemia	1.71
Hodgkin's disease	1.64
Bones and joints	1.61
Pancreas	1.49
Multiple myeloma	1.49
Non-Hodgkin's lymphoma	1.48
Brain and other nervous system	1.47
Other and unspecified cancers	1.45
Liver, gallbladder, and other biliary tract	1.40
Colon	1.34
Other endocrine glands	1.28
Eye	1.27
Connective tissue	1.24
	Ratios Less Than 1
Thyroid gland	0.79
Breast	0.01

*Based on annual rates per 100,000 person-years, age-adjusted using the 1970 U.S. population distribution

Source: S. S. Devesa et al., *Atlas of Cancer Mortality in the United States, 1950–94* (Rockville, Md.: National Institutes of Health, National Cancer Institute, 1999), 39.

TABLE 6-8   Cancer Mortality Rate, Male/Female Ratios;* Blacks, 1970–1994

Primary Site	Male/Female Ratios
	Ratios 3 or More
Larynx	6.53
Other oral cavity and pharynx	4.28
Esophagus	3.99
Lung, trachea, bronchus, and pleura	3.94
Nasopharynx	3.12
	Ratios 2–2.99
Nose, nasal cavity, and sinuses	2.76
Other skin	2.59
Stomach	2.37
Kidney, renal pelvis, and ureter	2.19
Lip	2.00
Salivary glands	2.00
	Ratios 1–1.99
Hodgkin's disease	1.98
Bladder	1.97
Liver, gallbladder, and other biliary tract	1.92
Non-Hodgkin's lymphoma	1.67
Bones and joints	1.66
Leukemia	1.64
Rectum	1.60
Other and unspecified cancers	1.59
Eye	1.50
Brain and other nervous system	1.50
Multiple myeloma	1.47
Pancreas	1.44
Melanoma of skin	1.27
Other endocrine glands	1.26
Colon	1.22
	Ratios Less Than 1
Connective tissue	0.94
Thyroid gland	0.60
Breast	0.01

*Based on annual rates per 100,000 person-years, age-adjusted using the 1970 U.S. population distribution

Source: S. S. Devesa et al., *Atlas of Cancer Mortality in the United States, 1950–94* (Rockville, Md.: National Institutes of Health, National Cancer Institute, 1999), 39.

TABLE 6-9   Cancer Mortality Rate, Black/White Ratios;* Males, 1970–1994

Primary Site	Black/White Ratios
	Ratios 3 or More
Esophagus	3.12
	Ratios 2–2.99
Penis	2.47
Prostate gland	2.14
Multiple myeloma	2.09
Other oral cavity and pharynx	2.08
Stomach	2.04
	Ratios 1–1.99
Larynx	1.99
Nose, nasal cavity, and sinuses	1.74
Breast	1.68
Other and unspecified cancers	1.59
Liver, gallbladder, and other biliary tract	1.54
Nasopharynx	1.51
Pancreas	1.37
Lung, trachea, bronchus, and pleura	1.36
Bones and joints	1.10
Connective tissue	1.08
Colon	1.07
Other endocrine glands	1.06
Rectum	1.01
	Ratios Less Than 1
Other skin	0.97
Kidney, renal pelvis, and ureter	0.88
Hodgkin's disease	0.86
Leukemia	0.86
Thyroid gland	0.85
Salivary glands	0.83
Bladder	0.83
Non-Hodgkin's lymphoma	0.70
Brain and other nervous system	0.58
Eye	0.43
Testis	0.41
Lip	0.18
Melanoma of skin	0.16

*Based on annual rates per 100,000 person-years, age-adjusted using the 1970 U.S. population distribution

Source: S. S. Devesa et al., *Atlas of Cancer Mortality in the United States, 1950–94* (Rockville, Md.: National Institutes of Health, National Cancer Institute, 1999), 39.

TABLE 6-10   Cancer Mortality Rate, Black/White Ratios;* Females, 1970–1994

Primary Site	Black/White Ratios
	Ratios 3 or More
Esophagus	3.02
	Ratios 2–2.99
Cervix uteri	2.68
Multiple myeloma	2.13
	Ratios 1–1.99
Stomach	1.85
Larynx	1.81
Corpus uteri and uterus NOS	1.75
Vagina	1.70
Bladder	1.48
Other and unspecified cancers	1.45
Pancreas	1.42
Connective tissue	1.42
Other oral cavity and pharynx	1.38
Nasopharynx	1.21
Nose, nasal cavity, and sinuses	1.21
Colon	1.19
Liver, gallbladder, and other biliary tract	1.12
Thyroid gland	1.12
Rectum	1.09
Other endocrine glands	1.08
Bones and joints	1.07
Breast	1.07
Vulva	1.03
Other skin	1.02
Lip	1.00
Lung, trachea, bronchus, and pleura	1.00
	Ratios Less Than 1
Salivary glands	0.94
Leukemia	0.90
Kidney, renal pelvis, and ureter	0.88
Ovary	0.81
Hodgkin's disease	0.72
Non-Hodgkin's lymphoma	0.62
Brain and other nervous system	0.57
Eye	0.36
Melanoma of skin	0.23

*Based on annual rates per 100,000 person-years, age-adjusted using the 1970 U.S. population distribution

Source: S. S. Devesa et al., *Atlas of Cancer Mortality in the United States, 1950–94* (Rockville, Md.: National Institutes of Health, National Cancer Institute, 1999), 39.

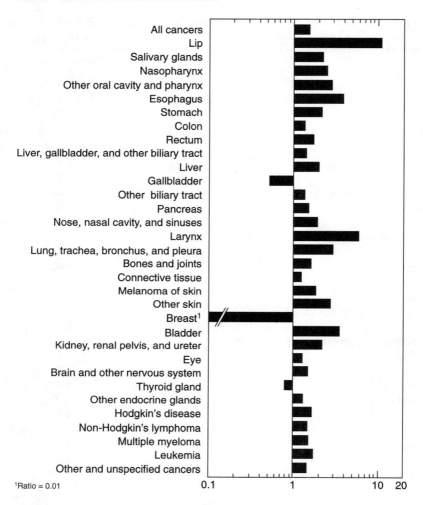

FIGURE 6-6 Male/Female Ratios of Cancer Mortality Rates among Whites in the United States, 1970–94. *Source:* S. S. Devesa et al., *Atlas of Cancer Mortality in the United States, 1950–94* (Rockville, Md.: National Institutes of Health, National Cancer Institute, 1999), 48.

For example, the greater occurrence of coronary heart disease in young men than in young women can be linked to some hormonal factors, perhaps protection of the women by estrogens before menopause.[8] Men and women also have different lifestyles, which may explain some differences. For instance, the greater incidence of lung cancer in males can be related to the fact that men smoke more cigarettes than women. However, these statistics are changing rapidly. The sex ratio in lung cancer should decrease as more women begin to feel the effects of long-term smoking. Similarly, the higher incidence of cirrhosis of the liver can be explained by the fact that men consume more alcohol than do women.

Finally, the higher morbidity and lower mortality in women can result in part from their lower case fatality rate; that is, some diseases have a less lethal effect on women than men. Because women consume more health services than men, however, it also can stem from the fact that women seek medical care at an earlier stage of a disease.[9] Depression provides a good example of contradictory sex differences in morbidity and mortality rates;[10] rates for many forms of depression are higher in women than in men, as is the rate of attempted suicide.[11]

Racial or Ethnic Origin

The examination of specific health statistics can be controversial, especially when related to ethnic or minority groups. Nevertheless, Haynes states:

> We should insist that adequate statistics be maintained so that health planners do not lose sight of special problems of minority groups. Only by such special focus will minority problems receive due attention. Representing a relatively small percentage of the total population, it is easy for minority problems to be ignored. This must not happen. We must oppose those within minority groups who wish to conceal special problems, and we must oppose those of the majority group who want to ignore these problems.[12]

Adequate health care for all is the goal of any health agency. To reach this goal, the agency must know the disease patterns that reflect the health status of the population it serves. Definite differences exist in mortality and morbidity among races. In some cases, such as sickle cell anemia, disease is determined genetically. In most instances, however, differences are related to socioeconomic status. Regrettably, socioeconomic data often is difficult to gather and is available only every ten years (census period). Even so, racial or ethnic origin can be useful as an indicator of groups with particular deficiencies in health care.

Table 6-11 shows variations across race groups in the ten leading causes of death. The four major race groups shown all share the eight leading causes in common. Heart disease and cancer rank first and second, respectively, for white, black, and American Indian populations. For the Asian/Pacific Islander population, cancer was the leading cause of death, with heart disease second. Stroke ranks third for the white, black, and Asian/Pacific Islander population, but ranks fifth for the American Indian population. For each of the four race groups, at least one of the ten leading causes is unique to that group. Cirrhosis/liver disease ranks sixth for the American Indian population, homicide and HIV ranks sixth and seventh, respectively, for the black population, and Alzheimer's ranks eighth for the white population.

TABLE 6-11 Causes of Death and the Percentage of Deaths for the Ten Leading Causes of Death by Race: U.S., 2000

Cause of Death (Based on the Tenth Revision, International Classification of Diseases, 1992)	White			Black			American Indian			Asian or Pacific Islander		
	Rank[1]	Deaths	Percentage of Total Deaths	Rank[1]	Deaths	Percentage of Total Deaths	Rank[1]	Deaths	Percentage of Total Deaths	Rank[1]	Deaths	Percentage of Total Deaths
All causes	...	2,071,287	100.0	...	285,826	100.0	...	11,363	100.0	...	34,875	100.0
Diseases of heart (I00–I09, I11, I13, I20–I51)	1	621,719	30.0	1	77,523	27.1	1	2,417	21.3	2	9,101	26.1
Malignant neoplasms (C00–C97)	2	480,011	23.2	2	61,945	21.7	2	1,914	16.8	1	9,221	26.4
Cerebrovascular diseases (I60–I69)	3	144,580	7.0	3	19,221	6.7	5	572	5.0	3	3,288	9.4
Chronic lower respiratory diseases (J40–J47)	4	112,840	5.4	8	7,607	2.7	7	429	3.8	5	1,133	3.2
Accidents (unintentional injuries) (V01–X59, Y85–Y86)	5	82,592	4.0	4	12,277	4.3	3	1,353	11.9	4	1,678	4.8
Influenza and pneumonia (J10–J18)	6	57,914	2.8	10	5,990	2.1	9	289	2.5	6	1,120	3.2
Diabetes mellitus (E10–E14)	7	55,561	2.7	5	12,021	4.2	4	616	5.4	7	1,103	3.2
Alzheimer's disease (G30)	8	46,460	2.2	...	2,728	1.0	...	95	0.8	...	275	0.8
Nephritis, nephrotic syndrome and nephrosis (N00–N07, N17–N19, N25–N27)	9	29,598	1.4	9	6,911	2.4	10	215	1.9	9	527	1.5
Intentional self-harm (suicide) (X6-X84, Y87.0)	10	26,475	1.3	...	1,962	0.7	8	297	2.6	8	616	1.8
Chronic liver disease and cirrhosis (K70, K73–K74)	...	22,982	1.1	...	2,737	1.0	6	534	4.7	...	299	0.9

TABLE 6-11 Causes of Death and the Percentage of Deaths for the Ten Leading Causes of Death by Race: U.S., 2000 (continued)

Cause of Death (Based on the Tenth Revision, International Classification of Diseases, 1992)	White			Black			American Indian			Asian or Pacific Islander		
	Rank[1]	Deaths	Percentage of Total Deaths	Rank[1]	Deaths	Percentage of Total Deaths	Rank[1]	Deaths	Percentage of Total Deaths	Rank[1]	Deaths	Percentage of Total Deaths
Certain conditions originating in the perinatal period (P00–P96)	...	8,532	0.4	...	5,021	1.8	...	124	1.1	10	392	1.1
Assault (homicide) (X85–Y09, Y87.1)	...	8,339	0.4	6	7,867	2.8	...	203	1.8	...	356	1.0
Human immunodeficiency virus (HIV) (B20–B24)	...	6,498	0.3	7	7,848	2.7	...	57	0.5	...	75	0.2

... Category not applicable

[1]Rank based on number of deaths

Source: Centers for Disease Control and Prevention, *National Vital Statistics Report* 50, no. 16 (2002):9.

Data for races other than white and black should be interpreted with caution because of inconsistencies between the reporting of race on death certificates and on censuses and surveys

TABLE 6-12 Infant Mortality* Rates and Ratios† among Black and White Births, by Year—U.S., 1980–2000

| | Infant Mortality | | | |
Year	Black	White	Ratio	All Races
1980	22.2	10.9	2.0	**12.6**
1981	20.8	10.3	2.0	**11.9**
1982	20.5	9.9	2.1	**11.5**
1983	20.0	9.6	2.1	**11.2**
1984	19.2	9.3	2.1	**10.8**
1985	19.0	9.2	2.1	**10.6**
1986	18.9	8.8	2.1	**10.4**
1987	18.8	8.5	2.2	**10.1**
1988	18.5	8.4	2.2	**10.0**
1989	18.6	8.1	2.3	**9.8**
1990	18.0	7.6	2.4	**9.2**
1991	17.6	7.3	2.4	**8.9**
1992	16.8	6.9	2.4	**8.5**
1993	16.5	6.8	2.4	**8.4**
1994	15.8	6.6	2.4	**8.0**
1995	15.1	6.3	2.4	**7.6**
1996	14.7	6.1	2.4	**7.3**
1997	14.2	6.0	2.4	**7.2**
1998	14.3	6.0	2.4	**7.2**
1999	14.6	5.8	2.5	**7.1**
2000§	14.0	5.7	2.5	**6.9**

*Number of infants born alive who died within the first year of life per 1,000 live births.

†Ratio of black to white infant mortality.

§ Preliminary data for infant mortality.

Source: National Center for Health Statistics. Mortality data based on race of infant as numerator and race of mother as denominator. Birth weight data based on birth certificate data and race of mother.

Despite substantial reductions in U.S. infant mortality during the past several decades, black-white disparities in infant mortality rates persist (Table 6-12). One of the *Healthy People 2010* national objectives for maternal and infant health is to reduce deaths among infants aged <1 year to ≤4.5 per 1,000 live births among all racial/ethnic groups. Important determinants of racial/ethnic differences in infant mortality are low birth weight (LBW), defined as <2,500 grams, and very low birth weight (VLBW), defined as <1,500 grams. High birth weight–specific mortality rates (BWSMRs) occur at these low birth weights. *Healthy People 2010* goals include reducing LBW to 5 percent and VLBW to 0.9 percent of live births.

Social Variables

In addition to personal attributes, a group of factors referred to as social variables also influences a population's health. These social variables include socioeconomic status, occupational exposures, other environmental health hazards, marital status, and other family-related characteristics.

Socioeconomic Status

Socioeconomic status, or social class, is a multidimensional construct that has long been used, often with quite a bit of controversy, to rank or stratify a population in terms of wealth (poverty and affluence), prestige, and power. There is extensive literature both on how to conceptualize and measure socioeconomic status and on its relationship to mortality and morbidity. It is generally believed that socioeconomic status is best measured by some mixture of income, education, and occupational data. In many instances it is appropriate to combine these variables into a socioeconomic status index, while at other times it is necessary to use them as single indicators. Because all these variables seem to be consistently related to health in the same manner, they are not distinguished here.

One review of the relationship between social class and health status: "Social class gradients of mortality and life expectancy have been observed for centuries, and a vast body of evidence has shown consistently that those in the lower classes have higher mortality, morbidity, and disability rates."[13] As is demonstrated, however, there are some specific exceptions to this general statement.

For both males and females, a lower educational level is associated with higher mortality. A significant difference in mortality can be seen among males (Table 6-13). The difference between the rates obviously favors females—the difference is rates drop from 353.8 for educated <12 years to 91.6 for educated 13 years or more. Clearly, education levels influence mortality patterns. The ratios range from 11.89 to 1.53, indicating the

TABLE 6-13   Age-adjusted Death Rates* for Persons 25–64 Years of Age, All Causes of Death, by Sex and Educational Attainment, U.S., 1999

Years of Educational Attainment	Both Sexes	Male	Female	Difference	Ratio
Less than 12 years	585.3	763.7	409.9	353.8	1.86
12 years	474.5	636.7	337.3	299.4	1.89
13 or more years	219.1	264.2	172.6	91.6	1.53

*Deaths per 100,000 standard population.

Source: Adapted from Table 35, National Center for Health Statistics, 2002. Health, United States, 2002: With Charbook on Trends in the Health of Americans, Hyattsville, MD.

mortality rates are higher for males compared to females across all education levels—with some trend upward.

Table 6-13 shows age-adjusted death rates for males and females as a function of educational attainment.

Table 6-14 shows the relationship between socioeconomic status (SES) and selected causes of death (again using the standardized mortality ratios). In this example, SES was measured on a scale of one to five. The standardized mortality ratios were age-adjusted to remove any effects of differing age distribution. The table demonstrates clearly that for all selected causes of death except coronary heart disease, the mortality ratios are progressively higher as the SES level decreases. For bronchitis, the mortality ratios in the lower class are seven times higher than in the higher class.

There is a substantial body of evidence that people of lower socioeconomic status have worse health than others. One measure of socioeconomic status that combines information regarding a number of relevant variables (such as income, education, and occupation) is the index of relative socioeconomic disadvantage of area. Best regarded as a measure of the economic and social characteristics of a person's local government, and to an extent indicative of individual socioeconomic status, the index is based on aggregate census data for small areas. Two national health surveys, in 1989/90 and 1995, confirmed that those in more disadvantaged areas scored more negatively than others on several health indicators.[14,15]

TABLE 6-14 Standardized Mortality Ratios: A Socioeconomic Status Example

Selected Causes of Death by Socioeconomic Status

	Socioeconomic Status				
	I	*II*	*III* *Skilled* *Labor*	*IV* *Semi-* *skilled*	*V* *Unskilled* *Labor*
Cause of Death	*Professionals*	*Intermediate*	*Labor*	*skilled*	*Labor*
Diabetes	28	41	90	110	176
Stomach cancer	21	52	111	121	143
Lung cancer	48	71	101	126	141
Coronary heart disease	91	90	104	95	118
Bronchitis	27	48	91	109	187
Accidents (excluding motor vehicle)	39	91	91	121	204
All other causes	70	85	105	106	139

Source: Adapted from Australian Bureau of Statistics, Australian Social Trends 1999; Health-Health Status: Health Socioeconomic Disadvantage of Area,
http://www.abs.gov.au/Ausstats/abs@.nsf/0/eaff36cce16dc3a5ca25699f0005d620?OpenDocument.

The same relationship holds true for morbidity. Higher rates of morbidity from a vast array of conditions have been observed in lower socioeconomic groups. Figure 6-7 shows the relationship between prevalence of hypertension and family income. Using either income or educational level,

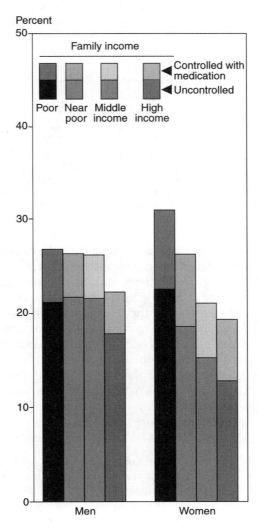

FIGURE 6-7 Hypertension among Adults 20 Years of Age and Over by Family Income and Sex: United States, average annual 1988–1994. *Source: Health, United States, 1998* with socioeconomic status and health chart book.

TABLE 6-15 Prevalence Rates of Asthma by Income and Educational Levels; U.S., 2002

Level	Prevalence Rate per 100	Standard Error	95% Confidence Interval
Income			
<$15,000	14.3	0.43	(13.5–15.2)
$15,000–$24,999	12.6	0.31	(12.0–13.2)
$25,000–$49,999	11.5	0.21	(11.1–11.9)
$50,000–$74,999	10.9	0.30	(10.4–11.5)
≥$75,000	10.8	0.27	(10.3–11.4)
Education			
Did not graduate	13.0	0.41	(12.2–13.8)
High school graduate	11.3	0.21	(10.8–11.7)
Some college	12.8	0.24	(12.4–13.3)
College graduate	11.0	0.19	(10.6–11.3)

Source: Adapted from Centers for Disease Control and Prevention, Table L7, Adult Self-Report Lifetime Asthma Prevalence Rate (Percent) and Prevalence (Number) by Income and State or Territory: BRFSS 2002, *http://www.cdc.gov/nceh/airpollution/asthma/brfss/02/lifetime/tableL7.htm.*

this example shows lower socioeconomic groups have higher prevalence rates of hypertension by controlled and uncontrolled status.

Further, in Table 6-15, the relativity of asthma to income and education is displayed. For instance as income increases the rates of asthma decrease. Notably the standard error and the 95 percent confidence interval are given, which are very small in the case of the standard error and very narrow in the case of the confidence interval. It will be noted later that the size of the standard error and the width of the confidence interval are very important in the interpretation of the results related to sample size and therefore power. Also, note in Table 6-15 that asthma and level of education do not exhibit a clear relationship.

It can be hazardous to try to explain the relationship between socioeconomic status and health. Syme and Berkman comment:

> There can be little doubt that the highest morbidity and mortality rates observed in the lower social class are in part due to inadequate medical care services as well as to the impact of a toxic and hazardous physical environment. There can be little doubt also that these factors do not entirely explain the discrepancy in rates between the classes. . . . That so many different kinds of diseases are more frequent in lower class groupings directs attention to generalized susceptibility to disease and to generalized compromises of disease defense systems.[16]

Life changes, life stresses, and particularly the way people cope with such stress probably are an important part of this negative social and psychological environment.

> Coping, in this sense, refers not to specific types of psychological responses but to the more generalized ways in which people deal with problems in their everyday life. It is evident that such coping styles are likely to be products of environmental situations and not independent of such factors. Several coping responses that have a wide range of disease outcomes have been described. Cigarette smoking is one such coping response that has been associated with virtually all causes of morbidity and mortality; obesity may be another coping style associated with a higher rate of many diseases and conditions; Pattern A behavior is an example of a third coping response that has been shown to have relatively broad disease consequences.[17]

Data on the socioeconomic level of their surrounding population thus can be helpful to health services managers. Even though the reasons might be poorly understood, lower socioeconomic groups do in fact have higher mortality and morbidity rates for the great majority of diseases. Dividing the population according to such levels would be helpful in identifying target groups, in planning the location of satellite or new facilities, and in tracing the general patterns of health and disease in a population. Data by census tract can be obtained from federal publications. Occupation, income, and education can be used as indicators, although education has been shown to be the best predictor.[18,19,20]

Occupational and Environmental Hazards

In addition to being an indicator of socioeconomic status, occupation is linked to health in other ways. Both the occupational environment and the everyday life environment can influence health through specific risks associated with noxious agents and general working or living conditions. It is important to stress at this point that the identification of occupational exposures and other environmental health hazards is an integral part of describing the "person" characteristics of health and disease in a population.

Marital Status, Family-Related Variables

Family-related variables have been the subject of many epidemiological studies.[21] Among such variables, marital status often is linked to mortality and morbidity. The overall mortality rate in both men and women is higher (in decreasing order) among the divorced, the widowed, and the single; it is lowest among married persons.[22] This trend is also true for admission

TABLE 6-16   Two- and Four-Year Incidence of a Depressive Episode by Sex and Marital Status; Canada, 1994–1995

	Males			Females		
Incidence	Married	Never Married	Previously Married	Married	Never Married	Previously Married
Two-Year	2.6	2.3	—	3.7	6.3	3.4
Four-Year	2.0	2.4	—	3.8	5.0	4.0

Source: Adapted from Statistics Canada, *Health Reports* 11, no. 3 (1999):72–73

rates to psychiatric hospitals for males, whereas the widowed female shows the highest rate for admission.

Table 6-16 illustrates the impact of marital status by sex. Canadian females who were never married were significantly more likely to experience a depressive episode in a two-year period than married females.

Historically, the variable between single and married status is evident in mortality rates. MacMahon and Tichopoulos suggest three explanations of the relationship between marital status and mortality rates.[23]

1. Persons in poor health, or in the presymptomatic stages of ill health, tend to remain single.
2. Persons who "live dangerously" and are consequently exposed to a wide variety of disease-producing agents and situations tend to remain single.
3. Differences in the way of life of single and married persons result from the presence or absence of the married state and are causally related to certain diseases. For example, there is more interpersonal contact and life is more routine in a family (married state). A spouse and other family members can provide psychological and physical support, perhaps contributing to better health.

For women, marital status can also be related to health through differences in sexual exposure, pregnancy, childbearing, and lactation.[24] This explains why cancer of the cervix is more common in married rather than single women. Early sexual experience and frequency of intercourse appear to be decisive factors in the emergence of cervical cancer. By contrast, breast cancer is more frequent in single rather than married women: In married women, hormonal balance, ensured by early age at first pregnancy and artificial menopause before the age of 40, seems to lower the risk of breast cancer.

Although the relationship between marital status and health is well documented, it should weaken somewhat because most characteristics of married life—possibly responsible for the positive impact on health—seem to be spreading out to other lifestyles (such as unmarried individuals living together) and becoming less specific to the wedded role. Early sexual experience and frequency of intercourse (as well as lack of multiple partners) no longer are characteristic of married life. Similarly, with the emergence of the extended family, as opposed to the nuclear family (as predicted by Toffler),[25] psychological and physical support should not be characteristics specifically restricted to married life.

Family Size, Birth Order, and Maternal Age Other variables associated with health status are family size, birth order, and maternal age. These variables refer to the "family of origin," or the family into which a person is born or spends the formative years, as opposed to the "family of procreation," in the case of marital status.[26]

Family size is associated first with health through the impact of multiple pregnancies on a woman's condition. Family size is also linked to contagious diseases because the concentration of persons and subsequent multiple contacts facilitate disease propagation. Finally, family size is highly correlated with socioeconomic status, large families being more common among the poor. This can also work in the opposite direction: Large family size can influence the socioeconomic status and, consequently, the health status, nutrition of all members, and children's growth and development.

Maternal age is strongly involved with infants' health. Very young mothers (ages 10–14 and 15–17, black and white) have a greater incidence of producing fetal deaths (Table 6-17). Another peak occurs in the 35–39 and 40–44 age groups. This high incidence can be explained by both biological and socioeconomic factors.[27] In general, very young teenage mothers are both physiologically immature and of low socioeconomic status. Older mothers (over 40) with no previous pregnancies, or very few, also are more likely to have a high fetal death rate.

The greatest problem associated with older mothers, however, is congenital malformation. Many congenital malformations, including anencephalus, hydrocephalus, and clubfoot are more frequent in both younger and older mothers. Some other malformations, such as those of the circulatory system and Down's syndrome, are more frequent in older mothers. Further, the relationship between maternal age and Down's syndrome is indeed striking. It is a direct relationship.

Birth order is a variable that is thought to influence infants' health. Although almost everything, including intelligence,[28] is related to birth order, studies of the subject have many biases.[29,30,31]

TABLE 6-17   *Fetal Death Rates by Race and Age of the Mother*

	Number			Rate		
	Total	White	Black	Total	White	Black
All ages	1120	491	610	8.8	6.0	14.4
10–14 yrs	7	0	7	16.4	0.0	23.6
15–17 yrs	80	22	58	12.7	7.1	18.5
18–19 yrs	105	39	64	8.9	6.0	12.2
20–24 yrs	298	114	182	8.7	5.7	13.2
25–29 yrs	254	121	126	7.4	5.2	12.6
30–34 yrs	213	110	98	8.2	5.9	15.1
35–39 yrs	127	69	56	10.6	8.2	17.8
40–44 yrs	36	16	19	18.0	11.8	33.7
45–55 yrs	0	0	0	0.0	0.0	0.0

Age-specific rates per 1,000 women in age group

Fetal deaths ≥20 weeks of gestation

Source: Planning Information Report 1999, Georgia Department of Public Health.

Family-related variables, mostly marital status and maternal age, thus are significant personal characteristics to be investigated in describing the health problems of a population.

Lifestyle Variables

Lifestyle is an important determinant of health and should be an integral part of the epidemiological framework. Lifestyle variables can be used in the same way as demographic and social variables to describe the personal aspects of the distribution of health in a population. These can also be a focus for intervention: Some lifestyle variables are so closely associated with mortality and morbidity that they represent a very real potential for effective and efficient health services action.

Lifestyle refers to the individual and societal behavior patterns that are at least partly under individual control and that demonstrably influence personal health.[32] Somers writes that the rationale for linking health and lifestyle can be summarized in three statements:[33]

1. The major causes of death, serious illness, and disability in the developed nations today are chronic disease and violence.
2. Behind most chronic disease, disability, and premature death are many environmental and behavioral factors, potentially amend-

TABLE 6-18   Major Causes and Actual Causes of Death and Risk Factors, U.S., 2000.

Major Causes of Death, 2000		
Cause	Percentage of All Deaths	Risk Factor
Heart disease	30	Smoking,* hypertension,* elevated serum cholesterol* (diet), lack of exercise, diabetes, stress, family history
Cancer	23	Smoking,* worksite carcinogens,* environmental carcinogens, alcohol, diet
Stroke	7	Hypertension,* smoking,* elevated serum cholesterol,* stress
Chronic lower respiratory disease	5	Smoking, vaccination status, heart disease, diet, exercise
Unintentional injuries	4	Alcohol,* drug abuse, smoking (fires), product design, handgun availability
Diabetes	3	Obesity*
Pneumonia and influenza	3	Smoking, vaccination status*
Alzheimer's disease	2	
Kidney disease	2	Alcohol, smoking, hypertension
Motor vehicle accidents	2	Alcohol,* no seat belts,* speed,* roadway design, vehicle engineering

*Major risk factors

Source: Adapted from "Deaths: Final Data for 2000" by A. M. Miniño et al., *National Vital Statistics Report* 50, no. 15 (2002):1–120.

able to prevention. (This is illustrated in Tables 6-1, 6-18, and 6-19, which list the risk factors for the major causes of death and disease.)

3. A few individual and societal lifestyle patterns constitute the major behavioral risk factors involved in chronic disease and severe disability.

Contrary to popular belief, the number of serious behavioral risk factors is limited. Those of major importance include cigarette smoking, alcohol and drug abuse, inadequate nutrition, lack of adequate physical activity, irresponsible use of motor vehicles, and irresponsible use of guns and other manifestations of violence.

Cigarette Smoking

In 2000, the most common actual causes of death in the United States were tobacco (435,000), poor diet and physical inactivity (400,000), alcohol consumption (85,000), microbial agents (e.g., influenza and pneumonia, 75,000), toxic agents (e.g., pollutants and asbestos, 55,000), motor vehicle

TABLE 6-19   Actual Causes of Death in the United States, 2000

Actual Causes of Death	Percentage of All Deaths
Tobacco	18.1
Poor diet/physical inactivity	16.6
Alcohol consumption	3.5
Microbial agents (e.g., influenza, pneumonia)	3.1
Toxic agents (e.g., pollutants, asbestos)	2.3
Motor vehicles	1.8
Firearms	1.2
Sexual behavior	0.8
Illicit drug use	0.7

Source: Adapted from "Actual Causes of Death in the United States, 2000," by A. H. Mokdad et al., *JAMA* 291, no. 10 (2000):1238–1246.

accidents (43,000), firearms (29,000), sexual behavior (20,000), and illicit use of drugs (17,000).[34,35]

Actual causes of death are defined as lifestyle and behaviors such as smoking and physical inactivity that contribute to this nation's leading killers, including heart disease, cancer, and stroke.

Contrary to what the cigarette industry might contend, the relationship between smoking and health has been documented ad nauseam. Scientific proof does not come from a perfect experiment but from a gradually evolving body of facts and knowledge. The cut-off point when something can be considered as proved is arbitrary.[36] In the case of the relationship between smoking and health, this point has long since been reached.

No single measure would lengthen life or improve the health of Americans more than eliminating cigarette smoking. This was clearly demonstrated in the previous chapter (see relative and attributable risks). In fact, one in five deaths in the United States is related to smoking.[37] Tobacco's contribution to cancer death rates is estimated at 30.5 percent.[38] Cigarette smokers' cancer death rates are more than double those of nonsmokers. Table 6-20 shows the expected deaths from cancer due to smoking.

Possible intervention strategies against cigarette smoking, including the marketing of cigarettes, are discussed in Chapter 9. It is important to stress at this point that smoking is one of the most important personal characteristics influencing health and that every health care provider, manager, and organization should make every effort to produce an impact on this habit.

A 2001 report issued by the National Cancer Institute states that people who smoke low-tar cigarettes are likely to inhale the same amount of cancer-causing substances as smokers of regular cigarettes, and they remain at high risk for developing smoking-related cancers and other dis-

TABLE 6-20 Cancer Deaths Caused by Smoking, U.S. Population 1994

ICD Code	Site	1994 Expected Cancer Deaths		Smoking Attributable Risk (%)		Estimated Deaths Due to Smoking	
		Male	Female	Male	Female	Male	Female
140–149	Oral	5,150	2,775	90	58.5	4,635	1,624
150	Esophagus	7,800	2,600	76.7	71.6	5,983	1,862
157	Pancreas	12,400	13,500	25.6	31.2	3,174	4,212
161	Larynx	3,000	800	79.3	86.9	2,379	695
162	Lung	94,000	59,000	89.2	78.5	83,848	46,315
180	Cervix	—	4,600	—	30.8	—	1,417
188	Bladder	7,000	3,600	43.1	34.3	3,017	1,235
189	Kidney	6,800	4,500	44.6	15.3	3,033	689
Total expected deaths due to cancer		283,000	255,000	—	—	106,069 (37.5%)	58,049 (22.8%)

Total male and female cancer deaths expected in 1994: 538,000

Total excess deaths due to cigarette smoking: 164,118

Percent attributed to cigarette smoking: 30.5%

Source: Based on data in Shopland et al., 1991, *http://seer.cancer.gov/publications/raterisk/risks69.html.*

eases. Although earlier studies of people smoking low-tar cigarettes suggested a reduction in cancer risks compared to people who smoke regular cigarettes, this has not been the case and the incidence of cancer deaths has increased in the early 1990s.

Even after many years of cigarette smoking, a person who stops reduces risks substantially compared with continuing users. The more years individuals refrain from smoking after stopping, the greater the reduction in excess cancer risk. Ten to fifteen years after stopping, lung cancer risk is reduced to nearly the level of nonsmokers. The same reduction in risk is observed for other cancer sites associated with smoking.

Alcohol and Drug Abuse

An estimated fourteen million Americans—one in every thirteen adults—abuse alcohol or are alcoholic. In addition, 53 percent of men and women in the United States report that one or more of their close relatives have a drinking problem.[39] Furthermore, the effects of alcohol abuse on health are severe. Somers reports that alcoholism is "the most devastating sociomedical problem short of war and malnutrition." Alcohol is a major factor in liver disease, peptic ulcer and other gastrointestinal disorders, nervous system damage, heart disease, nutritional disorders, motor vehicle accidents, homicides, and suicides. It is also a factor in child abuse, battered spouses, and in the outcome of pregnancy (low birth weight, fetal alcohol syndrome).

Drug abuse involves legal and illegal drugs, prescribed and nonprescribed. Although medical problems, including mortality, related to heroin and barbiturates, are declining, the use of cannabinoids (marijuana, hashish) has been increasing with unclear health consequences. An increasing use of amphetamine derivatives MDMA, also known as Ecstasy, and Phencyclidine also known as PCP, has become a significant problem in recent years. The use of central nervous system stimulants, including amphetamines and cocaine, as well as caffeine in cola beverages, coffee, tea, and cocoa, can represent an even greater health hazard. Stimulants of the central nervous system have an effect on the cardiovascular system and on the metabolic rate. Caffeine has also shown to interfere with normal hormonal secretions, is associated with bladder cancer, and is thought to be associated with pancreatic cancer, although the latter has yet to be demonstrated conclusively.

Drugs prescribed by physicians, such as hypnotics, tranquilizers, stimulants, and sleeping pills, also are often abused, leading to psychological and physical dependence, and some drugs are often used to commit date-rape. Many over-the-counter drugs such as aspirin, cold remedies, and even laxatives, largely among the older adult population, tend to be abused, with potentially damaging health consequences.

Nutritional Inadequacies—Obesity

There is increasing evidence that nutritional habits are strongly related to health and disease, most notably coronary heart disease and cancer. Obesity might be the most prevalent form of malnutrition in the industrialized countries and is associated with many health problems, including heart disease. It was estimated that 38.8 million American adults were obese in the year 2000.[40] Furthermore, juvenile-onset obesity, which is particularly serious, is increasingly prevalent. The results of the National Health and Nutrition Examination Survey (1999) showed that 13 percent of children and adolescents were overweight.

The most common health problem in the world might be high consumption of sugar, long associated with dental disease. The heavy use of salt is associated with hypertension. Heavy consumption of fat, particularly saturated, leads to high cholesterol with atherosclerosis and coronary heart disease.

Less well known is the significant relationship between nutrition and many forms of cancer. A recent study estimates that about 32 percent of cancer is avoidable by changes in diet; however, it now seems unlikely that less than 20 percent or more than 42 percent of cancer deaths would be avoidable by dietary change.[41] Diet can act not only as a primary causative factor and an enhancer of tumor growth, but also as a protective factor in preventing some types of cancers.

Fat intake (usually estimated as exceeding 45 percent of total calories) is associated with cancers of the colon, prostate, breast, and large bowel. High protein intake is linked to an increased risk of breast, endometrium, ovary, prostate, large bowel, pancreas, and kidney cancer. In addition, low-protein diets have been shown in animal studies to inhibit tumor development. Low fiber consumption is thought to be associated with colon-rectal cancer.

There is, finally, some concern that chemical carcinogens are present in food additives and in industrial food preparation (such as chemical decaffeination). Nitrosamines, aflatoxins, and polycyclic hydrocarbons, among others, are potentially carcinogenic. Some studies suggest that Vitamin A (more specifically, beta carotene), Vitamin C, and Vitamin E are potentially protective against chemical carcinogens.

Inadequate Physical Activity

Lack of adequate physical activity is related to health and disease in several ways. Recent research suggests the following:

> Significant health benefits can be obtained by including a moderate amount of physical activity (e.g., 30 minutes of brisk walking or raking leaves, 15 minutes of running, or 45 minutes of playing volleyball) on

most, if not all, days of the week. Through a modest increase in daily activity, most Americans can improve their health and quality of life. Additional health benefits can be gained through greater amounts of physical activity. People who can maintain a regular regimen of activity that is of longer duration or of more vigorous intensity are likely to derive greater benefit. Physical activity reduces the risk of premature mortality in general, and of coronary heart disease, hypertension, colon cancer, and diabetes mellitus in particular. Physical activity also improves mental health and is important for the health of muscles, bones, and joints.[42]

Conversely, lack of physical exercise seems to aggravate coronary problems and also leads to obesity and its associated health problems.

Physical activity appears to improve health-related quality of life by enhancing psychological well-being and by improving physical functioning in persons compromised by poor health. Physical activity appears to relieve symptoms of depression and anxiety and improve mood. Regular physical activity can reduce the risk of developing depression.[43] Another study on the benefits of regular exercise in the elderly shows an improvement in social and cultural life, fewer physician visits, and fewer medications for those who undertake regular exercise. As Berg writes, "Few interventions offer as much in the prevention of disability as the use of regular, properly planned physical exercise for the elderly."[44]

Irresponsible Use of Motor Vehicles

Motor vehicle accidents are a critical public health problem because they are the leading cause of death in children, adolescents, and young adults and are a consistently important health hazard among all ages. Most of this mortality, as well as correspondingly high morbidity, can be related to irresponsible use.

The single most important human factor identified with fatal motor accidents is the use of alcohol. In 2000, 16,653 people died in alcohol-related motor vehicle crashes. That's 40 percent of the year's total traffic deaths. Approximately 1.5 million drivers were arrested in 2000 for driving under the influence of alcohol or narcotics. That's just over 1 percent of the estimated 120 million or more episodes of impaired driving that occur among U.S. adults each year.[45]

Another aspect of irresponsible vehicular usage is that only 75 percent of drivers in the United States use seat belts.[46] It has been shown conclusively that the use of seat belts reduces significantly the injury rates from car accidents. Motorcycle helmets were used by only 58 percent of motorcycle riders in the year 2002. Even more striking, in the year 2000, more than two-thirds of the children fatally injured were not in age-appropriate restraints or were completely unrestrained.[47]

A final aspect of irresponsible use of motor vehicles is driving speed. In 2001, speeding was a contributing factor in 30 percent of all fatal crashes, and 12,850 lives were lost in speeding-related crashes.[48]

Irresponsible Use of Guns and Other Manifestations of Violence

Deaths related to violence account for a large proportion of total deaths in the nation. Homicide victimization rates are higher for very young children than older children, who have the lowest rates of all age groups. Older teens and young adults have the highest rates of victimization.[49] This is shocking especially because it serves as merely one measurable indicator of child abuse and child neglect. The United States has one of the highest homicide rates in the industrialized world—more than five times the rate for most European nations.[50] An association is found between firearm ownership and both suicide and homicide. High rates are found when comparing levels for whole countries,[51] though such studies have important limitations. High rates are also found when comparing individuals in households that did or did not have a firearm.[52] As Somers writes:

> It is often said that "violence as a way of life" or "violence as a way of problem solving" are normal aspects of American life. It is difficult to distinguish between deliberate violence and irresponsibility. In any case, the results are frequently disability, psychological suffering, and premature death.[32]

Summary

This concludes the discussion of some of the major lifestyle factors associated with health and disease. Even though it can be difficult at times to see the importance of some of these factors to health services management, their impact on a population's disease pattern is sufficient to warrant the attention and concern of all those involved in health care delivery. These lifestyle factors should be considered in describing the health problems of a community. This chapter reviewed demographic, social, and lifestyle variables that describe those affected by the diseases prevalent in a population. The information can help health services managers to gain a better understanding of the problems faced by their populations of interest and to develop comprehensive programs to solve them. The lifestyle variables are the major areas where institutions can become actively involved in setting up prevention programs.

The health field concept treats lifestyle as a major determinant of health that must undergo change if improvements in physical and mental status are to occur. Descriptive epidemiology (person) is the cornerstone of analysis for health services managers. The multiple variables considered are most important to the subsequent utilization of services, but are also critical for the use of market analysis in view of health promotion and disease prevention.

References

1. T. C. Timmreck, *An Introduction to Epidemiology*, 3d ed. (Boston: Jones and Bartlett Publishers, 2002), 2–3.
2. L. Gosdis, *Epidemiology*, 2d ed. (Philadelphia: W. B. Saunders Company, 2000), 131–138.
3. L. E. Daly and G. J. Bourke, *Interpretation and Uses of Medical Statistics*, 5th ed. (Oxford: Blackwell Sciences Ltd., 2000), 168–169.
4. W. H. Frost, "The Age Selection of Mortality from Tuberculosis in Successive Decades," *American Journal of Hygiene* 30 (1939):91–96.
5. Timmreck, *An Introduction to Epidemiology*, 48–49.
6. Bureau of the Census, *Social Indicators III*, U.S. Department of Commerce (Washington, D.C.: U.S. Government Printing Office, December 1980), 59.
7. Pennsylvania Department of Health, "Health Statistics—Technical Assistance, Tools of the Trade," *http://www.health.state.pa.us/hpa/stats/techassist/sexratio. htm.*
8. B. B. Kalben, *Why Men Die Younger: Causes of Mortality Differences by Sex* (Chicago: Society of Actuaries, 2001), 22–23, 29–30.
9. Kalben, *Why Men Die Younger*, 11.
10. Mood Disorders Society of Canada et al., *A Report on Mental Illness in Canada* (Ottawa, Canada): (Health Canada, 2002), 32.
11. Mood Disorders Society of Canada et al., *A Report on Mental Illness in Canada*, 26.
12. A. M. Haynes, Minorities and Health Statistics, *Urban Health* (June 1975), 14.
13. S. L. Syme and L. F. Berkman, "Social Class, Susceptibility, and Sickness," *American Journal of Epidemiology* 104, no. 1 (July 1976):1.
14. C. Mathers, "Health Differential among Adult Australians Aged 25–64 Years," *Health Monitoring Series*, no. 1 (1994):296–297.
15. Australian Bureau of Statistics, Australian Social Trends 1999; Health-Health Status: Health Socioeconomic Disadvantage of Area, *http://www.abs.gov.au/ Ausstats/abs@.nsf/0/eaff36cce16dc3a5ca25699f0005d620?OpenDocument.*
16. Syme and Berkman, "Social Class," 4–5.
17. Syme and Berkman, "Social Class," 5.
18. Henrik L. Blum, *Planning for Health* (New York: Human Sciences Press, Inc., 1981), 23.
19. M. H. Naji and E. H. Stockwell, "Socioeconomic Differentials in Mortality by Cause of Health," *Health Services Reports* 88, no. 5 (1973):449–456.
20. Victor R. Fuchs, "The Economics of Health in a Postindustrial Society," *Public Interest* 56 (Summer 1979): 3–20.
21. B. Macmahon and D. Tichopoulos, *Epidemiology: Principles and Methods*, 2d ed. (Boston: Little, Brown, 1996).
22. S. Mani and G. F. Cooper, "A Study in Causal Discovery from Population-Based Infant Birth and Death Records," *Proceedings of the AMIA Annual Fall Symposium* (Philadelphia: Hanley and Belfus Publishers, 1999):315–319.

23. B. McMahon, T. F. Pugh, and J. Ipsen, *Epidemiologic Methods* (Boston: Little, Brown, & Co., 1960):135.
24. J. S. Mausner and A. K. Bahn, *Epidemiology: An Introductory Text*, (Philadelphia: W. B. Saunders Company, 1974), 56.
25. A. Toffler, *The Third Wave* (New York: Bantam Books, 1980).
26. Mausner and Bahn, *Epidemiology: An Introductory Text*, 57.
27. J. C. Kleinman, "Trends and Variations in Birth Weight," *Health, United States*, (Hyattsville, MD: U.S. Department of Health and Human Services, 1981):135.
28. L. Belmont and F. A. Marola, "Birth Order, Family Size, and Intelligence," *Science* 182 (1973):1096–1101.
29. Mausner and Bahn, *Epidemiology: An Introductory Text*, 58.
30. C. Schooler, "Birth Order Defects: Not Here, Not Now," *Psychological Bulletin* 78 (1972):161.
31. J. R. Huguenard and G. E. Sharples, "Incidence of Congenital Pyloric Stenosis in Birth Series," *Journal of Chronic Diseases* 35 (1972):727.
32. A. R. Somers, "Life Style and Health," *Maxcy-Roseneau Public Health and Preventive Medicine*, 11th ed., ed. John M. Last (New York: Appleton-Century-Crofts, Inc. 1980), 1047.
33. Somers, "Life Style and Health," 1047.
34. J. R. Richmond, "Health for the Future" (speech presented to Women's National Democratic Club, Washington, D.C., February 19, 1980, quoted in *Health, United States, 1980*, U.S. Department of Health and Human Services, Public Health Service [Washington, D.C.: U.S. Government Printing Office, December 1980], 294).
35. G. B. Gori, unpublished data, National Cancer Institute, 1977, quoted in Somers, "Life Style and Health," 1049.
36. K. Popper, *The Logic of Scientific Discovery*, 3d ed. (London: Hutchinson, 1972).
37. Centers for Disease Control and Prevention, "Smoking-Attributable Mortality and Years of Potential Life Lost—United States, 1990," *Morbidity and Mortality Weekly Report* 42, no. 33 (1993):645–648.
38. National Cancer Institute, "Surveillance, Epidemiology, and End Results," *http://seer.cancer.gov/publications/raterisk/risks69.html*.
39. NIAAA, "Alcoholism, Getting the Facts, a National Institute on Alcohol Abuse and Alcoholism," NIH Publication No. 96–4153, revised 2001 *http://www.niaaa.nih.gov*.
40. CDC, "Nutrition and Physical Activity, Obesity and Overweight, Obesity Trends," *http://www.cdc.gov/nccdphp/dnpa/obesitv/trend/index.htm*.
41. W. C. Willett, "Diet, Nutrition, and Avoidable Cancer," *Environmental Health Perspectives* 103 Suppl 8(November 1995):165–70.
42. CDC, Physical Activity and Health, "A Report of the Surgeon General," *http://www.cdc.gov/nccdphp/sgr/sgr.htm*.
43. CDC, "Report of the Surgeon General."
44. R. L. Berg, "Prevention of Disability in the Aged," *Maxcy-Roseneau Public Health and Preventive Medicine*, 11th ed., J. L. Last (New York: Appleton-Century-Crofts, Inc., 1980), 1295.

45. CDC, "Quick Facts about Impaired Driving," *http://www.cdc.gov/ncipc/duip/spotlite/3d.htm*.

46. National Highway Traffic Safety Administration, "NHTSA Safety Belt and Helmet Use in 2002," NOPUS report, September 2002, *http://www-md.nhtsa.dot.gov/pdf/md30/NCSAIRpts/2002/809–500.pdf*.

47. CDC, "Quick Facts," *http://www.cdc.gov/ncipc/duiu/spotlite/childseat.htm*.

48. U.S. Department of Transportation National Highway Traffic Safety Administration, "Traffic Safety Facts 2001 Overview," *http://www-nrd.nhtsa.dot.gov/pdf/nrd-30/NCSA/TSF2001/2001overview.pdf*.

49. U.S. Department of Justice, Bureau of Justice Statistics, "Homicide Trends in the United States," *http://www.ojp.usdoj.gov/bis/homicide/teensani.htm*.

50. World Policy Institute, "Comparative Homicide Rates in English-speaking Developed Countries," *http://www.worldpolicy.org/americas/usa/firearms-homicides.html*.

51. M. Killias, "International Correlations between Gun Ownership and Rates of Homicide and Suicide," *Canadian Medical Association Journal* 148 (1993):1721–1725.

52. D. A. Brent et al., "The Presence and Accessibility of Firearms in the Homes of Adolescent Suicides: A Case-control Study," *Journal of the American Medical Association* (1992). Volume 266 (1998):2899–2995. And A. L. Kellerman et al., "Suicde in the Home in Relation to Gun Ownership," *New England Journal of Medicine*, vol. 327 (1992):467–472. And A. L. Kellerman et al., "Gun Ownership as a Risk Factor for Homicide in the Home," *New England Journal of Medicine*, vol. 329 (1993):1084–1091.

7

Descriptive Epidemiology: Place and Time

Place: Where Disease Occurs

The preceding chapter dealt with the characteristics that can affect disease patterns—as they relate to the person. Disease occurrence can also be characterized in terms of where it occurs (place) and when (time).

Therefore, the second major issue in descriptive epidemiologic studies of a community is: Where does disease occur? As in person-related characteristics, the quest again is for a pattern of disease occurrence, this time in relation to geography.

The method of analysis involves mapping disease patterns and making comparisons between geographic areas in tables, graphs, and charts. Relationships between location and disease have long been used as a basis for hypotheses of the etiology of diseases. Another objective is to assist health services managers in identifying problem areas.

Differences in occurrence of a disease between places can be caused by many factors, such as the physical and biological environment inherent in the areas compared or in the characteristics of the inhabitants.[1] Epidemiologists concerned with the biology of disease are, or at least traditionally have been, mostly concerned with the physical and biological environment causative factors.

Those that depend on specific environmental factors and conditions are called place diseases.[2] Obvious examples are parasitic and infectious diseases; less-well-known ones[3] include endemic goiter in iodine-deficient inland regions, histoplasmosis in inland river valleys where humidity is high, and mottled dental enamel, a condition related to the fluoride content of water and whose geographical pattern of occurrence led to the identification of the role of fluoride in preventing dental caries.

Multiple sclerosis also shows a distinctive geographical distribution pattern, with rare incidence between the equator and 30 to 35 degrees latitude, increasing with distance from the equator in both northern and southern hemispheres.[4] The prevalence rate of multiple sclerosis is six times higher in Winnipeg, Manitoba, than in New Orleans, and 2.4 times higher in Halifax, Nova Scotia, than in Charleston, South Carolina.[5]

Further, ethnic background can play a role because the highest rates of multiple sclerosis are in areas populated by those with a northern European/Scandinavian background. Also, clusters and epidemics of the disease have been reported in Canada, Norway, and Florida. Epidemics have occurred in the Faroe Islands and in Iceland. No cases of MS were apparent before 1945. Since then cases have been reported with peaks in 1945, 1955, and 1965.[6]

Relationships between place and disease also can result from the personal characteristics of the inhabitants. There are numerous examples of this. The lower cardiovascular death rate in Japan as compared to the United States has been related to diet (intake of cholesterol). The overall lower mortality rate in Utah, in reference to heart disease and cancer, has been associated with the particular lifestyle of the large Mormon population. A somewhat more "exotic" example is the geographical pattern of kuru, a rapidly fatal neurologic disease. This is limited to one area of New Guinea among one tribal group and results from cannibalistic practices. As the area has come under control of the Australian government and as cannibalism has been discouraged, kuru has been disappearing.[7]

The importance of location of disease for administrative, as opposed to biologic, purposes stems from the fact that, as Donabedian writes, "Certain features of social organization conspire to concentrate particularly vulnerable populations in certain areas, notably the urban ghetto and some rural sections of the country. The association is often so close that mere residence in certain areas may constitute presumptive evidence of unmet need."[8]

In other words, there tend to be clusters of person factors (as described in Chapter 6) in certain places. In this sense, the location or place of disease is particularly relevant to health services managers because they can use it as an aggregate indicator of multiple risk factors in a particular population subgroup. Mortality differences between places also can be caused by differences in survivorship, that is, in the case where fatality rates result from differences in medical services and facilities.[9] Mortality and morbidity differences can be artifactual (nonreal), stemming from differences or errors in reporting and diagnosis (errors in the numerators) or in the population census (errors in the denominators).

Analysis of disease patterns by place can be done using either natural or political boundaries. Natural boundaries are likely to be more useful when investigating environmental causative factors, including climate, water, or soil.[10,11] However, it often is more convenient to use political boundaries, either on an international, national, state, or local level. This is most essential if the expected results are to be used for the allocation of resources and money.

International Comparisons

International comparison of disease serves several purposes. It allows the monitoring of each country's health status. It is used in etiologic studies to look at associations between disease and environmental conditions as well as person factors. It also provides some estimate of potential improvement in the countries that do not have the lower rates.

Interpretation of differences among countries can be hazardous, however, as major variances in reporting and diagnosis are likely. Small differences in specific causes of death probably are insignificant, but it is hard to discuss very large differences such as can be observed for several diseases.

Table 7-1 shows the overall mortality rates among men and women in selected countries. Because all of these countries have reasonably good

TABLE 7-1 Mortality among Males and Females in Selected Countries, 2000 Estimates

| | *Average Annual Death Rate per 1,000 Population* | | | | | |
| | *Male* | | | *Female* | | |
Country	*Deaths*	*Crude*	*ASR(W)**	*Deaths*	*Crude*	*ASR(W)**
United States	30,150	219.46	161.80	268,965	190.51	116.43
Canada	35,303	229.05	160.49	30,400	193.21	116.69
Denmark	8,013	306.12	184.88	7,531	281.48	144.04
Norway	5,672	256.29	155.65	4,886	216.97	113.08
Sweden	11,626	263.10	137.93	10,250	228.23	104.02
Netherlands	21,425	274.06	181.98	17,296	217.06	120.03
United Kingdom	84,722	296.29	171.02	76,923	256.89	128.05
Belgium	16,697	335.52	198.06	12,151	234.35	113.44
France	92,541	321.34	201.50	59,296	195.82	98.03
Germany	118,899	295.28	176.57	107,213	255.55	116.94
Switzerland	9,822	269.00	171.01	7,479	200.32	103.33

*Age-Standardized Rate: An age-standardized rate (ASR) is a summary measure of a rate that a population would have if it had a standard age structure. Standardization is necessary when comparing several populations that differ with respect to age because age has such a powerful influence on the risk of cancer. The most frequently used standard population is the world standard population. The calculated incidence of mortality rate is then called world standardized incidence of mortality rate. It is also expressed per 100,000.

Source: J. Ferlay et al., GLOBOCAN 2000: Cancer Incidence, Mortality and Prevalence Worldwide, Version 1.0, IARC Cancer Base No. 5 (Lyon, France: IARC Press, 2001), *http://www-dep.iarc.fr/globocan/globocan.html.*

vital statistics systems, the differences are interesting. These death rates have been age-adjusted to control for the effect of varying age composition.

In 2000 estimates show that mortality rates among men and women were lowest in the Scandinavian countries and The Netherlands, followed in order by Canada, the United States, and the northwestern European countries. The order varies somewhat for specific age groups. At ages under 25, lower rates were observed in the Scandinavian countries and The Netherlands, followed by the northwestern European countries, then Canada and the United States. At ages 65 and over, the lowest mortality among men, the leader was Canada, followed by the United States, the Scandinavian countries and The Netherlands, and the northwestern European countries. Among women 65 and older, the United States had the lowest rate.[12]

The international differences are sometimes very wide for specific diseases and causes of death. The incidence of infectious and parasitic diseases of course varies strikingly between tropical and temperate areas. There are many less easily explainable differences in chronic, noninfectious diseases.[13]

Table 7-2 shows the ranking of various countries in terms of several cancer sites. The top rates range from 6.8 to 267.9 times higher than the lowest. Some countries—Ireland, Denmark, and Hungary—have high cancer rates for many different sites. Others such as China and Colombia have low rates for almost all sites, with Mauritians at the bottom (best) in almost every category listed here. Still others have a low rate for certain causes of death and a very high one for others.[14] For example, Japan has low rates for male colon and female breast cancer, as well as for male prostate, but it has relatively high rates for male lung cancer. Although not listed, Japan has the highest rate in the world for stomach cancer.

Rates for the United States and Canada are exactly the opposite of Japan: among the higher ones for male colon and female breast cancer and among the lowest for male stomach cancer.[15,16] Some countries such as Canada and Australia, geographically far apart but sharing a common heritage as well as comparable industrialization and lifestyles, have almost identical rates for all causes of death listed in Table 7-2.

As noted earlier, international comparisons often are used to study the etiology of diseases. For example, international comparisons show that the incidence of colon, rectum, stomach, and breast cancer is high where there is a low level of selenium in the soil.[17,18,19] A useful etiologic tool when lifestyle or environmental factors are suspected is the study of migrants. Studies of Japanese migrants to Hawaii and California show that they soon are likely to have the high breast cancer rates of women in the United States.[20,21,22] Studies of immigrants also have been used to implicate dietary practices in many forms of cancer.[23,24]

TABLE 7-2 Death Rates per 100,000 Population for 45 Countries, 2000

Country	All Sites		Colon and Rectum		Breast	Prostate	Lung and Bronchus	
	Male	Female	Male	Female	Female	Male	Male	Female
United States	161.8 (22)	116.4 (10)	15.9 (27)	12.0 (20)	21.2 (12)	17.9 (18)	53.2 (13)	27.2 (1)
Australia	150.9 (28)	103.2 (25)	20.1 (12)	14.4 (12)	19.7 (18)	18.0 (17)	36.2 (31)	14.0 (10)
Austria	168.6 (20)	113.8 (12)	23.0 (8)	14.9 (10)	23.3 (9)	18.9 (12)	41.8 (25)	10.8 (16)
Azerbaijan	114.2 (41)	61.8 (45)	6.4 (40)	4.8 (42)	8.8 (43)	4.3 (43)	25.5 (37)	4.5 (42)
Bulgaria	150.3 (29)	89.4 (35)	17.8 (20)	12.0 (21)	16.7 (31)	9.0 (34)	43.7 (22)	7.1 (32)
Canada	160.5 (23)	116.7 (9)	16.4 (26)	11.6 (23)	22.7 (10)	17.1 (21)	50.4 (14)	25.0 (3)
Chile	141.2 (34)	108.7 (18)	7.0 (39)	7.1 (37)	12.7 (37)	19.9 (9)	20.3 (40)	7.0 (33)
China	143.3 (33)	76.9 (43)	7.2 (38)	5.3 (41)	4.5 (45)	1.0 (45)	33.2 (32)	13.5 (11)
Colombia	116.1 (40)	106.5 (19)	5.8 (41)	6.1 (39)	10.6 (40)	15.1 (27)	17.0 (43)	8.5 (24)
Croatia	230.1 (2)	105.4 (21)	24.8 (6)	13.0 (16)	19.9 (17)	15.3 (25)	70.3 (3)	9.4 (20)
Cuba	141.0 (35)	104.0 (23)	11.4 (32)	12.4 (18)	15.6 (35)	22.1 (5)	42.8 (23)	15.6 (8)
Czech Republic	222.2 (3)	127.6 (6)	34.2 (1)	18.5 (3)	21.0 (13)	15.7 (23)	65.3 (5)	11.5 (14)
Denmark	184.9 (14)	144.0 (2)	23.8 (7)	18.5 (4)	29.2 (1)	23.1 (4)	50.0 (15)	26.7 (2)
Estonia	201.5 (9)	104.8 (22)	16.7 (24)	12.0 (22)	19.3 (19)	15.3 (26)	64.5 (6)	8.6 (23)
Finland	145.8 (32)	92.5 (32)	12.5 (30)	9.5 (32)	17.9 (26)	19.1 (11)	41.2 (26)	7.4 (28)
France	201.5 (10)	98.0 (30)	18.3 (17)	12.1 (19)	21.4 (11)	19.2 (10)	48.5 (19)	6.7 (35)
Germany	176.6 (16)	116.9 (8)	21.7 (11)	17.0 (6)	23.7 (8)	18.4 (15)	46.2 (20)	9.6 (18)
Greece	149.5 (31)	81.8 (42)	8.4 (37)	6.7 (38)	16.7 (32)	10.7 (33)	50.0 (16)	7.4 (29)
Hungary	272.3 (1)	147.4 (1)	33.5 (2)	20.9 (1)	25.3 (7)	17.9 (19)	86.2 (1)	20.0 (5)
Ireland	170.2 (19)	127.8 (5)	22.6 (9)	15.4 (8)	25.8 (6)	21.6 (6)	38.3 (30)	17.3 (7)
Israel	135.1 (38)	111.4 (15)	19.7 (13)	15.3 (9)	26.2 (4)	14.2 (30)	27.5 (36)	9.3 (21)
Japan	159.5 (24)	83.1 (41)	17.6 (21)	11.0 (28)	7.7 (44)	5.5 (40)	33.1 (33)	9.6 (19)
Kazakhstan	201.9 (8)	102.6 (27)	12.2 (31)	8.6 (33)	13.3 (36)	5.2 (41)	59.5 (9)	8.3 (25)
Kyrgyzstan	185.6 (13)	112.6 (14)	10.9 (35)	7.9 (35)	17.0 (29)	6.4 (39)	40.7 (27)	7.3 (30)
Latvia	196.7 (11)	102.8 (26)	17.9 (19)	13.3 (15)	18.1 (24)	13.0 (31)	59.1 (10)	6.3 (37)

TABLE 7-2 (continued)

Country	All Sites		Colon and Rectum		Breast	Prostate	Lung and Bronchus	
	Male	Female	Male	Female	Female	Male	Male	Female
Lithuania	195.9 (12)	97.0 (31)	18.0 (18)	10.7 (29)	19.0 (20)	15.6 (24)	56.5 (11)	5.5 (39)
Macedonia	140.1 (36)	85.5 (38)	11.2 (34)	7.8 (36)	17.2 (28)	6.8 (37)	39.8 (28)	6.6 (36)
Mauritius	79.6 (45)	66.3 (44)	5.8 (42)	3.9 (45)	9.2 (41)	7.3 (36)	16.7 (44)	4.2 (44)
Mexico	112.5 (42)	106.3 (20)	4.7 (44)	4.6 (43)	12.2 (38)	16.6 (22)	22.1 (39)	8.2 (26)
Netherlands	182.0 (15)	120.0 (7)	19.0 (14)	14.0 (13)	27.8 (2)	20.0 (8)	59.7 (8)	14.8 (9)
New Zealand	167.2 (21)	131.1 (3)	25.7 (4)	20.2 (2)	25.9 (5)	21.2 (7)	39.3 (29)	18.7 (6)
Norway	155.7 (27)	113.1 (13)	22.0 (10)	18.0 (5)	20.7 (14)	26.8 (3)	31.7 (34)	12.8 (12)
Poland	205.2 (6)	111.4 (16)	16.6 (25)	11.6 (24)	16.8 (30)	11.2 (32)	71.5 (2)	11.3 (15)
Portugal	157.1 (26)	89.1 (37)	18.5 (16)	11.3 (26)	18.4 (22)	17.9 (20)	29.5 (35)	4.8 (40)
Rep. of Moldova	157.8 (25)	89.4 (36)	15.8 (28)	10.6 (30)	18.5 (21)	5.0 (42)	42.1 (24)	6.2 (38)
Romania	150.0 (30)	90.0 (34)	11.4 (33)	8.2 (34)	16.2 (34)	8.3 (35)	45.1 (21)	7.3 (31)
Russian Fed.	211.2 (5)	100.6 (29)	17.5 (22)	12.7 (17)	16.7 (33)	6.8 (38)	68.2 (4)	6.8 (34)
Slovakia	217.8 (4)	108.8 (17)	28.0 (3)	16.1 (7)	18.4 (23)	14.3 (29)	60.7 (7)	7.8 (27)
Slovenia	203.1 (7)	115.9 (11)	25.1 (5)	14.6 (11)	20.3 (16)	18.8 (13)	55.3 (12)	10.1 (17)
Spain	176.1 (17)	85.0 (40)	17.3 (23)	11.1 (27)	18.1 (25)	15.0 (28)	49.4 (17)	4.2 (45)
Sweden	137.9 (37)	104.0 (24)	14.4 (29)	11.5 (25)	17.5 (27)	27.3 (2)	22.6 (38)	12.6 (13)
Trinidad & Tobago	103.5 (44)	101.9 (28)	8.5 (36)	9.7 (31)	20.6 (15)	32.3 (1)	13.2 (45)	4.3 (43)
Turkmenistan	117.7 (39)	85.2 (39)	4.7 (45)	4.1 (44)	9.2 (42)	1.8 (44)	18.9 (42)	4.6 (41)
United Kingdom	171.0 (18)	128.0 (4)	18.7 (15)	13.8 (14)	26.8 (3)	18.5 (14)	48.6 (18)	21.1 (4)
Venezuela	104.1 (43)	91.8 (33)	5.8 (43)	6.1 (40)	11.6 (39)	18.2 (16)	19.4 (41)	9.2 (22)

Note: Figures in parentheses are order of rank within site and sex group.

Source: Adapted from the American Cancer Society, Cancer Facts and Figures 2003 (Atlanta, Ga.: American Cancer Society, 2003), 30–31.

Variation within Countries

As opposed to international comparisons, which are useful mainly for etiologic purposes, variations within countries are most appropriate for administrative purposes, although as is noted later, they can and have often been used in analyzing the etiology of diseases. Variations within a country, on a national, state, or local level, can be used advantageously in the management and planning of health services.

Variations between U.S. States   There are many geographic differences in mortality patterns within the United States.[25,26,27] In general, mortality rates are higher in the East, particularly the Southeast. For blacks and for white males, the highest rate areas for all natural causes are largely in the Southeast. For white females, they more often are in the Middle Atlantic States and in the Chicago area. The Southeast has a particularly high incidence of cardiovascular diseases and stroke (Figure 7-1).[28,29,30]

Heart disease is one of the most significant and persistent public health problems in the United States, causing a tremendous burden of premature mortality and disability. It is the leading cause of death for men of all racial and ethnic groups, and although about half of all heart disease deaths occur among men and half among women, over 70 percent of premature (i.e., before age 65) heart disease deaths occur among men. From the mid-1960s to the mid-1980s, Americans experienced significant declines in heart disease mortality. However, recent studies show that from the mid-1980s to the present, those declines have slowed considerably and have even stopped for some population groups. In addition, there are recent findings, reported in several scientific studies, that numerous community-based public health programs to reduce heart disease risk factors and prevent onset of the disease have had only limited effectiveness. Both of these trends have created a renewed sense of urgency in the public health community to develop and implement better and more effective programs and policies to reduce the burden of heart disease in the United States.

Why is it critical to understand local geographic disparities in the burden of heart disease among men? Health disparities among places reflect underlying inequalities in local social environments that make some communities more health-promoting than others. The social environment provides the context within which individuals are exposed to structural risk factors (e.g., poverty, social isolation, and lack of economic opportunity) that contribute to adoption of disadvantageous behaviors (e.g., cigarette smoking, physical inactivity, poor diet). Understanding the health-promoting characteristics of local communities, and the barriers to change, is a critical first step in designing effective programs and policies. In addition, identifying the places that bear the greatest burden of heart disease mortality will permit the targeting of appropriate resources to improve the

FIGURE 7-1   Death Rates for Stoke, Whites Ages 35 Years and Older, 1991–1998*

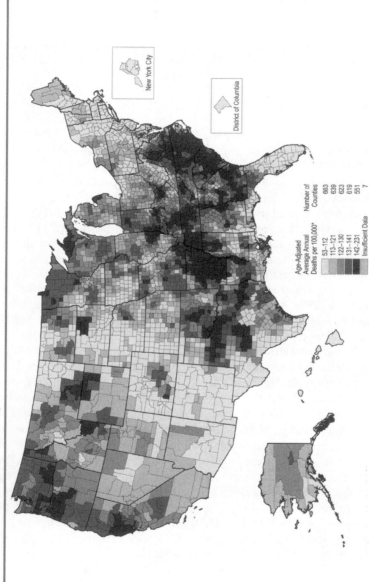

Age-Adjusted
Average Annual
Deaths per 100,000*

	Number of Counties
53–112	663
113–121	639
122–130	623
131–141	619
142–231	551
Insufficient Data	7

*Stroke deaths are spatially smoothed to enhance the stability of rates in countries with small populations.

Source: Caspers, M.L. et al. 2003. *Atlas of Stroke Mortality: Racial, Ethnic, and Geographic Disparities in the United States.* Atlanta, GA: Department of Health and Human Services, Centers for Disease Control and Prevention, p. 57.

local social environment and health outcomes in those communities. A challenge for health service is that ameliorating the social environment in local communities requires structural and institutional changes, improvements in community social relations, and reductions in inequalities within those communities.

Most contemporary heart disease prevention efforts focus on changing the behavior of individuals regarding lifestyle factors: dietary habits, leisure-time physical activity, and tobacco use.[31] Health promotion programs that focus on behavioral risk factors have been effective among adults who are highly educated, fully employed, and highly motivated to improve their health. The lifestyle approach to heart disease prevention is for people who are at highest risk: namely, rural residents, the working class, and the poor. These groups of signified importance tend to have greater exposure to risk factors such as cigarette smoking, physical inactivity, high-fat diets, and psychologic stress. These groups also face substantial social, economic, and geographic barriers to risk factor reduction.

A holistic approach to heart disease prevention focuses on broad improvements in local social environments, recognizing that the social environment provides the context within which individuals are exposed to structural risk factors (poverty, social isolation, stressful working environments) and adopt detrimental behaviors (cigarette smoking, physical inactivity, poor diets).[32,33] Under this model, primary prevention of heart disease can be achieved through community-wide improvements in the social environment, including full employment in healthy work environments, access to affordable healthy foods and recreational facilities, freedom from bigotry and discrimination, and opportunities for social interaction and participation in civic life.[34]

There are dramatic patterns of spatial concentration of racial and ethnic minorities in particular localities and regions within the United States. Geographic segregation and concentration of particular racial and ethnic groups are important predictors of access to economic opportunities, social services, and medical care resources.[35]

In 1999, stroke was the third leading cause of death in the United States and a leading cause of serious, long-term disability, placing an enormous burden on the public's health. Approximately 600,000 U.S. residents suffer a new or recurrent stroke each year, and roughly 167,000 die of a stroke each year.[36] In 1999, a total of 1.1 million U.S. adults reported functional limitations and difficulty with activities of daily living resulting from a stroke.[37] Substantial disparities in the health and economic burden of stroke among racial and ethnic populations have been documented, with African Americans far more likely to die of stroke than members of other racial and ethnic groups in the United States.[38]

In addition, an alarming trend has been observed in stroke mortality rates during the past decade. Although stroke mortality declined substantially for many racial and ethnic groups during the 1970s and early 1980s, little improvement was made during the 1990s.[39] Equally as disturbing, stroke hospitalizations actually increased 18.6 percent from 1988 through 1997.[40] These observations have raised awareness within the public health and medical professions that new and innovative efforts are needed to more effectively prevent stroke. In addition, there is increased appreciation of the need for public health agencies and other institutions to act locally to provide more targeted and culturally appropriate stroke prevention programs and policies.

Substantial geographic disparities in stroke mortality have been observed in the United States for decades.[41,42,43,44,45,46,47,48] Early on, the term "stroke belt" was coined to describe the concentration of high stroke mortality rates in the southeastern United States. The first study that examined the geographic pattern of stroke mortality used the state as the unit of analysis.[49] Later studies report more detailed patterns in the geographic disparities in stroke mortality by using smaller units of analysis (i.e., health service areas, state economic areas, and counties).[50,51,52,53,54,55]

Existing studies of the geographic disparities in stroke mortality confirm a concentration of high stroke mortality rates in the Southeast for all persons ages 35 and older, for blacks as well as whites, and for both women and men. Hypotheses regarding the determinants of the loosely defined stroke belt have evolved through the years. Initially, researchers believed the stroke belt was a fixed geographic entity, promoting geologic hypotheses on the deficiency of trace elements (e.g., selenium) and the hardness of the water.[56] However, evidence exists that the geographic pattern of the stroke belt has changed substantially in only twenty-five years.[57]

In 1962, a large concentration of counties with high stroke death rates was reported in the coastal states of North Carolina, South Carolina, and Georgia. By 1988, this concentration had diminished, and a new concentration of counties with high rates was observed in the Mississippi Delta. This observation shifted the hypotheses away from properties of the physical environment and focused researchers' attention on the possibility that differential trends in social conditions—including the prevalence of risk factors, the social environment, access to care, and migration patterns—could be contributing to the observed geographic disparities in stroke mortality.[58,59] Although geographic bias in the accuracy of stroke diagnosis and/or death certificate reporting can also contribute to the observed geographic disparities in stroke mortality, no studies have confirmed this hypothesis to date.[60,61,62]

A few studies have examined the associations of geographic disparities in stroke risk factors with geographic disparities in stroke mortality. A 1977 study of blacks and whites in three geographically diverse communities with different rates of stroke mortality (low, medium, and high) reported that only blood glucose levels were correlated with stroke mortality for both blacks and whites. Blood pressure levels correlated only with stroke mortality rates for black women and with men across the three communities, and no consistent patterns were observed for the other risk factors included in the study (i.e., serum cholesterol, weight and height measurements, and cigarette smoking).[63]

Similarly, data from the first National Health and Nutrition Examination Survey (NHANES I) Epidemiologic Follow-up Study indicated that, even after adjusting for the leading stroke risk factors (i.e., age, smoking, diabetes, history of heart disease, education, systolic blood pressure, alcohol use, and physical activity), people living in the Southeast still had the highest risk for stroke.[64] In 1997, the contribution of socioeconomic status (SES), as measured by education and family income, to the geographic disparities in stroke mortality was evaluated using the National Longitudinal Mortality Study (NLMS).[65] Although individual SES was strongly associated with the risk for stroke, it did not contribute substantially to the geographic patterns of stroke mortality reported in the NLMS.

Two studies have examined the role of characteristics other than stroke risk factors. A study of the effect of interstate migration patterns on geographic disparities in stroke mortality from 1979 to 1981 reported that stroke mortality rates in several states were strongly influenced by the patterns of people migrating into the states and that these patterns differed for blacks and whites.[66] Although the rates for whites in three states (Florida, Arizona, and Colorado) and the District of Columbia were lower because of immigration, rates for blacks were lower in only one state (Colorado), but were higher in twenty-one states.

Another study examined the association between occupational structure (a measure of the social and economic resources available to residents of a community) and stroke mortality rates in communities in the South. The results indicated that communities with the lowest levels of occupational structure (e.g., the fewest resources) experienced the highest rates of stroke mortality.[67]

Ameliorating the negative social environment factors in local communities requires structural and institutional changes, improvements in community social relations, and reductions in inequalities within those communities. Identifying the places that bear the greatest burden of stroke mortality is a necessary first step to target appropriate resources for improving the local social environment and health outcomes in those communities.

An important strength of this publication is the examination of geographic disparities in stroke mortality for the five leading racial and ethnic groups in the United States. Previous reports focused predominantly on blacks and whites.

Several other factors from a historical perspective can explain these geographic differences within the United States. Many counties classified as mining areas and/or as having a history of mining have high rates for all causes of death and all natural causes. However, because these rates are high for both males and females, they cannot be attributed solely to the occupational risks of mining.

Various hypotheses have been proposed[68] to explain this association between mining and mortality rates. They illustrate the use of the geographic description of disease patterns in etiologic reasoning. One hypothesis is that the presence of large coal or metal ore deposits, and particularly the mining of them, in some way disturbs the environment sufficiently to increase the risk of dying in middle age. The causal factor could be the exposure to the coal or metal itself or, possibly more likely, to by-products or waste substances (such as sulfur), including trace substances (possibly arsenic) in the ores. The mode of transmission might be through water, especially drinking water, or air pollution. In some areas, mine waste is used to surface country roads, thereby increasing the potential for air pollution in contrast to places where the waste is simply dumped in huge piles. Cultural or socioeconomic factors can also be considered. Individuals who move into mining counties are not necessarily at the same risk as individuals who pursue other occupations or work in other industries. Further, mining tends to be a boom-or-bust type of economy, which may have stressful effects on humans.

An alternate hypothesis can be proposed for some "history of mining" counties, particularly those with substantial outmigration over the years: that the able-bodied, more aggressive individuals tend to move away in search of employment and that the remaining persons ages 35 to 74 include a higher than usual proportion of those with chronic diseases or vague ill health that detracted from their willingness to look elsewhere for jobs. Thus, in some instances it is appropriate to consider the hypothesis that the high rates in counties with a history of mining result largely from selective outmigration.[69]

Another factor that seems related to the geographic distribution of diseases is altitude. Elevation above sea level is associated to a moderate but statistically significant extent with death rates for various diseases, but especially for cancer. The lowest rate areas to a large extent are in high plains areas.

Another factor related to the geographic distribution of disease is the degree of urbanization. (Urban-rural differences are examined next.)

As an example of the use of this type of analysis, it should be noted that this information could have been included in the example in Chapter 4 on the identification of health problems in a Georgia county. That example calculated the standardized mortality ratios for the leading causes of death in County A using the state of Georgia as the "standard." The southeastern states, including Georgia, have high rates of cerebrovascular and ischemic heart diseases. Consequently, because Georgia rates are problematic, it would be interesting to use another standard, such as the United States rate, for the identification of a cerebrovascular disease or ischemic heart disease problem in a particular county.

In other words, a standardized mortality ratio of 100 in a Georgia county for cerebrovascular disease or ischemic heart disease, when using that state as standard, still indicates a problem. Similarly, the problem identified in County A (SMR for cerebrovascular disease = 130) is even more important than previously thought.

Variations within States There are wide variations in disease patterns within many of the states. However, contrary to variations between states, those within a state probably are more associated with differences in clustering of "person" factors, with degree of urbanization, and with availability of health care resources than with physical and biologic environmental conditions. As an example of within-state variations, Figure 7-2 shows the distribution of infant mortality in Georgia.

Trends in infant mortality suggest that achievement of the Year 2000 Objective of 7 deaths per 1,000 live births will require substantial new efforts to improve perinatal health. This is particularly evident in Figure 7-2, which shows the infant mortality rate in Georgia from 1990 to 1994. Fifteen counties have lowered their infant mortality rates below the Year 2000 Objective of 7 deaths per 1,000 live births. At the other end of the yardstick, fifteen counties have rates in the 17 to 26 per 1,000 range—nearly twice the state average.

An important component of variations in disease patterns is the difference between urban and rural areas. Urbanization has long been associated with higher mortality rates. This characterization of cities as notoriously unhealthy places[70] came about in the early days of modern public health practice when the high population density in urban areas made their inhabitants particularly vulnerable to epidemic diseases.

With the shift in disease patterns from infections to chronic diseases, urban-rural differences seem to have become less pronounced and more specific. An analysis of urban and rural mortality from all causes in Georgia showed rates in rural counties were 29 percent higher than in urban counties.[71] This difference was even greater in younger age groups, diminishing with age. In the over-64 population, the urban mortality rate was significantly higher than the rural rate.

Although much of the rural-urban difference in overall mortality is attributed to the larger proportion of older rural residents, the age-race adjusted rural rate still is significantly higher than the urban rate. Furthermore, specific differences in the United States for rural health problems are displayed in Table 7-3. Problems include risk factors such as adolescent and adult smoking, alcohol consumption, female obesity, and physical inactivity. Urban-rural variation in mortality patterns shows higher infant mortality rates in the southern rural areas, and death rates for children and young adults (ages

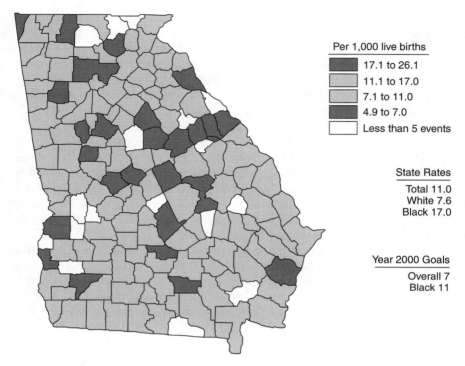

Per 1,000 live births

- 17.1 to 26.1
- 11.1 to 17.0
- 7.1 to 11.0
- 4.9 to 7.0
- Less than 5 events

State Rates

Total 11.0
White 7.6
Black 17.0

Year 2000 Goals

Overall 7
Black 11

FIGURE 7-2   Infant Mortality Rate, Georgia, 1990–1994. *Source:* Perinatal Epidemiology Unit, Epidemiology and Prevention Branch, Division of Public Health, Georgia Department of Human Resources, and March of Dimes Defects Foundation, "The Challenge of Change: A Mid-Decade Look at Maternal and Child Health in Georgia," *http://health/state.ga.us/pdfs/epi/mch1999.pdf.* Accessed 4/26/04.

1–24) are highest in most rural areas. Other diseases such as ischemic heart disease and chronic obstructive pulmonary diseases reflect considerable variation by region in the United States. Also, deaths due to unintentional injuries and motor vehicle accidents are at least twice as high in rural areas. Finally, homicide rates are higher in urban areas. Suicides are highest in rural areas. Specific urban health problems include homicides and cancer.

Other studies show higher infant and maternal mortality rates in rural areas.[95,96] Higher cancer rates in urban areas are documented in several studies[97,98] and often are related to exposure to industrial pollutants.[99,100] The

TABLE 7-3 Urban and Rural Health Issues—Selected Highlights

Urban-Rural Health Risk Factors *Improving health behaviors to reduce the risk of disease and disability poses distinct challenges for central counties of large metro areas, with their ethnically diverse and large economically disadvantaged populations. Equally difficult but different challenges confront the most rural counties with more dispersed and older populations.*	▪ Nationally, **adolescents** living in the most **rural counties** are the most likely to smoke and those living in central counties of large metro areas are the least likely to **smoke**. In 1999 for the United States as a whole, 19 percent of adolescents in the most rural counties smoked compared with 11 percent in central counties.[72] ▪ Nationally, **adults** living in the most **rural counties** are most likely to **smoke** and those living in large metro (central and fringe) counties are least likely to smoke (27 compared with 20 percent of women and 31 compared with 25 percent of men, in 1997–98). Regionally, the largest urban-rural increases in smoking are seen for women in the Northeast and for men and women in the South.[73] ▪ Nationally and regionally, men are twice as likely as women to consume five or more drinks in one day in the last year. In the Northeast, adults 18–49 years in central counties were less likely to report this level of alcohol consumption than those living in other urbanization levels. In the West, prevalence of this level of **alcohol consumption** was higher among adults living in nonmetro counties than other urbanization levels.[74] ▪ Self-reported **obesity** varies more by urbanization level for women than for men. Nationally, women living in fringe counties of large metro areas have the lowest prevalence of obesity and women living in the most rural counties have the highest (16 compared with 23 percent in 1997–98). Self-reported obesity among men ranges from 18 percent in central counties of large metro areas to 22 percent in the most rural counties.[75] ▪ **Physical inactivity** during leisure time varies substantially with level of urbanization, but the patterns differ by region. In 1997–98 the proportion of the population physically inactive during leisure time was highest in nonmetro counties in the South (56 percent of women and 52 percent of men) and in central counties of large metro areas of the Northeast (51 percent of women and 47 percent of men).[76]
Urban-Rural Mortality	▪ For the United States as a whole and within each region, **infant mortality rates** are lowest in fringe counties of large metro areas. In the Northeast and Midwest, central counties of large metro areas had the highest infant mortality rates in 1996–98 (45 percent higher than in fringe counties), while in the South and West, nonmetro counties had the highest rates (24 and 30 percent higher than in fringe counties).[77]

TABLE 7-3   (continued)

Urban-Rural Mortality (continued)	

Urban-Rural Mortality (continued)

- For the United States as a whole, **death rates for children and young adults** (ages 1–24) are lowest in fringe counties of large metro areas and highest in the most rural counties. In all regions except the Northeast, 1996–98 death rates in the most rural counties were over 50 percent higher than rates in fringe counties. In the Northeast and for males in the Midwest, death rates in central counties are as high as those in the most rural counties.[78]

- Nationally and within each region, **death rates for working-age adults** (ages 25–64) are lowest in fringe counties of large metro areas. In the Northeast and Midwest, 1996–98 death rates were highest in central counties of large metro areas (34–53 percent higher than in fringe counties). In the South, death rates were highest in nonmetro counties (31–44 percent higher than in fringe counties).[79]

- Nationally, **death rates among seniors** (age 65 and over) are lower in large metro (central and fringe) counties than in nonmetro counties. Although in 1996–98 death rates for seniors varied by less than 10 percent across urbanization levels, this variation represents a large number of deaths.[80]

- For adults 20 years and over, **urbanization patterns in ischemic heart disease** (IHD) death rates differ by region. In the South, 1996–98 IHD death rates were lowest in fringe counties of large metro areas and over 20 percent higher in the most rural counties. In the Northeast and West, IHD death rates were highest in central counties of large metro areas.[81]

- For men 20 years and over, **death rates for chronic obstructive pulmonary diseases** (COPD) are lowest in large metro (central and fringe) counties and highest in nonmetro counties. For the nation as a whole, COPD rates among men were 30 percent higher in nonmetro counties than in large metro counties in 1996–98. Regionally, the urban-rural increase for men is largest in the Northeast, followed by the South. For women, COPD death rates vary little across urbanization levels, with an urban-rural increase found only in the Northeast.[82]

- Nationally and within each region, **death rates from unintentional injuries** increase markedly as counties become less urban (nationally, over 80 percent higher in the most rural counties than in fringe counties of large metro areas in 1996–98). Death rates for unintentional injuries were especially high in nonmetro counties of the South and West. Death rates for **motor vehicle traffic-related injuries** in the most rural counties are over twice as high as the rates in central counties of large metro areas.[83]

TABLE 7-3 (continued)

Urban-Rural Mortality (continued)

- For the United States as a whole and within each region, the highest **homicide rates** are found in central counties of large metro areas. In the Northeast and Midwest, 1996–98 homicide rates for males in central counties were about 7 times as high as those in nonmetro counties, where rates were lowest. In the South and West, the lowest homicide rates were found in fringe counties of large metro areas.[84]
- Nationally and within each region, **suicide rates** for males 15 years and older are lowest in large metro (central and fringe) counties and increase steadily as counties become less urban. In 1996–98 the urban-rural increase in male suicide was steepest in the West, where the rate for the most rural counties was nearly 80 percent greater than the rate in large metro counties.[85]

Urban-Rural Health Care Access and Use

A community's health depends not only on the sociodemographic characteristics and risk factors of its residents, but also on their access to and use of health care services. Factors affecting access include health insurance coverage as well as provider supply.

- **Lack of health insurance** among nonelderly Americans is least common in fringe counties of large metro areas and most common in central counties and in the most rural counties. In 1997–98 lower-income nonelderly persons were over three times as likely to be uninsured as higher-income nonelderly persons at all urbanization levels. About one-third of lower-income residents of central and nonmetro counties were uninsured in 1997–98.[86]
- The urbanization pattern for **physician supply** depends on physician specialty. In 1998 the supply of family and general practice physicians rose slightly as urbanization decreased. By contrast, the supply of all other types of physicians decreased markedly as urbanization decreased, nationally and in all regions.[87]
- Nationally and in each region, **dentist supply** decreased markedly as urbanization decreased. Compared with other regions, the South had the fewest dentists per 100,000 population in 1998 at each level of urbanization.[88]
- The urbanization pattern for **dental care use** is similar to that for dentist supply. In 1997–98 for the United States as a whole, only 57 percent of adults (ages 18–64 years) in the most rural counties reported having a dental visit within the past year compared with 71 percent in fringe counties of large metro areas. Residents of nonmetro counties in the South were less likely to have had a **dental visit** in the past year than nonmetro residents of other regions.[89]

TABLE 7-3 (continued)

Urban-Rural Health Care Access and Use (continued)	▪ **Inpatient hospital discharge rates** among adults (ages 18–64) are higher in nonmetro than in metro counties. Higher hospital use in nonmetro areas results in part from delays in seeking care for conditions that could have been treated in ambulatory settings if detected earlier.[90] ▪ Admission rates to substance **abuse treatment programs** vary by primary substance and urbanization level of the county where the program is located. Nationally, alcohol treatment admission rates are higher in small metro and nonmetro counties with a city of 10,000 than in counties at other urbanization levels. Admission rates for opiates and cocaine tend to decrease as urbanization decreases.[91]
Other Urban-Rural Health Measures *Other important health indicators include adolescent childbearing, health-related activity limitations, and total tooth loss.*	▪ The **birth rates for adolescents** ages 15–19 are lowest in fringe counties of large metro areas. In the Northeast and Midwest, adolescent birth rates are substantially higher in central counties of large metro areas than in other urbanization levels. In the South and West, adolescent birth rates in small metro and nonmetro counties were similar to those in central counties (all more than 30 percent higher than rates in fringe counties).[92] ▪ For the United States as a whole, **limitation in activity due to chronic health conditions** among adults is more common in nonmetro counties than in large metro counties. This urban-rural difference in activity limitation rates is most marked in the Northeast and South, where rates in nonmetro counties were more than 40 percent higher than those in large metro counties in 1997–98.[93] ▪ For the United States as a whole, **total tooth loss** among seniors generally increases as urbanization declines. In 1997–98, almost one-half of lower-income seniors living in nonmetro counties had lost all their natural teeth.[94]

Source: M. S. Eberhardt et al., *Urban and Rural Health Chartbook* (Hyattsville, Md.: National Center for Health Statistics, 2001), 3–5.

evidence concerning heart disease, however, is more contradictory. Some studies show higher urban disease rates[101,102] involving the "stress of urban living" as a causative factor, whereas other studies report higher rural disease rates.[103] However, recently the geographic studies for men and women on heart disease and the *Atlas of Stroke Mortality* have expanded the environmental hypothesis to include lifestyle and the structure of the culture as having a preferred influence on the variation in rates.[104,105,106]

Local Variations   Health services managers, as noted, need data on local patterns of disease occurrence. Local variations in noninfectious disease incidence primarily reflect differences in person-related factors, notably socioeconomic status. Place of disease patterns in small areas is best analyzed using census divisions because denominator data is available and rates can be computed; socioeconomic information also is available. Mapping by census tracts can help health services managers target specific populations and areas in need and allocate resources and provide facilities accordingly.

Analysis by place on a local level also is most appropriate when dealing with outbreaks of infectious diseases. A classic example of an epidemiologic analysis by place is John Snow's study of cholera in London in 1848 to 1854. Snow mapped the exact location of cholera deaths occurring during a ten-day period in 1848 (Figure 7-3). Through visual analysis of the distribution of cases, Snow noted the clustering of deaths around the Broad Street pump, from which residents received their water supply. After removal of the pump handle, no new cholera cases were reported. This fact, coupled with Snow's earlier work, suggested that cholera was transmitted by contaminated water.

By determining the relationship between location and disease, many place-related studies attempt to accomplish the same thing Snow did: discover the etiological factors of a disease.

An example of this is the outbreak of Legionnaires' disease in Philadelphia in July 1976, when 182 persons attending an American Legion convention were affected by pneumonia caused by a previously unrecognized bacterium. It is worthwhile to quote at length from the investigators' report to examine how they went about trying to ascertain the place of occurrence:

> The place of exposure cannot be defined with certainty, but the most reasonable hypothesis is that exposure occurred within or in the immediate vicinity of Hotel A. Such a hypothesis is consistent with the observation that of delegates, those who stayed at Hotel A had a significantly higher rate of illness than those who did not, and that of the delegates who did not stay at Hotel A, those who fell ill spent more time on the average in Hotel A than those who stayed well.
>
> The fact that cases occurred in persons who had been near, but not in, Hotel A shows that in at least some cases, exposure occurred outside Hotel A, and suggests that exposure could have occurred on the streets or sidewalks around that hotel. Other evidence of exposure outside the hotel comes from the observation that serologically confirmed cases in delegates occurred more frequently in those who watched the parade from the sidewalk in front of Hotel A and that the length of time spent on the sidewalk was associated with illness. Exposure might well have occurred within Hotel A also. In the delegate group, there was a strong association between time spent in the lobby of Hotel A and risk of contracting the disease.

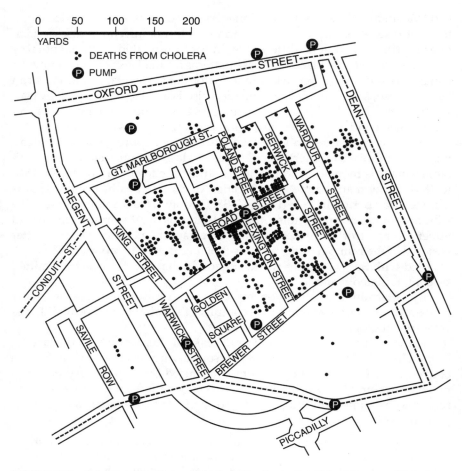

FIGURE 7-3 John Snow's Map of Cholera Deaths in the Soho District of London, 1848. *Source:* Reprinted from *Health Care Delivery: Spatial Perspectives* by Gary Shannon and G. E. Alan Dever with permission of McGraw-Hill Book Company, ©1974, 3; based on *Some Aspects of Medical Geography* by L. D. Stamp with permission of Oxford University Press, ©1964, 16.

It is unlikely that the place of exposure was in any of the main convention function rooms in Hotel A because attendance at those functions was not associated with illness. Similarly, bedrooms were unlikely places of exposure since roommates of patients were not at increased risk of illness and because there was no geographic clustering of bedrooms of cases in Hotel A. Because no hospitality room was said to have been visited by more than half the patients and because there was no striking association between attendance or food consumption and illness, the rooms are unlikely to have been the sites of exposure.

If the exposure was airborne, the association of illness and time spent in the lobby might be explained. An airborne agent might also have affected non-Legionnaires who were in the hotel only transiently and had no other apparently noteworthy exposure; it might also have exposed persons who walked near the hotel but did not enter it.[107]

It was shown later that the main mode of transmission of the Legionnaires' disease bacterium was indeed through the air (airborne). A more recent example is the SARS epidemic that occurred in Hong Kong and Toronto.

Severe acute respiratory syndrome (SARS) was first recognized in Toronto in a woman who returned from Hong Kong on February 23, 2003.[108] Transmission to other persons resulted subsequently in an outbreak among 257 persons in several Greater Toronto Area (GTA) hospitals. After implementation of province-wide public health measures that included strict infection-control practices, the number of recognized cases of SARS declined substantially, and no cases were detected after April 20. On April 30, the World Health Organization (WHO) lifted a travel advisory issued on April 22 that had recommended a limitation on travel to Toronto. This report describes a second wave of SARS cases among patients, visitors, and health care workers (HCWs) that occurred at a Toronto hospital approximately four weeks after SARS transmission was thought to have been interrupted. The findings indicate that exposure to hospitalized patients with unrecognized SARS after a province-wide relaxation of strict SARS control measures probably contributed to transmission among HCWs. The investigation underscores the need for monitoring fever and respiratory symptoms in hospitalized patients and visitors, particularly after a decline in the number of reported SARS cases.

From February 23 to June 7, the Ontario Ministry of Health and Long-Term Care received reports of 361 SARS cases (suspect: 136 [38%]; probable: 225 [62%]) as shown in Figure 7-7a). As of June 7, a total of 33 persons (9%) had died. Of 74 cases reported from April 15 to June 9 to Toronto Public Health, 29 (39%) occurred among HCWs, 28 (38%) occurred as a result of exposure during hospitalization, and 17 (23%) occurred among hospital visitors (Figure 7-7b). Of the 74 cases, 67 (90%) resulted directly from exposure in hospital A, a 350-bed GTA community hospital.

The majority of cases were associated with a ward used primarily for orthopedic patients (fourteen rooms) and gynecology patients (seven rooms). Nursing staff members used a common nursing station, shared a washroom, and ate together in a lounge just outside the ward. SARS attack rates among nurses assigned routinely to the orthopedic and gynecology sections of the ward were approximately 40 percent and 25 percent, respectively.

During early and mid-May, as recommended by provincial SARS-control directives, hospital A discontinued SARS expanded precautions (i.e., routine contact precautions with use of an N95 or equivalent respirator) for non-SARS patients without respiratory symptoms in all hospital areas other than the emergency department and the intensive care unit (ICU). In addition, staff no longer were required to wear masks or respirators routinely throughout the hospital or to maintain distance from one another while eating. Hospital A instituted changes in policy on May 8; the number of persons allowed to visit a patient during a four-hour period remained restricted to one, but the number of patients who were allowed to have visitors was increased.

On May 20, five patients in a rehabilitation hospital in Toronto were reported with febrile illness. One of these five patients was determined to have been hospitalized in the orthopedic ward of hospital A from April 22 to 28, and a second was found on May 22 to have SARS-associated coronavirus (SARS-Co V) by nucleic acid amplification test. On investigation, a second patient was determined to have been hospitalized in the orthopedic ward of hospital A from April 22 to April 28. After the identification of these cases, an investigation of pneumonia cases at hospital A identified eight cases of previously unrecognized SARS among patients.

On May 23, hospital A was closed to all new admissions other than patients with newly identified SARS. Soon after, new provincial directives were issued, requiring an increased level of infection-control precautions in hospitals located in several GTA regions. HCWs at hospital A were placed under a ten-day work quarantine and instructed to avoid public places outside work, avoid close contact with friends and family, and to wear a mask whenever public contact was unavoidable. As of June 9, of 79 new cases of SARS that resulted from exposure at hospital A, 78 appear to have resulted from exposures that occurred before May 23.

Several potential approaches for monitoring patients might improve recognition of SARS in hospitalized patients. A standardized assessment for SARS (e.g., clinical, radiographic, and laboratory criteria) might be used among all hospitalized patients with new-onset fever, especially for units or wards in which clusters of febrile patients are identified. In addition, some hospital computer information systems might allow review of administrative and physician order data to monitor selected observations that might serve as triggers for further investigation.

The Toronto investigation found early transmission of SARS to both patients and visitors in hospital A. In areas affected recently by SARS, clusters of pneumonia occurring in visitors to health care facilities or in HCWs should be evaluated fully to determine if they represent transmission of SARS. To facilitate detection and reporting, clinicians in these areas should be encouraged to obtain a history from pneumonia patients of whether they visited or worked at a health care facility and whether family members or close contacts also are ill. Targeted surveillance for community-acquired pneumonia in areas recently affected by SARS might provide another means for early detection of these cases.

The findings from the Toronto investigation indicate that continued transmission of SARS can occur among patients and visitors during a period of apparent HCW adherence to expanded infection-control precautions for SARS. Maintaining a high level of suspicion for SARS on the part of health care providers and infection-control staff is critical, particularly after a decline in reported SARS cases. The prevention of health care–associated SARS infections must involve HCWs, patients, visitors, and the community.[109]

Noninfectious causes of death also can be analyzed and mapped on a local level. Figure 7-4 illustrates the excess infant mortality in the 134 census tracts of Jefferson County, Colorado. Figure 7-5 shows the infant mortality rate for Jefferson County, Colorado. Specifically, this map presents the lower 95 percent confidence limits that are greater than zero indicating that these rates for the shaded areas are significant. Health services managers might find it valuable to map a number of variables to help them analyze local situations. For instance, Figure 7-5 illustrates the variation in outcomes related to infant birth statistics. Specifically, infant mortality rates, percentage of low birth weight babies, percentage of infants born to mothers with twelve or more years of education, and percentage of infants born to adolescent mothers (ages 15 to 19). The spatial variations of their outcome variables can be measured against the 2000 or 2010 *Healthy People* objectives or to determine progress in meeting the national standards. Further, the intra-urban variation highlights "highish pockets" by which to target health promotion and disease prevention programs.

Value, but with a Caution

The description of health and disease by place can help health services managers to identify the problems of their population, develop programs, and focus on high-risk areas for specific ailments. It also is used in epidemiology to study the etiology of disease.

Place can be associated with health and disease through physical and biologic environmental variables. However, as the areas examined get smaller, the relationship of place and disease occurrence most often is caused by the clustering of personal characteristics (demographic, social, lifestyle) of the inhabitants. In this sense, place is a good preliminary indicator of factors affecting health and disease. An important corollary of locating health problems by geographic area is the spatial distribution of services.[110,111] As is described in subsequent chapters, health services managers can also analyze the utilization of services by place, as well as the allocation of resources.

A word of caution is necessary. Analysis by place can lead to ecologic fallacy. As explained in Chapter 4, it is not possible to make assertions about individuals based only on examination of geographic areas. Analysis should be based on consistent factors. For example, the correlation between two attributes of a set of areas is not necessarily the same as that between the same attributes of individuals within the areas.[112]

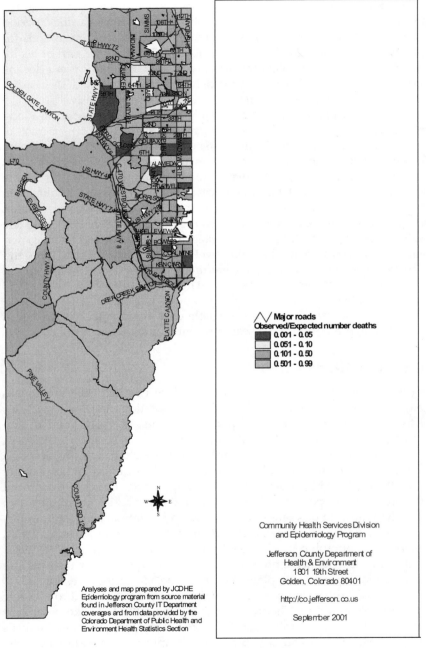

FIGURE 7-4 Infant Mortality: Probabilities of Observed Number of Infant Deaths Relative to Expected Number of Deaths—Jefferson County, 1999–2000

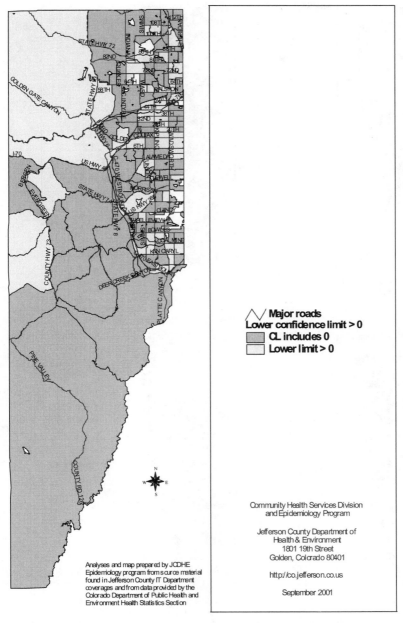

Major roads
Lower confidence limit > 0
CL includes 0
Lower limit > 0

Community Health Services Division
and Epidemiology Program

Jefferson County Department of
Health & Environment
1801 19th Street
Golden, Colorado 80401

http://co.jefferson.co.us

September 2001

Analyses and map prepared by JCDHE
Epidemiology program from source material
found in Jefferson County IT Department
coverages and from data provided by the
Colorado Department of Public Health and
Environment Health Statistics Section

FIGURE 7-4 (continued)   Infant Mortality Rates with Lower 95 Percent
Confidence Limit >0—Jefferson County, 1990–2000. *Source:* Community Health
Services Division and Epidemiology Program, Jefferson County Department of
Health and Environment, *http://co.jefferson.co.us.*

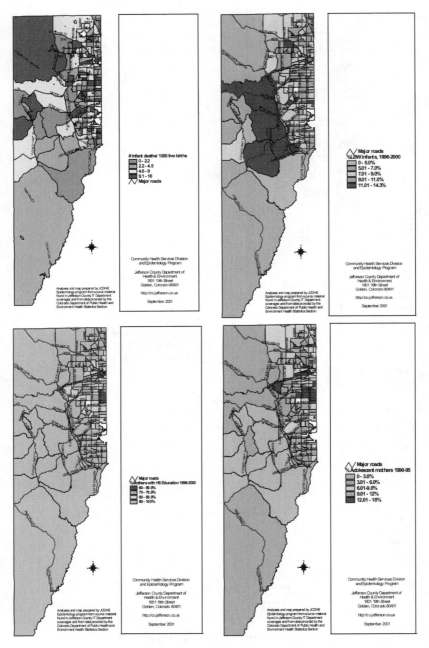

FIGURE 7-5 Plotting Vital Statistics. *Source:* Community Health Services Division and Epidemiology Program, Jefferson County Department of Health and Environment, *http://co.jefferson.co.us.*

Time: When Disease Occurs

A final element in describing a disease is its time of occurrence. The distribution in time of a disease refers to trends in its incidence and prevalence as well as its fluctuations around this trend.[113] The variations in the incidence and prevalence of a disease over time can be informative because they reflect temporal differences in the factors affecting health and disease (whether biologic, environmental, lifestyle, or medical care organization).

Time in epidemiology can be expressed either in hours, days, months, or years, depending on the disease studied. This analysis is in terms of three major kinds of time changes: short-term variations, secular trends, and cyclical trends. Although the focus is on time patterns of disease occurrence separate from person and place patterns, it is evident that to examine variations in time, the population of concern has to have been defined previously at least by place. In other words, the variation in time of a disease cannot be examined without consideration of its place. The last section of this chapter examines a particular type of interaction—time-space clusters.

Short-Term Variations

Short-term variations are found mostly, although not exclusively, in infectious diseases. This short time can vary from hours to months. Several epidemiologic concepts are of particular importance when discussing short-term variations. An epidemic occurs when the incidence of a disease is unusually high at a given time. An epidemic therefore refers to an excess incidence of disease over what normally would be expected, no matter whether that incidence is, in absolute terms, high or low.

The level after which incidence can be considered in excess is called the epidemic threshold. When an epidemic is not restricted to a given place but occurs simultaneously at many points, such as often is the case with influenza, it is referred to as pandemic. The usual frequency of occurrence of a disease regularly and continuously present is referred to as its endemic level. The term *outbreak* is used when speaking of an epidemic, probably because it sounds less alarming, especially when dealing with an incidence that in absolute terms is not very high.

The two main types of epidemics are common source and propagated (or progressive). The difference is in the mode of transmission of the disease agent. Common source epidemics involve exposure of a group of persons to a common, noxious influence.[114] All noninfectious disease epidemics technically are from a common source. Infectious disease epidemics in which the mode of transmission of the causal agent is food, air, water, ice, tobacco, or alcohol are common source epidemics. When the mode of transmission is from person to person, or more generally from host to host (from animals to people), the epidemic is propagated, or progressive.

Another important concept related to short-term variations is the incubation period. This refers to the interval between involvement of an etiologic agent and onset of illness. Although this term most often refers to infectious diseases, it also can apply to noninfectious etiologic agents as well. As discussed later, the incubation period is not necessarily short. For example, many chronic diseases are characterized by long latency (incubation) periods and indefinite onset. This is the case when lifestyle, such as smoking, is the etiologic factor, or when occupational or environmental exposure to hazardous substances (such as Agent Orange) lead to chronic illnesses years or decades later. The incubation period for some infectious diseases such as syphilis and tuberculosis also can be long.

Short-term variations are best analyzed with graphs by plotting (either on a histogram or a frequency polygon) the distribution of cases by time of onset. When dealing with epidemics, this distribution is referred to as the epidemic curve. Figure 7-6 shows the epidemic curve of an outbreak of food poisoning. In this case, the time units of importance are hours. Figure 7-7a shows the epidemic curve of the outbreak of severe acute respiratory syndrome (SARS) by date of illness in the most identifiably probable and suspect travel and nontravel categories. In addition, Figure 7-7b illustrates the source of infection and date of illness onset for hospital visitors, hospital patients, and health care workers. The incubation period of the coronavirus can be estimated from this graph as approximately ten days.

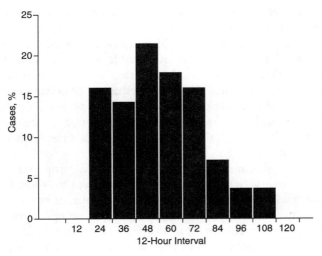

FIGURE 7-6   Fifty-nine Cases of Botulism, by Interval between Eating at a Restaurant and Onset of First Neurologic Symptom—Michigan, 1977. *Source:* S. S. Arnon et al., "Botulinum Toxin as a Biological Weapon," *JAMA* 285, no. 8 (2001): 1059–1070.

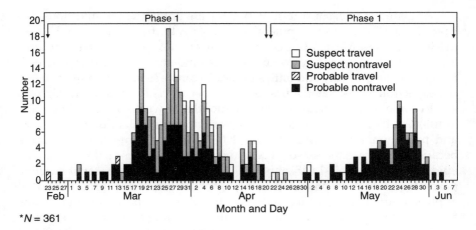

N = 361

FIGURE 7-7A Number of Reported Cases of Severe Acute Respiratory Syndrome, by Classification and Date of Illness—Ontario, February 23–June 7, 2003. *Source:* Centers for Disease Control and Prevention, *http://www.cdc.gov/mmwr/preview/mmwrhtml/mm5223a4.htm*.

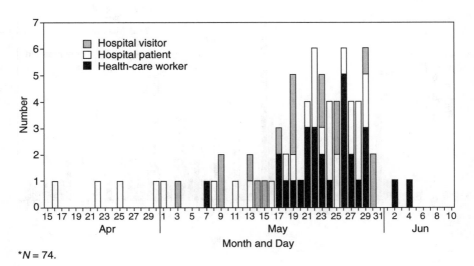

N = 74.

FIGURE 7-7B Number of Reported Cases of Severe Acute Respiratory Syndrome, by Source of Infection and Date of Illness Onset—Toronto, Canada, April 15–June 9, 2003. *Source:* Centers for Disease Control and Prevention, *http://www.cdc.gov/mmwr/preview/mmwrhtml/mm5223a4.htm*.

As stated earlier, short-term variations are not limited to infectious diseases. Figure 7-8 shows the epidemic curve of deaths from heat-related illness in Missouri, New Mexico, Oklahoma, and Texas in August 2001 when record-breaking high temperatures occurred. The epidemic threshold can be estimated to be in mid-July and until August. As can be seen, a definite epidemic of deaths from heat-related illness occurred between July 19 and July 25, 2001.

In some other infectious diseases, months or weeks are the time units of interest. Figure 7-9 shows the time variation of deaths due to influenza and pneumonia between 2000 and 2003. This is an interesting example because this shows the seasonal baseline and the epidemic's threshold. The epidemic threshold is 1.645 standard deviations and the seasonal baseline percentage which is projected using a robust regression procedure that applies a periodic regression model to the observed percentage of deaths from pneumonia and influenza during the preceding five years. The results in this case indicate at least two past epidemic periods—early 2000 and early 2002.

Cyclical Trends

Cyclic trends refer to recurring patterns of disease over time. This regular pattern can consist of cycles that last several years, as in the four- to six-year cycle

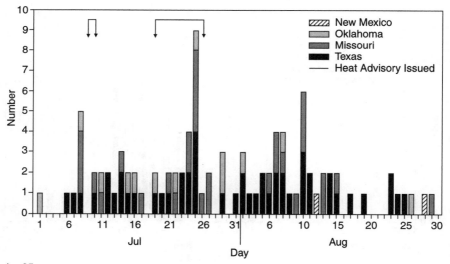

*n=95.

FIGURE 7-8   Reported Cases of Heat-related Deaths, by Date and Site—Missouri, New Mexico, Oklahoma, and Texas, August 2001. *Source:* Centers for Disease Control and Prevention, *http://www.cdc.gov/mmwr/preview/mmwrhtml/mm5126a2.htm.*

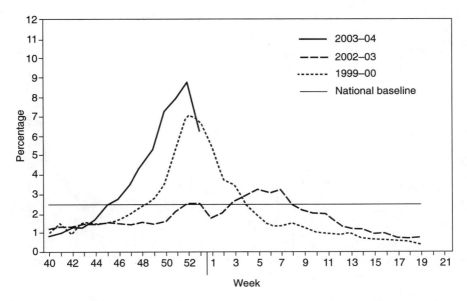

FIGURE 7-9   Percentage of Visits for Influenza-like Illness Reported by Sentinel Provider Surveillance Network, by Week—United States, 1999–00, 2002–03, and 2003–04 Influenza Seasons. *Source:* Department of Health and Human Services, Centers for Disease Control and Prevention, "Influenza Activity—United States, December 21, 2003–January 3, 2004," *Morbidity and Mortality Weekly Report* 52, no. 53 (2004 update):1288–1290.

of influenza Type B, or the two- to three-year cycle of influenza Type A. A common cyclic pattern can be observed in the incidence of diseases or deaths related to seasonal changes. Seasonal variations have long been a favorite topic of epidemiologists. As a 1945 article reported:

> Seasonal fluctuation is not only a very general epidemiologic principle, but for a given disease is one of its most constant epidemiologic characteristics. Most infectious diseases exhibit marked variations with season and these are remarkably constant from year to year. The influence of season is most strikingly evident in the variation in seasonal curves at different latitudes amounting to a complete reversal of months of prevalence in corresponding latitudes in the northern and southern hemispheres.[115]

Many diseases, both infectious and noninfectious, exhibit seasonal fluctuations. Figure 7-10 demonstrates that even the overall death rate (all causes) fluctuates seasonally, higher in winter and lower in summer. Figure 7-11 shows clearly the seasonal pattern of encephalitis. The summer increases from 1992 to 2001 definitely can be considered as an epidemic or

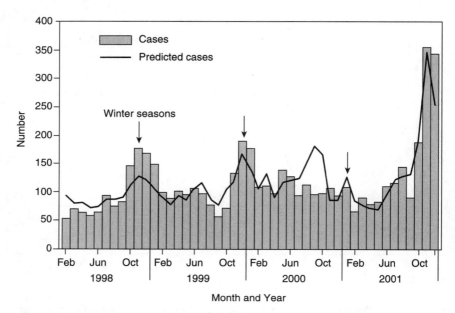

FIGURE 7-10 Number of Predicted Coccidioidomycosis Cases Compared with Actual Cases, by Month and Year—Arizona, 1998–2001. *Source:* Department of Health and Human Services, Centers for Disease Control and Prevention, "Increase in Coccidioidomycosis—Arizona, 1998–2001," *Morbidity and Mortality Weekly Report* 52, no. 6 (2003):109–112.

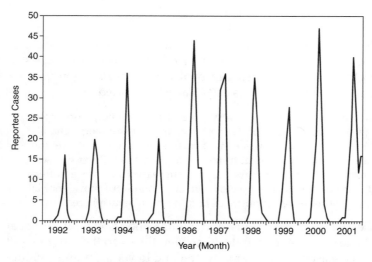

FIGURE 7-11 Encephalitis: Reported Cases Caused by California Serogroup Viruses, by Month of Onset—United States, 1992–2001. *Source:* Centers for Disease Control and Prevention, *http://www.cdc.gov/mmwr/preview/mmwrhtml/mm5053a1.htm.*

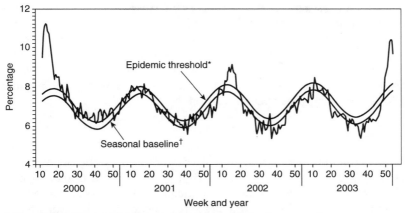

* The epidemic threshold is 1.645 standard deviations above the seasonal baseline percentage.

†The seasonal baseline is projected by using a robust regression procedure that applies a periodic regression model to the observed percentage of deaths from P&I during the preceding 5 years.

FIGURE 7-12   Percentage of Deaths Attributed to Pneumonia and Influenza (P&I) Reported by 122 Cities Mortality Reporting System, by Week and Year—United States, 2000–2004. *Source:* Department of Health and Human Services, Centers for Disease Control and Prevention, "Influenza Activity—United States, January 18–24, 2004," *Morbidity and Mortality Weekly Report* 53, no. 3 (2004 update):63–66.

quite possibly endemic, given the cyclical nature of the disease as reported for California. Deaths attributed to pneumonia and influenza also exhibit a seasonal cyclic pattern (Figure 7-12) even though, as said earlier, particular types of influenza can exhibit longer cyclic patterns. The increase in drownings in the summer or skiing accidents in winter are other examples of seasonal fluctuations.

Finally, other diseases and causes of death show cyclic patterns over very short periods. For example, deaths from motor vehicle accidents exhibit weekly cycles, peaking on weekends. Folklore has it that births—or is it fecundity?—follow monthly (lunar) cycles, peaking on the full moon.

Several reasons might explain cyclic trends in disease incidence. There is no doubt that climate and other biometeorologic factors, including temperature and precipitation, affect both infectious and noninfectious diseases. Another factor is the length of the day: It has been shown, for example, that the incidence of neurosis increases during the long polar night in Norway.[116]

In a number of diseases, it is clear that seasonal variation is determined by corresponding changes in the opportunities for transmission of the infectious agent, as influenced by the bionomics of the vector.[117] In other words, the warm weather multiplication of insects, ticks, mites, and other pests brings a corresponding increase in the incidence of infectious diseases transmitted to humans from those hosts.

Cyclic changes in activities, whether social, recreational, or even occupational/professional, have an easily understandable impact on disease incidence. Swimming in summer and skiing in winter are obvious examples. In certain areas, hunting brings people in unusual contact with some hosts such as rabbits. The seasonal increase in farming accidents is a factor. Similarly, an increase in the cholesterol level of accountants as the income tax deadline approaches has been reported.[118]

Secular Trends

Secular trends refer to changes that take place over a long period of time, such as years or decades, involving both infectious and noninfectious diseases. Figure 7-13 shows the trends in the overall death rate and the infant mortality rate between 1977 and 1981. As the preceding section noted, the death rate

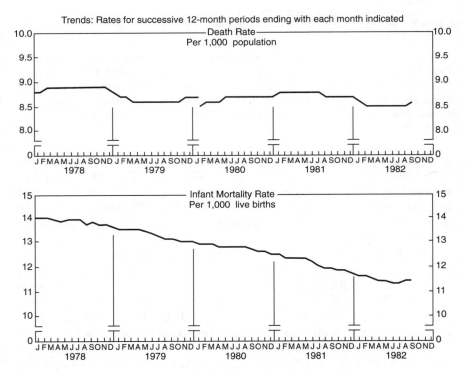

FIGURE 7-13 Secular Trends in Death and Infant Mortality Rates, U.S., 1978–1982. *Source:* Reprinted from U.S. Department of Health and Human Services, Public Health Service, National Centers for Health Statistics, *Monthly Vital Statistics Report*, 30, no. 12 (March 18, 1982):3.

follows a yearly cyclic pattern. In such cases, secular trends are best shown in using moving averages so as to smooth out short-term variations. In Figure 7-13, this is done by using rates for successive twelve-month periods, with the ending of each month plotted. This shows that the death rate was very stable between 1977 and 1981, whereas infant mortality declined.

Tracing secular trends for particular diseases and causes of death can be illuminating. Figure 7-14 shows the trends in some important causes of death. Most have declined between 1950 and 2000, with the exception of lung cancer, which has been increasing steadily, and cirrhosis of the liver, which rose between 1950 and 1970 but has been slowly declining since.

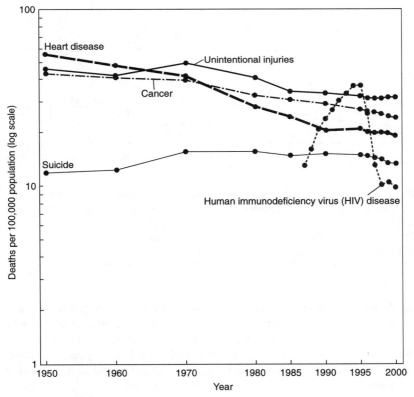

NOTES: Death rates are age adjusted.
Causes of death shown are the five leading
causes of death among persons 25–44 years
of age in 2000.

FIGURE 7-14 Secular Trend and Death Rates for Leading Causes of Death among Persons Ages 25–44—United States, 1950–2000. *Source:* Centers for Disease Control and Prevention, National Center for Health Statistics, National Vital Statistics System. Freid, V. M. et al., 2003. *Chartbook on Trends in the Health of Americans. Health, United States, 2003.* Hyattsville, MD: National Center for Health Statistics, 52.

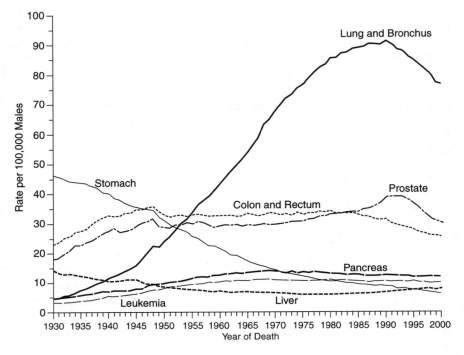

FIGURE 7-15 Annual Age-adjusted Center Death Rates* among Males for Selected Cancer Types—United States, 1930–2000. *Rates are age-adjusted to the 2000 U.S. standard population. *Source:* U.S. Mortality Public Use Data Tapes, 1960–2000, U.S. Mortality Volumes, 1930 to 1959, National Center for Health Statistics, Centers for Disease Control and Prevention.

Figure 7-15 illustrates secular trends for various cancers in females and males. In both sexes, stomach cancers have been declining substantially while lung cancer has been soaring since the 1930s in males and since the late 1960s in females. Uterine cancer in females and, to a smaller extent, liver cancer in both sexes also have been declining. The incidence of most other cancers has been fairly stable. Although not illustrated, deaths from all cancers have been slightly increasing.

As an example of secular trends in relation to person-characteristics (and place, of course), even though cancer death rates for the whole population have been increasing slightly Figure 7-16 shows they have been declining in populations younger than 65 and have shown slight increases in the over-65 age group (1975–2000).[119]

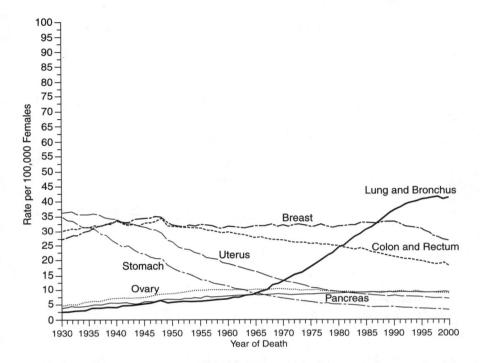

FIGURE 7-15 (continued) Annual Age-adjusted Death Rates* among Females for Selected Cancer Types—United States, 1930–2000. *Rates are age-adjusted to the 2000 U.S. standard population. *Source:* U.S. Mortality Public Use Data Tapes, 1960 to 2000, U.S. Mortality Volumes 1930 to 1959, National Center for Health Statistics, Centers for Disease Control and Prevention.

Infectious diseases also evidence marked secular trends. Figure 7-17 shows the virtual elimination of anthrax; however, with bioterrorism threats related cases in early 2001 showed a spike—up to 25 cases from a long-time previous low of only 1 or no cases (1951–2001). Figure 7-18 indicates a decrease in gonorrhea for black, non-Hispanic populations and constant rate noted for the other groups (1986–2001).[120]

Many factors influence the secular trends in many diseases. One is whether the changes are real or artifactual—that is, resulting from errors in the numerator or the denominator. Errors in the numerator can be caused by changes in the recognition of disease, in the rules and procedures for classifications of causes of death, or in accuracy of reporting, even in

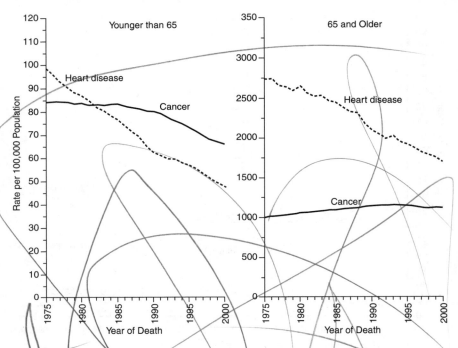

FIGURE 7-16   Death Rates* from Cancer and Heart Diseases for Ages Younger than 65, and 65 and Older. *Rates are age-adjusted to the 2000 U.S. standard population. *Source:* U.S. Mortality Public Use Data Tapes, 1960 to 2000, National Center for Health Statistics, Centers for Disease Control and Prevention, 2003.

reporting age at death.[121] Errors in the denominator can stem from mistakes in the numeration of the population.

Real changes can result from shifts in the age distribution of the population (this can be controlled through the age adjustment of rates), in survivorship and medical care organization, or from genetic, environmental, or lifestyle factors.

Time-Place Clusters

The clustering in time and place of some diseases has been a topic of considerable interest in recent years among epidemiologists. A 1982 editorial in the *American Journal of Public Health* commented, "The greatest potential for geographic analysis of mortality lies in the examination of time-space interactions."[122]

The notions of time and place of occurrence of a disease are related conceptually. Although until now they have been dealt with separately, the notion of time is always present in the consideration of place, and vice

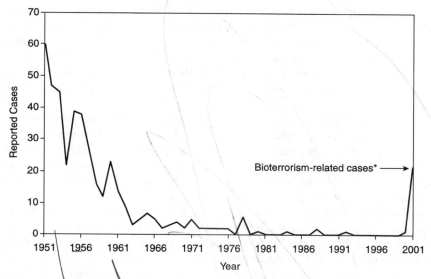

*One epizootic-associated cutaneous case was reported in 2001 from Texas.

FIGURE 7-17   Anthrax, Reported Cases, by Year—United States, 1951–2001. *Source:* Centers for Disease Control and Prevention, h*ttp://www.cdc.gov/mmwr/ preview/mmwrhtml/mm5053al.htm.*

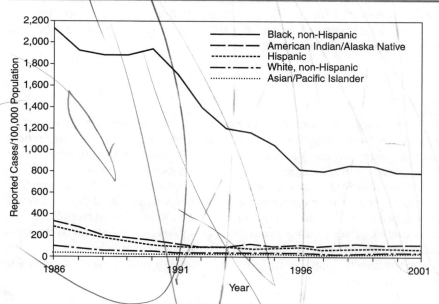

FIGURE 7-18   Gonorrhea, Reported Cases per 100,000 Population, by Race and Ethnicity—United States, 1986–2001. *Source:* Centers for Disease Control and Prevention, *http://www.cdc.gov/mmwr/preview/mmwrhtml/mm5053al.htm.*

versa. For example, the concept of epidemics is related not only to the time of occurrence but also to the place. An epidemic is in fact a clustering of a disease in both time and place. When dealing with usual, classic infectious disease epidemics, the focus concentrates on the time variations, in a restricted place. This can be done because there are enough cases, even in such a restricted area, to demonstrate significant abnormally high levels of incidence.

When considering rare diseases, the additional information concerning the place of occurrence is vital. It is possible that some rare diseases might cluster in several different times and places in unusually high levels, but at too low levels for the usual consideration of time in a restricted place to be able to detect. Special techniques therefore have been developed to examine possible space-time clustering of rare diseases.

All of these techniques aim to answer the following question: When mapping a case of a rare disease, whose date and place of onset are known, will cases that follow it closely tend to be relatively nearby on the map compared with other cases that occur more distantly in time?[123] In other words, will there be a clustering in time and place of cases of the disease? If there is time-place clustering, those cases will be close both in time and space, whereas unrelated cases will tend to have a larger average separation in time and space.[124]

The demonstration of time-space clusters is important because it indicates a common source, perhaps infectious, for disease. Such clusters have been demonstrated for rubella syndrome, thalidamide deformity, and tracheoesophageal fistula.[125] Some reports suggest that leukemia in children can also appear in time-space clusters.[126]

Summary

The distribution and variation in time of a disease is a fundamental feature of classic epidemiology. Short-term variations, cyclic and secular trends, and time-place clusters all provide important clues as to causation. Once again, however, the danger of ecologic fallacy is ever present.

Time variations and trends are of major concern to health services managers. They are an essential part of the assessment and description of the health problems in a population. Trends can be extrapolated, so knowledge of the irregular occurrence of a disease is essential to the provision of efficient standby capacity. These trends can also assist health care managers to plan for future needs and to identify new markets for expansion.

References

1. T. C. Timmreck, *An Introduction to Epidemiology*, 3d ed. (Sudbury, Mass.: Jones and Bartlett Publishers, 2002), 15.
2. P. Elliott et al., *Spatial Epidemiology: Methods and Applications* (Oxford: Oxford University Press, 2000).
3. Centers for Disease Control and Prevention, "Summary of Notifiable Diseases—United States, 2002," *Morbidity and Mortality Weekly Report* 51, no. 53 (2003):1–13.
4. J. C. Torner and R. B. Wallace, "Neurological Disorders," in *Maxcy-Roseneau—Last Public Health and Preventive Medicine*, 14th ed., eds. R. B. Wallace and B. N. Doebbeling, 1019–1029 (Stamford, Conn.: Appleton & Lange, 1998).
5. D. C. Poskanzer, "Neurologic Disease," in *Maxcy-Roseneau Public Health and Preventive Medicine*, 11th ed., ed. J. M. Last, 1258 (New York: Appleton-Century-Crofts, Inc., 1980).
6. Torner and Wallace, "Neurological Disorders," 1019–1029.
7. A. Donabedian, *Aspects of Medical Care Administration: Specifying Requirements for Health Care* (Cambridge, Mass.: Harvard University Press, 1973), 84.
8. Donabedian, *Aspects of Medical Care Administration*, 60.
9. V. Carstairs, "Socio-Economic Factors at Area Level and Their Relationship with Health," in *Spatial Epidemiology: Methods and Applications*, ed. P. Elliott et al. (Oxford: Oxford University Press, 2000), 51–67.
10. E. M. Kilbourne, "Illness Due to Thermal Extremes," in *Maxcy-Roseneau—Last Public Health and Preventive Medicine*, 14th ed. (Stamford, Conn.: Appleton & Lange, 1998), 607–617.
11. J. B. Conway, "Water Quality Management," in *Maxcy-Roseneau—Last Public Health and Preventive Medicine*, 14th ed. (Stamford, Conn.: Appleton & Lange, 1998), 737–763.
12. J. Ferlay et al., GLOBOCAN 2000: Cancer Incidence, Mortality and Prevalence Worldwide, Version 1.0, IARC Cancer Base No. 5 (Lyon, France: IARC Press, 2001), *http://www-dep.iarc.fr/globocan.html*.
13. Ferlay et al., GLOBOCAN 2000.
14. American Cancer Society, *Cancer Facts and Figures 2003* (Atlanta, Ga.: American Cancer Society, 2003), 30–31.
15. L. Gordis, *Epidemiology*, 2d ed. (Philadelphia: W. B. Saunders Company, 2000), 233–235.
16. Gordis, *Epidemiology*, 233–235.
17. R. J. Shamberger, "Relationship of Selenium to Cancer. I. Inhibitory Effect of Selenium on Carcinogenesis," *Journal of the National Cancer Institute* 44 (1970):931–936.
18. B. Janson et al., "Geographical Distribution of Gastrointestinal Cancer and Breast Cancer and Its Relation to Selenium Deficiency," in *Prevention and Detection of Cancer, Part 1. Prevention, vol. 1, Etiology*, ed. H. E. Nieburgs (New York: Marcel Dekker Inc., 1977), 1161–1178.
19. J. LaDou, *Occupation and Environmental Medicine*, 2d ed. (Stamford, Conn.: Appleton & Lange, 1997), 427–428.

20. B. E. Henderson, "Descriptive Epidemiology and Geographic Pathology," in *Cancer: Achievements, Challenges, and Prospects for the 1980s,* vol. 1, eds. J. H. Burchenal and H. F. Oettgen (New York: Grune & Stratton, Inc., 1980), 51–69.

21. P. Buell, "Changing Incidence of Breast Cancer in Japanese–American Women," *Journal of the National Cancer Institute* 51 (1973):147.

22. W. Haenszel and M. Kurihara, "Studies of Japanese. I. Mortality from Cancer and Other Diseases among Japanese in the United States," *Journal of the National Cancer Institute* 51 (1973):1765–1779.

23. W. Haenszel et al., "Large-Bowel Cancer in Hawaiian Japanese," *Journal of the National Cancer Institute* 51 (1973):1765–1779.

24. B. Armstrong and R. Doll, "Environmental Factors and Cancer Incidence and Mortality in Different Countries, with Special Reference to Dietary Practices," *International Journal of Cancer* 15 (1975):617–631.

25. M. L. Casper et al., *Atlas of Stroke Mortality: Racial, Ethnic, and Geographic Disparities in the United States* (Atlanta: Department of Health and Human Services, Centers for Disease Control and Prevention, 2003).

26. E. Barnett et al., *Men and Heart Disease: An Atlas of Racial and Ethnic Disparities in Mortality,* 1st ed. (Morgantown: Office for Social Environment and Health Research, West Virginia University, 2001).

27. M. L. Casper et al., *Women and Heart Disease: An Atlas of Racial and Ethnic Disparities in Mortality,* 2d ed. (Morgantown: Office for Social Environment and Health Research, West Virginia University, 2000).

28. M. L. Casper et al. *Atlas of Stroke Mortality: Racial, Ethnic and Geographic Disparities in the United States* (Atlanta: Department of Health and Human Services, Centers for Disease Control and Prevention, 2003), 57.

29. American Heart Association, *2002 Heart and Stroke Statistical Update* (Dallas: American Heart Association, 2001), 9.

30. K. J. Mertz et al., *Cardiovascular Disease in Georgia, 2002* (Atlanta: Georgia Department of Human Resources, Division of Public Health, and the American Heart Association, Southeast Affiliate, 2002), 10.

31. U.S. Department of Health and Human Services, *Healthy People 2000: National Health Promotion and Disease Prevention Objectives,* DHHS Pub. No. (PHS) 91–50212 (Washington, D.C.: U.S. Government Printing Office, 1991).

32. E. D. Sclar, "Community Economic Structure and Individual Well-being: A Look Behind the Statistics," *International Journal of Health Services* 10 (1980): 563–579.

33. D. Armstrong, E. Barnett, M. Casper, and S. Wing, "Community Occupational Structure, Medical and Economic Resources, and Coronary Mortality among U.S. Blacks and Whites, 1980–1988," *Annals of Epidemiology* 8, no. 3 (1998):184–191.

34. S. Wing, "Social Inequalities in the Decline of Coronary Mortality," *American Journal of Public Health* 78 (1988): 1415–1416.

35. Casper et al., *Women and Heart Disease,* 37.

36. American Heart Association, *2002 Heart and Stroke Statistical Update.*

37. American Heart Association, *2002 Heart and Stroke Statistical Update.*

38. C. Ayala, K. J. Greenlund, J. B. Croft, et al., "Racial/Ethnic Disparities in Mortality by Stroke Subtype in the United States, 1955–1998," *American Journal of Epidemiology* 154, no. 11(2001): 1057–1063.

39. R. Cooper, J. Cutler, P. Desvigne-Nickens, et al., "Trends and Disparities in Coronary Heart Disease, Stroke and Other Cardiovascular Disease in the United States: Findings of the National Conference on Cardiovascular Disease Prevention," *Circulation* 102, no. 25 (2000):3137–3147.
40. J. Fang and M. H. Alderman, "Trend of Stroke Hospitalization, United States, 1988–1997," *Stroke* 32 (2001):2221–2226.
41. N. O. Borhani, "Changes and Geographic Distribution of Mortality from Cerebrovascular Disease," *American Journal of Public Health* 55 (1965):673–681.
42. H. I. Sauer, "Geographic Patterns in the Risk of Dying and Associated Factors, Ages 35–74 Years: United States, 1968–1972," *Vital and Health Statistics: Series 3, Analytic Studies* 18 (1980):1–120.
43. R. Fabsitz and M. Feinleib, "Geographic Patterns in County Mortality Rates from Cardiovascular Diseases," *American Journal of Epidemiology* 111, no. 3 (1980):315–328.
44. S. Wing, M. Casper, W. B. Davis, A. Pellom, W. Riggan, and H. A. Tyroler, "Stroke Mortality Maps United States Whites Aged 35–74 Years, 1962–1982," *Stroke* 19, no. 12 (1988):1507–1513.
45. D. J. Lanska, "Geographic Distribution of Stroke Mortality in the United States: 1939–1947 to 1979–1981," *Neurology* 43, no. 9 (1993):1839–1851.
46. M. L. Casper, S. Wing, R. F. Anda, M. Knowles, and R. A. Pollard, "The Shifting Stroke Belt: Changes in the Geographic Pattern of Stroke Mortality in the United States, 1962 to 1988," *Stroke* 26, no. 5 (1995):755–760.
47. L. W. Pickle, M. P. Mungiole, and R. F. Gillum, "Geographic Variation in Stroke Mortality in Blacks and Whites in the United States," *Stroke* 28, no. 8 (1997):1639–1647.
48. G. Howard, V. J. Howard, C. Katholi, M. K. Oli, and S. Huston, "Decline in U.S. Stroke Mortality: An Analysis of Temporal Patterns by Sex, Race, and Geographic Region," *Stroke* 32, no. 10 (2001):2213–2220.
49. N. O. Borhani, "Changes and Geographic Distribution of Mortality from Cerebrovascular Disease," *American Journal of Public Health* 55 (1965):673–681.
50. H. I. Sauer, "Geographic Patterns in the Risk of Dying and Associated Factors, Ages 35–74 Years: United States, 1968–1972," *Vital and Health Statistics: Series 3, Analytic Studies* 18 (1980):1–120.
51. Fabsitz and Feinleib, "Geographic Patterns in County Mortality Rates from Cardiovascular Diseases," 315–328.
52. S. Wing, M. Casper, W. B. Davis, A. Pellom, W. Riggan, H. A. Tyroler, "Stroke Mortality Maps United States Whites Aged 35–74 Years, 1962–1982," *Stroke* 19, no. 12 (1988):1507–1513.
53. Wing et al., "Stroke Mortality Maps United States Whites Aged 35–74 Years, 1962–1982," *Stroke* 1988; 1507–1513.
54. L. W. Pickle, M. P. Mungiole, and R. F. Gillum, "Geographic Variation in Stroke Mortality in Blacks and Whites in the United States," *Stroke* 28, no. 8 (1997):1639–1647.
55. Howard et al., "Decline in U.S. Stroke Mortality," 2213–2220.
56. Sauer, "Geographic Patterns in the Risk of Dying and Associated Factors," 18:1–120.
57. Wing et al., "Stroke Mortality Maps United States Whites Aged 35–74 Years, 1962–1982," 1507–1513.

58. Wing et al., "Stroke Mortality Maps United States Whites Aged 35–74 Years, 1962–1982," 1507–1513.

59. G. Howard, "Why Do We Have a Stroke Belt in the Southeastern United States? A Review of Unlikely and Uninvestigated Potential Causes," *American Journal of the Medical Sciences* 317, no. 3 (1999):160–167.

60. L. Kuller, H. Anderson, D. Peterson, et al., "Nationwide Cerebrovascular Disease Morbidity Study," *Stroke* 1, no. 2 (1970):86–99.

61. M. D. Nefzger, R. M. Acheson, and A. Heyman, "Mortality from Stroke among U.S. Veterans in Georgia and 5 Western States. I. Study Plan and Death Rates," *Journal of Chronic Diseases* 26, no. 7 (1973):393–404.

62. D. J. Lanska and P. M. Peterson, "Geographic Variation in Reporting of Stroke Deaths to Underlying or Contributing Causes in the United States," *Stroke* 8, no. 5 (1977):551–557.

63. P. D. Stolley, L. H. Kuller, M. D. Nefzger, et al., "Three-Area Epidemiological Study of Geographic Differences in Stroke Mortality. II. Results," *Stroke* 8, no. 5 (1977):551–557.

64. R. F. Gillum and D. D. Ingrum, "Relationship between Residence in the Southeast Region of the United States and Stroke Incidence, the NHANES I Epidemiologic Followup Study," *American Journal of Epidemiology* 144, no. 7 (1996):665–673.

65. G. Howard, R. Anderson, N. J. Johnson, P. Sorlie, G. Russell, and V. J. Howard, "Evaluation of Social Status as a Contributing Factor to the Stroke Belt Region of the United States," *Stroke* 28, no. 5 (1997):936–940.

66. D. J. Lanska and P. M. Peterson, "Effects of Interstate Migration on the Geographic Distribution of Stroke Mortality in the United States," *Stroke* 26, no. 4 (1995):554–661.

67. M. Casper, S. Wing, and D. Strogatz, "Variation in the Magnitude of Black-White Differences in Stroke Mortality by Community Occupational Structure," *Journal of Epidemiology and Community Health* 45, no. 4 (1991):302–306.

68. A. Yassi, *Basic Environmental Health* (Oxford: Oxford University Press, 2001), 340–341.

69. U.S. Department of Health and Human Services, *Geographic Patterns in the Risk of Dying and Associated Factors—Ages 35–74 Years—U.S., 1968–1972*, Vital and Health Statistics Analytical Studies Series 3, No. 18 (Hyattsville, Md.: National Center for Health Statistics, September 1980), 120.

70. J. P. Fox, C. E. Hall, and L. R. Elveback, *Epidemiology—Man and Disease* (London: MacMillan Company, 1970), 233.

71. J. S. Wright et al., "A Comparative Analysis of Rural and Urban Mortality in Georgia, 1979," *American Journal of Preventive Medicine*, no. 1 (1985):22–29.

72. M. S. Eberhardt et al., *Health, United States, 2001: Urban and Rural Health Chartbook* (Hyattsville, Md.: National Center for Health Statistics, 2001), 3, 32–33.

73. Eberhardt, *Health, United States, 2001*, 3, 34–35.

74. Eberhardt, *Health, United States, 2001*, 4, 36–37.

75. Eberhardt, *Health, United States, 2001*, 4, 38–39.

76. Eberhardt, *Health, United States, 2001*, 4, 40–41.

77. Eberhardt, *Health, United States, 2001*, 4, 42–43.
78. Eberhardt, *Health, United States*, 2001, 4, 44–45.
79. Eberhardt, *Health, United States*, 2001, 4, 46–47.
80. Eberhardt, *Health, United States*, 2001, 4, 48–49.
81. Eberhardt, Health, United States, 2001, 4, 50–51.
82. Eberhardt, Health, United States, 2001, 4, 52–53.
83. Eberhardt, Health, United States, 2001, 4, 54–55.
84. Eberhardt, Health, United States, 2001, 4, 56–57.
85. Eberhardt, Health, United States, 2001, 4, 58–59.
86. Eberhardt, Health, United States, 2001, 5, 66–67.
87. Eberhardt, Health, United States, 2001, 5, 68–69.
88. Eberhardt, *Health, United States*, 2001, 5, 70–71.
89. Eberhardt, *Health, United States*, 2001, 5, 72–73.
90. Eberhardt, *Health, United States*, 2001, 5, 74–75.
91. Eberhardt, *Health, United States*, 2001, 5, 76–77.
92. Eberhardt, *Health, United States*, 2001, 5, 60–61.
93. Eberhardt, *Health, United States*, 2001, 5, 62–63.
94. Eberhardt, *Health, United States*, 2001, 5, 64–65.
95. S. L. Gortmaker et al., "Reducing Infant Mortality in Rural America: Evaluation of the Rural Infant Care Program," *Health Services Research* 22, no. 1 (1987):91–116.
96. W. L. Larimore and A. Davis, "Relation of Infant Mortality to the Availability of Maternity Care in Rural Florida," *Journal of the American Board of Family Practice* 8, no. 5 (1995):392–399.
97. I. S. Silva, *Cancer Epidemiology: Principles and Methods* (Lyon, France: International Agency for Research on Cancer, 1999).
98. S. S. Devesa et al., *Atlas of Cancer Mortality in the United States, 1950–94* (Bethesda, Md.: National Institute of Health, National Cancer Institute, 1999).
99. W. J. Blot and J. F. Fraumani, "Geographic Patterns of Lung Cancer: Industrial Correlations," *American Journal of Epidemiology* 103 (1976):539–550.
100. W. J. Blot et al., "Geographic Patterns of Breast Cancer in the United States" *Journal of the National Cancer Institute* 59 (1977):1407–1411.
101. Casper et al., *Atlas of Stroke Mortality*, 2–14.
102. Barnett et al., *Men and Heart Disease*, 16–25.
103. Casper et al., *Women and Heart Disease*, 16–24.
104. Casper et al., *Atlas of Stroke Mortality*, 2–14.
105. Barnett et al., *Men and Heart Disease*, 16–25.
106. Casper et al., *Women and Heart Disease*, 16–24.
107. D. W. Fraser et al., "Legionnaires' Disease: Description of an Epidemic of Pneumonia," *New England Journal of Medicine* 297, no. 22 (December 1, 1977):1189–1197.
108. S. M. Poutanen, D. E. Low, B. Henry, et al., "Identification of Severe Acute Respiratory Syndrome in Canada," *New England Journal of Medicine* 348 (2003):1995–2005.
109. Centers for Disease Control and Prevention, "Update: Severe Acute Respiratory Syndrome—Toronto, Canada, 2003," *MMWR* 52, no. 23 (2003): 547–550.

110. C. L. Schlo and S. J. Franco, "Access to Health Care," in *Rural Health in the United States*, ed. T. C. Ricketts III, 25–37 (New York: Oxford University Press, 1999).

111. R. A. Rosenblatt and L. G. Hast, "Physicians and Rural America," in *Rural Health in the United States*, ed. T. C. Ricketts III, 38–51 (New York: Oxford University Press, 1999).

112. W. Robinson, "Ecological Correlations and the Behavior of Individuals," *American Sociological Review* 15 (June 1950):351–357.

113. Timmreck, *An Introduction to Epidemiology*, 277–287.

114. Timmreck, *An Introduction to Epidemiology*, 14.

115. W. L. Aycock, G. E. Lutman, and G. E. Foley, "Seasonal Prevalence as a Principle in Epidemiology," *American Journal of Medical Sciences* 209 (March 1945):396.

116. M. Jenicek, *Introduction a l'epidemiolojie* (St. Hyacinthe, Que.: Ediserne Inc., 1976), 106.

117. Aycock et al., "Seasonal Prevalence as a Principle in Epidemiology," 396.

118. Jenicek, *Introduction a l'epidemiolojie*, 106.

119. National Center for Health Statistics, Centers for Disease Control and Prevention, U.S. Mortality Public Use Data Tapes, 1960–2000.

120. Centers for Disease Control and Prevention, *http://www.cdc.gov/mmwr/preview/mmwrhtml/mm5053al.htm*.

121. A. M. Lilienfeld, *Foundations of Epidemiology* (New York: Oxford University Press, 1976), 68.

122. J. C. Kleinman, "The Continued Vitality of Vital Statistics," *American Journal of Public Health* 72, no. 2 (1982):126.

123. E. G. Knox, "Epidemics of Rare Diseases," *British Medical Bulletin* 27, no. 1 (1971):45.

124. N. Mantel, "The Detection of Disease Clustering and a Generalized Regression Approach," *Cancer Research* 27, no. 2 (1967):209.

125. Knox, "Epidemics of Rare Diseases," 47.

126. E. G. Knox, in *Current Research in Leukemia*, ed. F. G. J. Hayhoe, 274 (Cambridge: Cambridge University Press, 1965).

8

Demographics: Epidemiological Tools

The Study of Populations

Proceeding from the fundamentals of epidemiology as essential tools of health services management, this chapter examines demography. This topic often is neglected in the training of health administrators and community health specialists. For that reason, the chapter will discuss it at length.

Demography, or the study of human populations, is a scientific discipline closely related to epidemiology. It is the study of the size, composition, distribution, density, growth, and other demographic and socioeconomic characteristics of the population, as well as of the causes and the consequences of changes in those factors.[1]

As discussed in Chapter 3, the contributions of epidemiology to health services management start with a description of the population of interest to the institution. Demographic data is almost always prerequisite for epidemiological measurements. Analysis of utilization (current, ideal, or expected) also requires demographic information. (As Chapter 9 explains, so does marketing.) Finally, demographic trends directly influence health and disease patterns, as well as need for and use of health services.

Accompanying any demographic trend is a public and health policy implication. A basic understanding of demographic principles and techniques thus is required for the use of epidemiology in health services management. This chapter therefore reviews the basic tools of demography necessary in health services management and presents examples of their use by describing demographic trends in the United States, Canada, and populations around the world and the impact of these trends on utilization of the health care system.

Tools of Demographic Measurement

The principal tools of demographic measurement are the same as those of epidemiological measurement described in Chapter 4: crude counts, rates, ratios, proportions, cohort measures, and point and period measures. Demography includes an analysis of population, statics, and dynamics.[2] Population statics refers to the discipline dealing with the size, geographical distribution, and composition of a population at a fixed point in time. Population dynamics covers population changes and components of change.

Population Statics

Population statics were examined, in part, in Chapter 7 on descriptive epidemiology. The demographic study of the geographical distribution of the population is similar to the place description of health and disease patterns. The person characteristics used by demographers to describe the population composition are the same as those used in Chapter 5 (age, sex, race, marital status, and socioeconomic status).

This analysis therefore concentrates on population statics that reflect the most basic characteristics of population—its age and sex composition—and only briefly reviews the other components. Only a few examples of the use of these data in epidemiology and health services management are included because previous chapters extensively demonstrated the relationship between sociodemographic attributes and health, disease patterns, and service utilization.

Age and Sex Composition

Both age and sex influence disease patterns and utilization of health services. Analysis of the age-sex composition of the population of interest thus is a fundamental prerequisite of health planning and management.

A population's age and sex composition at any point is dependent on dynamic or demographic changes. As the next section indicates, births, deaths, and migration all influence population dynamics and, consequently, the composition of the group at any given time.

Median Age   The median age—that is, the age at which half the population is older and half is younger—is an indicator of the age composition of a population. For example, the median age of the U.S. population in 2000 was 35.3 years, whereas Iraq's was 18.3 (2000) and the German Democratic Republic's 40.0.[3] In 1980, the U.S. median age was 30.2 and in Germany it was 36. Two decades of change reflect an aging population, albeit a slow movement indicator of population aging.

Age-Dependency Ratio   Another indicator is the age-dependency ratio. This is the ratio of persons in what are termed the dependent ages (under 15 and over 64) to those in the economically productive ages (15–64). It is usually expressed as the number of persons in the dependent ages for every 100 persons in the productive ages as shown here:

$$Age\text{-}dependency\ ratio = \frac{Population\ under\ 15 + Population\ over\ 64}{Population\ aged\ 15\ to\ 64} \times 100$$

The age-dependency ratio indicates (with questionable validity) the economic burden the productive portion of a population must carry. The higher the age-dependency ratio, the heavier the economic burden. The United States age-dependency ratio in 1998 was 49.3 percent, meaning that there were approximately 49 persons in the dependent ages for every 100 persons in the employed or productive ages. By contrast, Mongolia's was 65 persons for every 100 in economically productive ages. In the late 1970s, the U.S. age-dependency rate was 54. The decrease from 54 to 49 reflects fewer dependents for every 100 in the working or productive ages.

The age-dependency ratio can be divided into old-age dependency (the ratio of those over 64 to those 15–64) and child-dependency (the ratio of those under 15 to those 15 to 64).[4]

Sex Ratio   The sex ratio, describing the gender composition of the group, is the ratio of males to females in a given population, also usually expressed per 100 (males per 100 females). As discussed in Chapter 5, the sex ratio at birth in any population is approximately 106 males per 100 females. Because of different mortality and migration patterns, however, this ratio subsequently varies between places and between age groups. The ratio can be particularly useful when analyzing small areas because they might have more significant variations in sex distribution.

Population Pyramids   The best way to illustrate age and sex composition graphically is the population pyramid. It shows the numbers or proportions of males to females in each age group and is a vivid picture of a population's composition. As discussed later, it also is useful in projecting trends.

The age-sex composition tends to fall into one of three general profiles,[5] as illustrated in Figure 8-1. Expansive populations have larger numbers of people in the younger age groups with each age cohort larger than the one born before it. Constrictive populations have smaller numbers of people in

Expansive

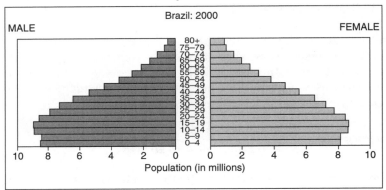

Constrictive

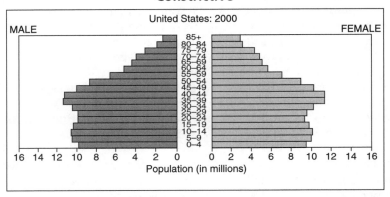

Near Stationary

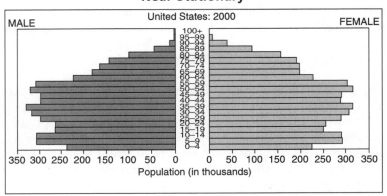

FIGURE 8-1   The Three General Profiles of Age Composition, 2000. *Source:* U.S. Census Bureau, International Data Base, *http://www.census.gov/ipc/www/idbnew.html.*

the younger ages, while stationary ones have roughly equal numbers in almost all age groups, tapering off gradually at older levels.

The most important factor influencing the shape of a population pyramid is the fertility rate.[6] The larger the number of children per each parent, the broader the base of the pyramid (and the younger the median). Mortality has a somewhat less simple influence on the age distribution. Contrary to what might be assumed, a population with lower mortality rates has a slightly younger age distribution;[7] differences in these rates are much more likely to result from variances in young age groups (mostly infants and children).[8]

Other Variables to Describe Composition

Other variables commonly used by demographers to describe the composition of a population include race, socioeconomic status, marital status, and other family-related variables. Race ratios similar to sex ratios can be calculated by (for example) dividing the number of whites by the number of blacks; as in sex ratios, the race ratio usually is expressed as the number of whites per 100 blacks.

Income, occupation, and education data indicates socioeconomic status. Theses variables can be used individually or combined into a socioeconomic index.

In addition to marital status, several other related characteristics can be examined. Marital history refers to the number of times a person married, when each marriage occurred, and when and how each previous one ended. Age at first marriage can be a good demographic and social indicator. The mean (average) size[9,10] of household and the mean size of family[11] as well as the number of children of dependent ages are also used as demographic indicators.

All of these social indicators can be used by health services managers to describe their population. As Chapters 4, 5, and 11 demonstrated, these social characteristics are closely associated with morbidity and health services utilization patterns.

Population Distribution

The last component of these statistics to be considered is the distribution of the population. This refers to pattern of settlement and dispersal of population within a country or other area.[12] The main descriptive concepts are urban versus rural, metropolitan status, population density, and population size.

There is surprisingly little agreement on the definition of urban. Various authors and publications offer different definitions based on any single criterion or a combination of the following criteria: population size, density, concentration, structure, types of occupation, sociocultural distinctions, ways of life, and states of mind.

In the United States census, urban areas are defined as incorporated and unincorporated places of 2,500 or more inhabitants, including the contiguous areas around cities of 50,000 or more. In Canada, the minimum size is 1,000 inhabitants, with a population density of at least 400 persons per square kilometer. In both the United States and Canada, as in most countries, the rural population is simply those residents living outside urban areas. The population in urban areas can be expressed as a percentage of the total population (percent urban). For example, in 2002 the population of the United States was 75 percent urban, whereas Singapore was 100 percent urban and Burundi was only 8 percent.[13]

The concept of metropolitan area is also used often in the description of population distribution. In general, a metropolitan area is defined as a large concentration of population (i.e., a large urban area), usually with 100,000 or more inhabitants and at least one city of 50,000 or more. Administrative areas bordering the city that are socially and economically integrated with it are included.[14]

In some countries, the term *large urban conglomerations* is used. In Canada, these are called Census Metropolitan Areas (CMA). In the United States, they are referred to as Metropolitan Statistical Areas (MSA). These are defined by the Office of Management and Budget using a large list of criteria supplied by the Bureau of the Census, including size, density, type of employment, and volume of commuting traffic.[15]

Population density is a concept much used in the study of distribution. Its usual measure is the number of people per unit of land area (population per square mile or kilometer). This is not always satisfactory, however, because it assumes that the population is dispersed evenly over the entire area under consideration.[16]

In some cases where the inhabitants are concentrated in a small portion of an area, the population density is very low, even though the people live in high-density areas. For example, Canada had a population density of only 8 per square mile in 2000, while the United States had 77 persons per square mile in the same year.[17] Consequently, other measures of population density have been used: percentage of population in multifamily dwellings and population per square mile for urbanized areas only.[18]

Population size is also used in analyzing distributions. The main advantage of crude size of locality is that a classification by multiple size categories can be used instead of the dichotomous urban-rural or MSA–non-MSA classification.

Interaction among Variables

It is important for health services managers to analyze the demographic makeup of their population because, as discussed in earlier chapters, the variables of age, sex, race, marital status, and socioeconomic position are related to health, disease, and utilization of services. When performing an analysis, however, managers should be aware that some demographic variables can interact with each other in such a way that a composite analysis (a combination of variables) might be more appropriate and yield results different from a study of each component alone.[19] In other words, the relationship between one demographic variable and health, disease, or utilization depends in part on another demographic variable.

For example, an analysis of utilization of health services might show no difference among age groups or incomes. However, a composite analysis by age and income may show that utilization is higher among both older age/lower income groups and younger age/higher income groups. This indicates that utilization is related not to age and income separately but to the composite of age and income variables.

Data to perform a composite analysis is not always available (e.g., when using published census data). However, when possible, it is always better to check for interaction between variables.[20]

Population Dynamics

In addition to the description of population composition (population statics), demography concerns population dynamics, or the changes in composition over time. Population change involves three components: births, deaths, and migration. Mortality measures were described in Chapter 4. This section reviews basic measures of fertility and migration and examines global measures of population change.

Natality   The term *natality* refers to the role of births in population change. Although some authors use the term *fertility* in this same broad sense, natality is restricted to actual birth performance, that is, to the intensity and tempo of births that actually occur in a population.[21] Fertility, therefore, refers to the production of live born *and* fecundity to the physiological capacity to reproduce (to give birth to a live child). Fecundity is a prerequisite for fertility. Infertile persons can either be infecund (sterile) or be using some form of birth control.

Although this was not always the case in the past, natality, fertility, and births have come to refer only to live births. Stillbirths, fetal deaths, and abortions are not included.

Crude Birth Rate   The most common measure of natality is the crude birth rate (CBR). It is simply the number of births in a year per 1,000 midyear population (the population as of July 1):

$$CBR = \frac{Number\ of\ live\ births}{Total\ midyear\ population} \times 1,000$$

The crude birth rate is a valid measure of the number of babies a population produces in a given year. However, it is not very useful for temporal or spatial comparisons, as it does not eliminate the impact of differential population structures. In other words, it does not tell much about the reproductive experience or about the intensity or tempo of births because it does not account for the age-sex composition of the population.

General Fertility Rate   The general fertility rate (GFR) is a more refined measure than the crude birth rate because it relates the number of births to the population at risk of giving birth—that is, the female population ages 15 to 44.[22] The general fertility rate is defined as the number of live births per 1,000 women ages 15–44:

$$GFR = \frac{Total\ live\ births}{Females\ ages\ 15\ to\ 44} \times 1,000$$

It should be noted that the total number of births, regardless of age of mother, is used in the numerator.[23] Some authors suggest using the population of women ages 15 to 49, but because women ages 45 to 49 contribute relatively few births to the total number, the general fertility rate is limited to those up to age 44. Contrary to the crude birth rate, the general fertility rate can be used for comparison purposes because it controls the age and sex composition of the populations involved. It thus is much more indicative of differences in reproductive behavior than is the crude birth rate.

The difference between these two rates is illustrated by the situation in the United States: Although the crude birth rate has been increasing in recent years, the general fertility rate has remained fairly constant. In other words, there are more babies born but not because women are having more babies but because there is now a larger pool of women in the reproductive age bracket due to the baby boom after the World War II.

Age-Specific Fertility   As described for mortality rates (Chapter 4), fertility rates can be made specific for any population subgroup. For example, it is possible to calculate the fertility for the black urban population in Georgia. Age-specific fertility rates are used for comparison over time and to detect differences in fertility behavior at different ages. An age-specific fertility rate (ASFR) is defined as the number of live births to women of a specified age group in one year per 1,000 women in that age group (at midyear):[24]

$$ASFR\ (15-19) = \frac{\textit{Live birth to women ages 15–19 in the year}}{\textit{Midyear population of women ages 15–19}} \times 1,000$$

The calculation of the age-specific rates for every five-year age group between 15 and 49 gives a complete picture of the fertility differences among these age groups. The rates provide a specific indication of the population at risk, which can be valuable for planning purposes. Fertility behavior of different populations can be examined. A standardized fertility rate can be calculated involving the same methods (direct and indirect adjustment) used to standardize mortality rates (Chapter 4).

These standardized rates indicate how many births per 1,000 there would have been in the population of interest if its age and sex composition were the same as in the standard (arbitrarily chosen) population. Fertility rates also can be adjusted (standardized) for other demographic variables such as marital status, race, urban-rural residence, duration of marriage, standard of education, or socioeconomic status.

Note that some authors refer to specific and standardized fertility rates as specific and standardized birth rates.[25,26] The use of the term *fertility*, however, seems more appropriate because the denominators are always limited to the female population at risk of childbearing, whereas the denominator of the crude birth rate is the total population. Furthermore, the general fertility rate is in fact a weighted average of these age-specific rates.

Total Fertility Rate   The total fertility rate (TFR) is a hypothetical measure (a synthetic estimate) of the average number of children that would be born alive to a woman during her lifetime if she were to pass through all her childbearing years conforming to the age-specific rates of a given year. The TFR is one of the most important fertility measures, as it indicates as nearly as possible how many children women are having.

Contrary to the general fertility rate, the total fertility rate is adjusted for age and sex composition of the population. The TFR is in fact a summary measure of the age-specific fertility rates over all ages of the childbearing period.

$$TFR = \frac{5\left(\sum_{a=15-19}^{a=45-49} fa\right)}{1,000}$$

where:

fa = an age-specific fertility rate per 1,000

Table 8-1 illustrates the calculation of total fertility rates. A TFR of 2.05 for the year 2000 means that if the 2000 age-specific fertility rates were to continue, United States women on the average would have 2.05 children per woman during their childbearing years.

A good example of the usefulness of the TFR is the comparison of the fertility rates for the United States and Canada. In the year 2000 the general fertility rate was 67.5 per 1,000 in the United States and 57.1 in Canada in 2003.[27] Likewise age-specific fertility rates show that fertility in the United States has been increasing on average while those rates of the Canadian women have been falling in the last decade or more.

Furthermore, the total fertility rates per woman (with controls for the age and sex composition) are 1.6 for Canada and 2.06 for United States for the year 2000. It can be concluded that in the year 2000 the United States had about a 22 percent higher fertility rate per woman than Canada. The gradual decline in fertility rate among the Canadian women of childbearing age has become apparent in the last decade or so.

TABLE 8-1 Calculation of a Total Fertility Rate (Data for United States, 2000)

Age Group	Age-Specific Fertility Rate per 1,000 Women
15–19	47.7
20–24	109.7
25–29	113.5
30–34	91.2
35–39	39.7
40–44	8.0
45–54	0.5
	$\Sigma fa = 410.3$

$$TFR = \frac{5 \times \Sigma fa}{1,000}$$

$$TFR = \frac{5 \times 410.3}{1,000} \times 2.05$$

Where: TFR = Total fertility rate
Σ = Summation
fa = Age-specific fertility
Σfa = Sum of all age-specific fertility rates

Note: In the formula, 5 is used because each age-specific group encompasses five years.

It should be noted that areas (two or more countries, districts, states, etc.) could be compared in like manner. This information should be most important if a health services manager or administrator was planning to build or expand obstetrical services for the institution. The demographic trend becomes critical to the needs and success of such ventures.

Although this now seems somewhat less relevant, demographers used to make a distinction between illegitimate and legitimate births.[28,29] An illegitimate birth was defined as a child born to a single, widowed, or divorced woman. The illegitimacy rate (IR) is the number of illegitimate live births per 1,000 unmarried women (single, widowed, or divorced) ages 15 to 44 in a given year. The illegitimacy ratio is the number of illegitimate live births per 1,000 live births (not women) in a given year. It is a measure of the proportion of births that are illegitimate. It is now preferable simply to use fertility rates specific to marital status (as in Table 8-2) or to study teenage fertility rates separately.

The most useful fertility measures for health services managers remain the age-specific fertility rates and the total fertility rates. As illustrated in Table 8-2, these can be specific to any population subgroups. Specific data provides valuable information for health services management, for example, in the planning of obstetrical services or family planning programs.

Migration   Migration is the third basic process that alters the size and composition of a population (with births and deaths). It refers to the geographic or spatial movement of population involving a change of usual places of residence between clearly defined geographic units.[30] This change of residence should not be considered if it is temporary (visiting, vacation, or business) but should be intended as permanent (for the purpose of residing).

Demographers usually distinguish between international and internal migration. The former refers to moves between countries and is designated as emigration from the nation left behind and as immigration to the receiving nation.[31] A country loses emigrants and receives immigrants. Internal migration refers to movements between different areas within a country. The terms *in-migration* and *out-migration* are used instead of immigration and emigration, respectively. In the United States and Canada, interstate (interprovincial) migration and intrastate (intraprovincial) migration also could be dealt with separately.

The immigration (or in-migration) rate is the number of immigrants (in-migrants) arriving at a destination per 1,000 population at that destination in a given year.[32]

$$Immigration\ rate = \frac{Number\ of\ immigrants\ in\ a\ year}{Total\ midyear\ population\ at\ destination} \times 1,000$$

TABLE 8-2   General Fertility Rates and Total Fertility Rates, United Statse, 2000 (Selected Groups/Characteristics)

Characteristics	General Fertility Rate per 1,000 Women	Total Fertility Rate per 1,000 Women
Total, 15 to 44 years old	64.6	1,218.0*
Age:		
15 to 19	59.7	131.0
20 to 24	91.8	572.0
25 to 29	107.9	1,049.0
30 to 34	87.9	1,549.0
35 to 39	45.1	1,839.0
Race:		
White	65.4	1,205.0
Black	63.2	1,350.0
Asian/Pacific Islander	54.6	966.0
Hispanic origin	95.1	1,510.0
Marital Status:		
Currently married	88.8	1,785.0
Married—husband present	90.8	1,782.0
Married—husband absent	64.5	1,821.0
Divorced or widowed	31.0	1,677.0
Never married	42.3	431.0
Education Attainment:		
Not a high school graduate	70.7	1,032.0
High school graduate	70.0	1,515.0
College, one or more years	59.0	1,130.0
Bachelor's degree	61.7	1,018.0
Graduate or professional degree	77.7	1,039.0
Labor Force Status:		
In labor force	49.5	1,167.0
Employed	47.7	1,171.0
Unemployed	79.4	1,088.0
Not in labor force	103.7	1,349.0
Annual Family Income:**		
Under $10,000	86.8	1,394.0
$10,000 to $19,999	74.8	1,413.0
$20,000 to $24,999	76.2	1,319.0
$25,000 to $29,999	78.9	1,243.0
$30,000 to $34,999	62.4	1,179.0
$35,000 to $49,999	64.9	1,227.0
$50,000 to $74,999	61.2	1,218.0
$75,000 and over	60.1	1,066.0

TABLE 8-2 (continued)

Characteristics	General Fertility Rate per 1,000 Women	Total Fertility Rate per 1,000 Women
Region of Residence:		
Northeast	60.8	1,126.0
Midwest	61.8	1,230.0
South	66.0	1,226.0
West	68.4	1,267.0

*May also be interpreted as 1.2 children per woman

**Data not shown for people with family income not reported

Source: U.S. Census Bureau, Current Population Survey, June 2000, *http://www.census.gov/population/www/socdemo/fertility.html.*

Similarly, the emigration (out-migration) rate is the number of emigrants departing an area of origin per 1,000 population at that area of origin in a given year.

$$Emigration\ rate = \frac{Number\ of\ emigrants\ in\ a\ year}{Total\ midyear\ population\ at\ destination} \times 1,000$$

Immigration and emigration (in-migration and out-migration) are more correctly referred to as gross immigration and gross emigration (gross in-migration and gross out-migration). The balance of the two for a given area during a given period (usually a year) is called net migration or net emigration, depending on which is larger. The net migration rate shows the net effect of immigration and emigration on an area's population, expressed as increase (+) or decrease (−) per 1,000 population of the area in a given year.[33]

$$Net\ migration\ rate = \frac{\begin{array}{c} Number\ of\ immigration - \\ Number\ of\ emigration \end{array}}{\begin{array}{c} Total\ midyear\ population \\ at\ destination \end{array}} \times 1,000$$

For example, in the year 2003, the United States had a net migration rate of +3.5 migrants per 1,000 population—a net increase of 3.5 persons per 1,000 population. Similarly, Canada had a net migration rate of +6.1 per 1,000 population—a net increase of 6.1 persons per 1,000 population for 2002.[34] Therefore, Canada experienced almost twice the increase in the number of immigrants per unit population than the United States.

Measures of Population Change

The relationship among the three components of population change—births, deaths, and migration—and population change over time can be expressed by the balancing equation:

$$P_2 = P_1 + (B - D) + (I - E)$$

where:

P_2 = population at the later date

P_1 = population at the earlier date

B = births

D = deaths between the two dates

I = immigration or in-migration

E = emigration or out-migration between the two dates

$(I - E)$ thus is the net migration. The difference between the number of births and deaths is the natural increase ($NI = B - D$). The rate of natural increase is the one at which a population is increasing (or decreasing) in a given year because of a surplus (or deficit) of births over (or under) deaths, expressed as a percentage of the base population:[35]

$$Rate\ of\ natural\ increase = \frac{Births - Deaths}{Total\ midyear\ population} \times 100$$

Or:

$$Rate\ of\ natural\ increase = \frac{Births - Deaths}{10} \times 100$$

For example, the rate of natural increase in the United States and Canada for the year 2002 was 0.6 and 0.3, respectively.[36]

The growth rate is the rate at which a population is increasing (or decreasing) in a given year because of a natural increase and net migration, expressed as a percentage of the base population:

$$Growth\ rate = \frac{(B - D) + (I - E)}{Total\ midyear\ population} \times 100$$

Or:

$$Growth\ rate = Rate\ of\ natural\ increase + Net\ migration\ rate$$

The growth rate takes into account all components of population change (births, deaths, and migration). It should not be confused with the rate of natural increase, which considers only births and deaths, or with the birth rate, which involves only births.

Another common way to measure population change is to calculate the intercensus change (IC). It is simply the difference between the population indicated in a previous census (P_1) and a subsequent census (P_2) of the same area:

$$IC = P_2 - P_1$$

The intercensus change in percentage (IC%) can be used to compare the growth of different populations.

$$IC\% = \frac{P_2 - P_1}{P_1} \times 100$$

These rates as they relate to population dynamics are important to health services managers. The increased need for services, the marketing of new ones, expansion into a new location, and the demand for care in the institution are dependent on a changing population structure. However, concepts of preventive medicine applied to these areas require knowledge about the lifestyles and environment in the existing structure. It certainly behooves health managers to use these techniques and tie them in directly with the material in earlier chapters.

Population Estimates

In the majority of countries, the most reliable and complete source of information on population composition is the national census. However, since population is changing constantly, population data for many purposes can soon be considered out of date. For this reason, demographers have developed several methods and techniques to estimate intercensus and postcensus (current) populations.

This section examines how to estimate current or postcensus population. The following portion deals with population projections, that is, the computation of future changes in population. Both of these topics can be complex and beyond the scope of this book, so this analysis is limited. Demography textbooks offer a more complete and detailed discussion on this subject. The publication *The Methods and Materials of Demography* offers an excellent discussion of population estimates and population projections.[37]

Estimation of population is of special importance for an epidemiological approach to health services management. As noted throughout this book, epidemiology offers various principles and methods to relate the occurrence of health and disease, as well as the utilization of health services, to the population. Valid estimates of population thus are needed constantly for the denominators of rates.

TABLE 8-3   Methods for Estimating Population

Demographic Methods	Statistical Methods
Component Methods	Ratio-Correlation Methods
Housing Unit Method	Censal Ratio Methods
Composite Methods	Extrapolation of Past Growth
Death Rate Methods (ASDR)*	Sample Surveys

*ASDR = age-specific death rate

Source: Adapted from "Estimating Population" by M. J. Batitus with permission of *American Demographics*, © April 1982, 3.

Techniques to estimate population fall into two broad categories (Table 8-3): demographic and statistical. Demographic techniques use data on any or all of the components of population change (births, deaths, migration). Statistical techniques, on the other hand, rely on predictors of population change, even though they might not be directly related to the three components of the population. It should be understood that there are many demographic vendors[38] who provide the basic methods for estimating population, but also provide the data for almost any geographical area for almost any variable. However, to understand their methods of estimation and projection, it is valuable to outline the basic methods used for projecting future population groups.

Component Methods

Component methods estimate the three components of population change separately. The estimation formula therefore is exactly the same as what was referred to previously as the balancing equation:

$$P_2 = P_1 + (B - D) + (I - E)$$

The population is estimated by adding natural increase and net immigration for the period since the last census to the latest census count. When data is available, this is without doubt the easiest way to estimate population. There usually is no problem getting data on births and deaths from vital statistics reports.

Net migration data can be much more difficult to obtain. Sometimes it is necessary to assume that the net migration rate for the years since the last census was the same as that reported in the last census or to extrapolate from past trends. If the net migration data is not available from the last census, it can be estimated by using figures from the two previous censuses (P_2 and P_1) and from vital statistics:

$$(I - E) = P_2 - P_1 - (B - D)$$

The Housing Unit Method

A second technique for estimating population relies on the net addition of housing. The housing unit method looks at the new additions to the housing stock and the loss of units from demolition. This data usually is available from municipal records of building permits. Next, the vacancy rate has to be determined. This usually is available from the last census or, again, from municipal building authorities. Finally, specifics on the average household size and on the number of households at the last census date are assembled from census data. The estimating formula is as follows:[39]

$$P_2 = [HH \text{ Census} + ((NHH - DHH) \times OR)] \times AHS$$

where:

P_2 = population estimate

HH = number of household units at last census date

NHH = new additions of housing units

DHH = number of household units lost through demolition

OR = occupancy rate $(1 -$ vacancy rate$)$

AHS = average household size

Composite Methods

Composite methods refer to a mixture of techniques to estimate population by broad age groups. For example, school enrollment can be used to estimate or measure changes in the population under age 18, income tax returns for the population ages 18 to 64, and Medicare enrollment for the population over 65. The total population estimate is calculated by adding the estimates for the different age groups.[40]

Age-Specific Death Rate Methods

A shortcut method to estimate population is the age-specific death rate (ASDR) method. This simple method divides the number of deaths in the postcensus year by the corresponding age-specific death rates for the census year. The result is an estimate of population in the postcensus year (P_2).

$$P_2 \sum_a^f \left(\frac{Deaths}{fa} \times 1,000 \right)$$

where:

fa = age-specific death rate per 1,000

This method of course has several limitations. First, it assumes that the death rates have remained stable between the census year and the post-census year of estimate. Furthermore, death rates in small areas tend to undergo considerable yearly fluctuations. Using an average of the death rates for a period of several years (see Chapter 4) can alleviate this problem. In any case, the populations by age group that are computed to obtain the total estimate should not be used as estimates of individual age groups. Overall, this method is quite accurate even for relatively small areas (county level). However, it should be used with great caution for very small areas, for example, less than 30,000 population.

The Statistical Methods

Several statistical methods also can be used to estimate population. The ratio correlation methods use regression techniques to relate changes in indirect indicators (such as automobile registration and school enrollment) to population change itself. The census-ratio methods project the ratio of such indirect indicators to the total population.[41] This ratio is calculated from the last census. Another statistical technique consists of simply extrapolating past growth—for example, the growth between the last three or four censuses. Finally, sample surveys are sometimes used.

Thus, many techniques to estimate population, mainly the statistical ones, can be complex and time consuming when applied to making estimates of small areas. Health services managers should first try to obtain estimates for their population from outside sources such as federal, state, county, or municipal governments. When these are not available, the component methods and the housing unit method can be used. The age-specific death rate method can be used, with caution, to estimate county or metropolitan population.

Population Projections

Whereas population estimates are used to determine the current number of people in a target area, population projections aim to determine what the total number will be in the future. A distinction can also be made between projections and forecasts. Population projections are based on certain assumptions about future trends in the rates of fertility, mortality, and migration. Demographers therefore usually make low, medium, and high projections of the same population based on different assumptions as to how these rates will change.[42] A forecast is a guess as to which of these projections is the most likely. To put it another way, all forecasts are projections, but not all projections are forecasts.[43]

There are five broad categories for projecting population:

1. Mathematical extrapolation methods

2. Ratio methods
3. Component and cohort component methods
4. Economy-based methods
5. Land-use methods.

These categories are far from mutually exclusive and a mix of principles and techniques from each is often used. Once again, these are described only briefly here; several specialized textbooks can provide further details.[44]

As with population estimates, past growth can simply be extended into the future. These mathematical extrapolations usually are not considered very valid, although large-scale applications of this method can become quite complex mathematically.[45] In general, however, mathematical extrapolation methods should be used only when rough approximation is required and only over a relatively short future.

Ratio Method—An Example

The ratio methods use an existing projection for a larger (parent) area and the ratio of the current population of the subareas to this parent group. The historical trend of the ratios is determined, projected into the future, and multiplied by the projection for the parent population.[46]

Table 8-4 illustrates the calculation of the ratio projection for a hypothetical county A. The projection of the future ratio is simply an extension

TABLE 8-4 Calculation of a Ratio Method of Population Projection for County A

	County A's Historical Population Ratio with the State		
Year	State Population	County A Population	County A as a State Ratio (population)
1980	5,462,982	483,024	0.0884
1985	5,962,000	536,580	0.0900
1990	6,478,149	546,171	0.0843
1995	7,192,305	583,172	0.0811
2000	8,186,453	665,865	0.0813
	Ratio Projection of County A's Population		
Year	State Projection	County A's Ratio	County A's Projection
2005	8413000	0.0812	683,135
2010	8824000	0.0820	723,568
2015	9200000	0.0815	747,040
2020	9552000	0.0812	775,622
2025	9869000	0.0815	804,323

Source: Projection calculated by the author, 2003.

of historical trends. As shown, the ratio of county population to state population had been increasing until 1985, then declined slowly from 1990 to 1995. It then increased slightly in 2000 and these fluctuations are expected to be maintained for the duration of the projected years ahead as shown. This ratio method is often used by government agencies and should be easy for health services managers to apply when population projections for larger (parent) areas are available.

Cohort Component Method—An Example

The component method and the cohort component method are similar except that the former uses total population whereas the latter subdivides the population into age groups (cohorts). In both methods, the components of population change (births, deaths, migration) are projected separately. In the cohort component method (also called cohort survival method), the population is carried forward by cohort, taking into account the survival rate and the migration rate of that age-specific group. The population of each age group is projected individually. For example, the population aged 10 to 14 in Table 8-5 (2000) is projected forward five years to 2005 by adjusting for deaths and migration. In 2005, this cohort became the 15 to 19 age group. The process is separated for every age group and for each future date desired.

Table 8-5 illustrates the calculation of a cohort component projection for a hypothetical county. Only calculations for females are shown. Projections for the male population are done the same way, except that the fertility rate columns would be excluded. Total population projections are obtained by summing the two.

The calculations in the table are based on the assumption that the fertility rates, survival rates, and net migration between 1991 and 1995 all remain unchanged in the succeeding time periods. If the person doing the projections has reason to believe that this would not be so, the rates can be altered accordingly.

The main advantage of the cohort component method is that it allows a detailed, age-specific analysis of future population trends. Births, deaths, and migration all are calculated and can be examined readily for each age group. An alternative is simply to calculate the overall growth rate for each cohort between two censuses and apply that rate to the new cohort for the same age group, and so on. The procedure is essentially the same except that births, deaths, and net migration are not considered separately but are combined into a single measure, the growth rate.

Economy-based methods of population projection use projected economic data for the projection of migration. Births and deaths are projected using other methods, and immigration and emigration are projected in relation to the future economy of an area (creation or loss of jobs). The land-

TABLE 8-5 Calculation of a Cohort Component Population Projection

Cohorts	Col. 1 1991	Col. 2 1991–1995	Col. 3 1991–1995	Col. 4 1991–1995	Col. 5 1991–1995	Col. 6 1996	Col. 7 1991–1995	Col. 8 1996–2000	Col. 9 2001	Col. 10 2001	Col. 11 2001–2005	Col. 12 2006	Col. 13 2006
Females	Actual Population	Survival Rates per 1,000	Fertility Rates per 1,000	Births	(Estimated 1996 Population)	Actual Population	Estimated Net Migration	Births	Survivors	Projection Estimate	Births	Survivors	Projection Estimate
0–4	1,290	982.2		1,044	1,025	1,115	+90	1,326	1,302	1,392	1,542	1,514	1,604
5–9	1,750	998.5			1,288	1,355	+67		1,113	1,180		1,390	1,457
10–14	1,870	998.5			1,747	1,730	−17		1,353	1,336		1,178	1,161
15–19	1,610	997.5	204.5	329	1,865	1,750	−115	357	1,726	1,611	352	1,337	1,222
20–24	1,135	997.5	599.0	680	1,606	1,390	−216	833	1,746	1,530	916	1,607	1,391
25–29	955	997.0	661.0	631	1,132	1,480	+348	978	1,386	1,734	1,146	1,525	1,873
30–34	980	996.0	340.0	333	951	1,160	+209	394	1,474	1,683	572	1,727	1,936
35–39	1,130	994.0	125.5	142	974	1,070	+96	134	1,153	1,249	157	1,673	1,769
40–44	1,220	990.1	28.0	34	1,119	1,190	+71	33	1,059	1,130	32	1,237	1,308
45–49	1,145	984.2	1.5	2	1,201	1,155	−46	2	1,171	1,125	2	1,112	1,066
50–54	850	975.9			1,117	1,125	+8		1,127	1,135		1,098	1,106
55–59	605	962.4			818	760	−58		1,083	1,025		1,092	1,034
60–64	420	943.0			571	565	−6		716	710		967	961
65–69	350	912.4			383	425	+42		516	558		648	690
70–74	270	862.6			302	340	+38		367	405		481	519
75–79	225	780.2			211	280	+69		265	334		316	385
80–84	140	648.1			146	190	+44		181	225		216	260
85 +	95	435.3			102	150	+48		148	196		183	231
	16,040			2,151	17,063	17,230	+672	2,731	17,886	18,558	3,177	19,301	19,973
				(× .4855)				(× .4855)			(× .4855)		

(continued)

TABLE 8-5 (continued)

Notes:

Column 2: Calculated using death rates. This is done by taking the average annual death rate for the five-year period compounded at a declining rate, the result of which is multiplied by 1,000. In mathematical terms:

$$SR = 1,000 \times \frac{1}{(1+i)^n}$$

where: SR = survival rate
i = annual average death rate
n = number of years

In essence, this rate states the probability that a person who is in a certain age bracket will live from the beginning to the end of the particular time period. Published life tables are often used to calculate survival rates.

Column 4: Column 3 times Column 1. The entry opposite 0–4 indicates the total of all births factored by the number who will be female (48.55%). An alternate approach for this calculation is to apply the same fertility rates to the average midyear population:

$$\frac{\text{Population 1991} + \text{Population 1996}}{2}$$

Column 5: Column 2 times Column 1 with its cohorts dropped one age bracket, that is, the survival rate for the next succeeding age bracket is applied to the number in the cohort. For example, the 955 women ages 25 to 29 in 1991 are multiplied by the survival rate for the age bracket 30 to 34 to obtain the 1996 estimate (migration held aside for the moment). The births calculated in Column 4 are factored by the 0–4 survival rate.

Column 7: Column 6 minus Column 5. The result is assumed to be net migration because Column 5 includes births and deaths of persons in 1991. This calculation also includes any error in census counts, fertility rate, and survival rate calculations of Columns 2 and 3. These errors are ignored, largely because they are impossible to measure. The calculation also includes births and deaths of migrants. With more work, the net migration can be recalibrated to extract these components, but [it was] decided to disregard this aspect.

Column 8: Column 3 times Column 6. The entry opposite 0–4 indicates the total of all births factored by the number who will be female (48.55%). Alternate calculation is possible, as noted for Column 4.

Column 9: Column 2 times Column 6 as for Column 5.

Column 10: The projection estimate calculated by taking Column 9 and adding Column 7. No survival rate or fertility rate calculations are made with the migration estimates because these are assumed to be part of the residually derived estimates. If the estimates had been derived using another method, then it might have been necessary to apply separate fertility rate and survival rate calculations (usually at half the rate).

Column 11: Column 3 times Column 10. The entry opposite 0–4 indicates the total of all births factored by the number who will be female (48.55%). Alternate calculation is possible, as noted for Column 4.

Column 12: Column 2 times Column 10 as for Column 5.

Column 13: Column 12 plus Column 7 with same assumptions as in Column 10.

Source: Abridged and adapted from *How Communities Can Use Statistics* by Statistics Canada, ©June 1981, 57.

use methods are similar to the housing unit methods of population estimates. By calculating how many housing units can be built and with a knowledge of the average household size, the likely additions to the population can be estimated, given a presumed rate of building to reach the saturation point.[47]

The ratio and the cohort component methods thus are probably the easiest population projection measures that health services managers can use. It is always advisable to use more than one method and to project the population under several different assumptions of birth, death, and migration rates.

The United States Census

Most of the data required for demographic analysis of the population comes from vital and health statistics and from the census. Census populations contain a wealth of information that too often is ignored by hospitals and other health institutions.[48]

To illustrate the kind of information collected in the census, the 2000 U.S. Census questionnaire is reproduced in Figure 8-2. All of this information is compiled and easily available for every area of the United States (equivalent data is available from Statistics Canada). There also exist private firms that supply demographic data (from the census).[49] These "demographic supermarkets" can compile all kinds of information for any given area and can provide computer graphics and population forecasts.

Health services managers thus can use the basic tools of demography to describe, estimate, and project their population of interest. Demographic characteristics are related not only to health and disease pattern but also to utilization of services. Demographic principles and techniques can also be used, for example, to analyze physician or nurse populations.

The purpose of the preceding section is to serve as a basic reference on demography. In the rest of the chapter, many of these techniques are applied to examine population trends and their impact on the health care system.

Population Trends

The World Population

In the mid-1980s, the world population was approximately 4.5 billion and growing at 1.7 percent per year. This growth rate meant that, if it remained constant, the world population would double in 41 years. This is amazing, considering that it took two million to five million years for the world population to reach its first billion. Table 8-6 shows that it took only until 1988 (thirteen years) for the total population to reach five billion.

PLEASE DO NOT FILL OUT THIS FORM.
This is not an official census form. It is for informational purposes only.

United States
Census 2000

U.S. Department of Commerce • Bureau of the Census

This is the official form for all the people at this address. It is quick and easy, and your answers are protected by law. Complete the Census and help your community get what it needs — today and in the future!

Start Here

Please use a black or blue pen.

1. How many people were living or staying in this house, apartment, or mobile home on April 1, 2000?

[   ] Number of people

INCLUDE in this number:
- foster children, roomers, or housemates
- people staying here on April 1, 2000 who have no other permanent place to stay
- people living here most of the time while working, even if they have another place to live

DO NOT INCLUDE in this number:
- college students living away while attending college
- people in a correctional facility, nursing home, or mental hospital on April 1, 2000
- Armed Forces personnel living somewhere else
- people who live or stay at another place most of the time

2. Is this house, apartment, or mobile home —
Mark [X] *ONE box.*
- [ ] Owned by you or someone in this household with a mortgage or loan?
- [ ] Owned by you or someone in this household free and clear (without a mortgage or loan)?
- [ ] Rented for cash rent?
- [ ] Occupied without payment of cash rent?

3. Please answer the following questions for each person living in this house, apartment, or mobile home. Start with the name of one of the people living here who owns, is buying, or rents this house, apartment, or mobile home. If there is no such person, start with any adult living or staying here. We will refer to this person as Person 1.

What is this person's name? *Print name below.*

Last Name
[   ]

First Name   MI
[   ] [   ]

OMB No. 0607-0856: Approval Expires 12/31/2000

Form **D-61A**

4. What is Person 1's telephone number? *We may call this person if we don't understand an answer.*
Area Code + Number
[   ] [   ] [   ] — [   ] [   ] [   ]

5. What is Person 1's sex? *Mark* [X] *ONE box.*
- [ ] Male   [ ] Female

6. What is Person 1's age and what is Person 1's date of birth?
Age on April 1, 2000
[   ] [   ]

Print numbers in boxes.
Month   Day   Year of birth
[   ] [   ] [   ] [   ] [   ]

→ **NOTE: Please answer BOTH Questions 7 and 8.**

7. Is Person 1 Spanish/Hispanic/Latino? *Mark* [X] *the "No" box if* **not** *Spanish/Hispanic/Latino.*
- [ ] **No,** not Spanish/Hispanic/Latino
- [ ] Yes, Mexican, Mexican Am., Chicano
- [ ] Yes, other Spanish/Hispanic/Latino — *Print group.*
- [ ] Yes, Puerto Rican
- [ ] Yes, Cuban

[   ]

8. What is Person 1's race? *Mark* [X] *one or more races* to indicate what this person considers himself/herself to be.
- [ ] White
- [ ] Black, African Am., or Negro
- [ ] American Indian or Alaska Native — *Print name of enrolled or principal tribe.*

[   ]

- [ ] Asian Indian [ ] Japanese   [ ] Native Hawaiian
- [ ] Chinese   [ ] Korean   [ ] Guamanian or Chamorro
- [ ] Filipino   [ ] Vietnamese [ ] Samoan
- [ ] Other Asian — *Print race.*   [ ] Other Pacific Islander — *Print race.*

[   ]

- [ ] Some other race — *Print race.*

[   ]

→ **If more people live here, continue with Person 2.**

FIGURE 8-2 The United States Census Questionnaire (Informational Copy).
Source: U.S. Census Bureau, *http://www.census.gov.*

Person 2

1. What is Person 2's name? *Print name below.*

Last Name

First Name   MI

2. How is this person related to Person 1? *Mark ☒ ONE box.*

☐ Husband/wife
☐ Natural-born son/daughter
☐ Adopted son/daughter
☐ Stepson/stepdaughter
☐ Brother/sister
☐ Father/mother
☐ Grandchild
☐ Parent-in-law
☐
☐ Other relative — *Print exact relationship.* →

If NOT RELATED to Person 1:

☐ Roomer, boarder
☐ Housemate, roommate
☐ Unmarried partner
☐ Foster child
☐ Other nonrelative

Son-in-law/daughter-in-law

3. What is this person's sex? *Mark ☒ ONE box.*

☐ Male ☐ Female

4. What is this person's age and what is this person's date of birth? *Print numbers in boxes.*

Age on April 1, 2000   Month   Day   Year of birth

→ **NOTE: Please answer BOTH Questions 5 and 6.**

5. Is this person Spanish/Hispanic/Latino? *Mark ☒ the "No" box if not Spanish/Hispanic/Latino.*

☐ No, not Spanish/Hispanic/Latino   ☐ Yes, Puerto Rican
☐ Yes, Mexican, Mexican Am., Chicano ☐ Yes, Cuban
☐ Yes, other Spanish/Hispanic/Latino — *Print group.* ⟋

6. What is this person's race? *Mark ☒ one or more races to indicate what this person considers himself/herself to be.*

☐ White
☐ Black, African Am., or Negro
☐ American Indian or Alaska Native — *Print name of enrolled or principal tribe.* ⟋

☐ Asian Indian ☐ Japanese ☐ Native Hawaiian
☐ Chinese   ☐ Korean   ☐ Guamanian or Chamorro
☐ Filipino   ☐ Vietnamese ☐ Samoan
☐ Other Asian — *Print race.* ⟋   ☐ Other Pacific Islander — *Print race.* ⟋

☐ Some other race — *Print race.* ⟋

→ **If more people live here, continue with Person 3.**

Person 3

1. What is Person 3's name? *Print name below.*

Last Name

First Name   MI

2. How is this person related to Person 1? *Mark ☒ ONE box.*

☐ Husband/wife
☐ Natural-born son/daughter
☐ Adopted son/daughter
☐ Stepson/stepdaughter
☐ Brother/sister
☐ Father/mother
☐ Grandchild
☐ Parent-in-law
☐
☐ Other relative — *Print exact relationship.* →

If NOT RELATED to Person 1:

☐ Roomer, boarder
☐ Housemate, roommate
☐ Unmarried partner
☐ Foster child
☐ Other nonrelative

Son-in-law/daughter-in-law

3. What is this person's sex? *Mark ☒ ONE box.*

☐ Male ☐ Female

4. What is this person's age and what is this person's date of birth? *Print numbers in boxes.*

Age on April 1, 2000   Month   Day   Year of birth

→ **NOTE: Please answer BOTH Questions 5 and 6.**

5. Is this person Spanish/Hispanic/Latino? *Mark ☒ the "No" box if not Spanish/Hispanic/Latino.*

☐ No, not Spanish/Hispanic/Latino   ☐ Yes, Puerto Rican
☐ Yes, Mexican, Mexican Am., Chicano ☐ Yes, Cuban
☐ Yes, other Spanish/Hispanic/Latino — *Print group.* ⟋

6. What is this person's race? *Mark ☒ one or more races to indicate what this person considers himself/herself to be.*

☐ White
☐ Black, African Am., or Negro
☐ American Indian or Alaska Native — *Print name of enrolled or principal tribe.* ⟋

☐ Asian Indian ☐ Japanese ☐ Native Hawaiian
☐ Chinese   ☐ Korean   ☐ Guamanian or Chamorro
☐ Filipino   ☐ Vietnamese ☐ Samoan
☐ Other Asian — *Print race.* ⟋   ☐ Other Pacific Islander — *Print race.* ⟋

☐ Some other race — *Print race.* ⟋

→ **If more people live here, continue with Person 4.**

FIGURE 8-2 (continued)

Person 4

Information about children helps your community plan for child care, education, and recreation.

1. What is Person 4's name? *Print name below.*

Last Name

First Name   MI

2. How is this person related to Person 1? *Mark ☒ ONE box.*

☐ Husband/wife
☐ Natural-born son/daughter
☐ Adopted son/daughter
☐ Stepson/stepdaughter
☐ Brother/sister
☐ Father/mother
☐ Grandchild
☐ Parent-in-law
☐ Son-in-law/daughter-in-law
☐ Other relative — *Print exact relationship.*

If NOT RELATED to Person 1:
☐ Roomer, boarder
☐ Housemate, roommate
☐ Unmarried partner
☐ Foster child
☐ Other nonrelative

Son-in-law/daughter-in-law

3. What is this person's sex? *Mark ☒ ONE box.*
☐ Male ☐ Female

4. What is this person's age and what is this person's date of birth? *Print numbers in boxes.*
Age on April 1, 2000   Month   Day   Year of birth

→ **NOTE: Please answer BOTH Questions 5 and 6.**

5. Is this person Spanish/Hispanic/Latino? *Mark ☒ the "No" box if not Spanish/Hispanic/Latino.*

☐ No, not Spanish/Hispanic/Latino   ☐ Yes, Puerto Rican
☐ Yes, Mexican, Mexican Am., Chicano   ☐ Yes, Cuban
☐ Yes, other Spanish/Hispanic/Latino — *Print group.*

6. What is this person's race? *Mark ☒ one or more races to indicate what this person considers himself/herself to be.*

☐ White
☐ Black, African Am., or Negro
☐ American Indian or Alaska Native — *Print name of enrolled or principal tribe.*

☐ Asian Indian ☐ Japanese ☐ Native Hawaiian
☐ Chinese ☐ Korean ☐ Guamanian or Chamorro
☐ Filipino ☐ Vietnamese ☐ Samoan
☐ Other Asian — *Print race.* ☐ Other Pacific Islander — *Print race.*

☐ Some other race — *Print race.*

→ **If more people live here, continue with Person 5.**

Person 5

Knowing about age, race, and sex helps your community better meet the needs of everyone.

1. What is Person 5's name? *Print name below.*

Last Name

First Name   MI

2. How is this person related to Person 1? *Mark ☒ ONE box.*

☐ Husband/wife
☐ Natural-born son/daughter
☐ Adopted son/daughter
☐ Stepson/stepdaughter
☐ Brother/sister
☐ Father/mother
☐ Grandchild
☐ Parent-in-law
☐ Other relative — *Print exact relationship.*

If NOT RELATED to Person 1:
☐ Roomer, boarder
☐ Housemate, roommate
☐ Unmarried partner
☐ Foster child
☐ Other nonrelative

Son-in-law/daughter-in-law

3. What is this person's sex? *Mark ☒ ONE box.*
☐ Male ☐ Female

4. What is this person's age and what is this person's date of birth? *Print numbers in boxes.*
Age on April 1, 2000   Month   Day   Year of birth

→ **NOTE: Please answer BOTH Questions 5 and 6.**

5. Is this person Spanish/Hispanic/Latino? *Mark ☒ the "No" box if not Spanish/Hispanic/Latino.*

☐ No, not Spanish/Hispanic/Latino   ☐ Yes, Puerto Rican
☐ Yes, Mexican, Mexican Am., Chicano   ☐ Yes, Cuban
☐ Yes, other Spanish/Hispanic/Latino — *Print group.*

6. What is this person's race? *Mark ☒ one or more races to indicate what this person considers himself/herself to be.*

☐ White
☐ Black, African Am., or Negro
☐ American Indian or Alaska Native — *Print name of enrolled or principal tribe.*

☐ Asian Indian ☐ Japanese ☐ Native Hawaiian
☐ Chinese ☐ Korean ☐ Guamanian or Chamorro
☐ Filipino ☐ Vietnamese ☐ Samoan
☐ Other Asian — *Print race.* ☐ Other Pacific Islander — *Print race.*

☐ Some other race — *Print race.*

→ **If more people live here, continue with Person 6.**

1042

FIGURE 8-2   (continued)

Person 6

Your answers help
your community plan
for the future.

1. **What is Person 6's name?** *Print name below.*
   Last Name

   First Name   MI

2. **How is this person related to Person 1?** *Mark ☒ ONE box.*

   - ☐ Husband/wife
   - ☐ Natural-born son/daughter
   - ☐ Adopted son/daughter
   - ☐ Stepson/stepdaughter
   - ☐ Brother/sister
   - ☐ Father/mother
   - ☐ Grandchild
   - ☐ Parent-in-law
   - ☐
   - ☐ Other relative — *Print exact relationship.* ➔

   If NOT RELATED to Person 1:
   - ☐ Roomer, boarder
   - ☐ Housemate, roommate
   - ☐ Unmarried partner
   - ☐ Foster child
   - ☐ Other nonrelative

3. **What is this person's sex?** *Mark ☒ ONE box.*
   - ☐ Male   ☐ Female

4. **What is this person's age and what is this person's date of birth?** *Print numbers in boxes.*
   Age on April 1, 2000   Month   Day   Year of birth

➔ **NOTE: Please answer BOTH Questions 5 and 6.**

5. **Is this person Spanish / Hispanic / Latino?** *Mark ☒ the "No" box if not Spanish/Hispanic/Latino.*
   - ☐ **No,** not Spanish/Hispanic/Latino
   - ☐ Yes, Mexican, Mexican Am., Chicano
   - ☐ Yes, Puerto Rican
   - ☐ Yes, Cuban
   - ☐ Yes, other Spanish/Hispanic/Latino — *Print group.* ➘

6. **What is this person's race?** *Mark ☒ one or more races to indicate what this person considers himself/herself to be.*
   - ☐ White
   - ☐ Black, African Am., or Negro
   - ☐ American Indian or Alaska Native — *Print name of enrolled or principal tribe.* ➘

   - ☐ Asian Indian
   - ☐ Chinese
   - ☐ Filipino
   - ☐ Other Asian — *Print race.* ➘
   - ☐ Japanese
   - ☐ Korean
   - ☐ Vietnamese
   - ☐ Native Hawaiian
   - ☐ Guamanian or Chamorro
   - ☐ Samoan
   - ☐ Other Pacific Islander — *Print race.* ➘

   - ☐ Some other race — *Print race.* ➘

➔ **If more people live here, list their names on the back of this page in the spaces provided.**

FIGURE 8-2 (continued)

Persons 7 – 12

If you didn't have room to list everyone who lives in this house or apartment, please list the others below. *You may be contacted by the Census Bureau for the same information about these people.*

Person 7 — Last Name

First Name   MI

Person 8 — Last Name

First Name   MI

Person 9 — Last Name

First Name   MI

Person 10 — Last Name

First Name   MI

Person 11 — Last Name

First Name   MI

Person 12 — Last Name

First Name   MI

The Census Bureau estimates that, for the average household, this form will take about 10 minutes to complete, including the time for reviewing the instructions and answers. Comments about the estimate should be directed to the Associate Director for Finance and Administration, Attn: Paperwork Reduction Project 0607-0856, Room 3104, Federal Building 3, Bureau of the Census, Washington, DC 20233.

Respondents are not required to respond to any information collection unless it displays a valid approval number from the Office of Management and Budget.

Thank you for completing your official U.S. Census 2000 form.

The "Informational Copy" shows the content of the United States Census 2000 "short" form questionnaire. Each household will receive either a short form (100-percent questions) or a long form (100-percent and sample questions). The short form questionnaire contains 6 population questions and 1 housing question. On average, about 5 in every 6 households will receive the short form. The content of the forms resulted from reviewing the 1990 census data, consulting with federal and non-federal data users, and conducting tests.

For additional information about Census 2000, visit our website at **www.census.gov** or write to the Director, Bureau of the Census, Washington, DC 20233.

FOR OFFICE USE ONLY

A. JIC1   **B.** JIC2   **C.** JIC3   **D.** JIC4

FIGURE 8-2 (continued)

TABLE 8-6 Estimated Timing of Each Billion of World Population

Population	Time Taken to Reach	Year Attained
First billion	2–5 million years	About 1800 A.D.
Second billion	Approx. 130 years	1930
Third billion	30 years	1960
Fourth billion	15 years	1975
Fifth billion	13 years	1988
Sixth billion	11 years	1999
PROJECTIONS:		
Seventh billion	14 years	2013
Eighth billion	15 years	2028
Ninth billion	20 years	2048

Source: Adapted from "World Population—1950 to 2050," United States Census Bureau, International Data Base, *http://www.census.gov.*

TABLE 8-7 Ten Largest Cities in the World in 1990, 2000, and 2010

1990	Population (in Millions)	2000	Population (in Millions)	2010 (Projected)	Population (in Millions)
1. Tokyo	25.1	1. Tokyo	26.4	1. Tokyo	26.4
2. New York	16.1	2. Mexico City	18.1	2. Bombay	23.6
3. Mexico City	15.1	3. Bombay	18.1	3. Lagos	20.2
4. Sao Paulo	15.1	4. Sao Paulo	17.8	4. Sao Paulo	19.7
5. Shanghai	13.3	5. New York	16.6	5. Mexico City	18.7
6. Bombay	12.2	6. Lagos	13.4	6. Dhaka	18.4
7. Los Angeles	11.5	7. Los Angeles	13.1	7. New York	17.2
8. Buenos Aires	11.2	8. Calcutta	12.9	8. Karachi	16.6
9. Osaka	11.0	9. Shanghai	12.9	9. Calcutta	15.6
10. Calcutta	10.9	10. Buenos Aires	12.6	10. Jakarta	15.3

Source: Adapted from *Trading Places on the Top 30 List*, United Nations World Urbanization Prospects, 1999.

Most of the current growth is taking place in the less developed regions of the world. Table 8-7 lists the ten largest cities in the world in 1990, 2000, and 2010. As can be seen, there was a clear shift in their ranking.

The difference in growth rate (mainly because of a difference in fertility behavior) also is evident when comparing the age pyramids of the developed (e.g., western Europe) and the developing (e.g., western Africa) regions of the world (Figure 8-3). The age profile of the developing nations clearly is expansive, whereas the developed regions are nearly stationary.

Table 8-8 summarizes many demographic indicators for the world's continents. Asia is by far the most populous, although its current rate of

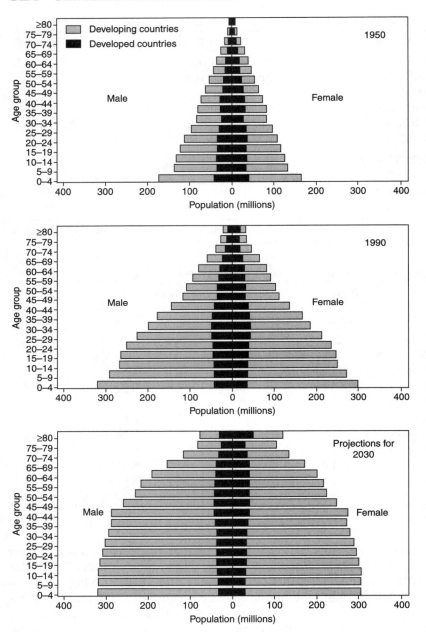

FIGURE 8-3 World Population Pyramids by Age and Sex Distribution, 1950, 1990, and 2030. *Source:* Adapted from Public Health and Aging: Trends in Aging—United States and Worldwide, CDC, *MMWR,* 52, no. 6 (2003):101–106.

TABLE 8-8 Estimated Annual World Population Increments and Distribution Areas, 1950 to 2000 (Millions)

Major Area	1950–1955	1955–1960	1960–1965	1965–1970	1970–1975	1975–1980	1980–1985	1985–1990	1990–1995	1995–2000
World	47.0	53.1	62.7	71.4	74.9	72.8	79.0	86.1	81.4	79.0
More developed regions	10.1	10.4	10.2	8.2	8.0	6.9	6.4	6.7	5.1	3.5
Less developed regions	37.0	42.7	52.5	63.2	66.9	65.9	72.5	79.4	76.3	75.5
Least developed countries	4.0	4.9	6.0	7.1	8.0	9.0	10.5	12.4	14.7	15.5
Less developed regions w/o the least developed countries	33.0	37.8	46.4	56.1	58.9	57.0	62.0	67.0	61.6	60.0
Europe	5.6	5.8	5.9	4.4	3.9	3.4	2.7	3.1	1.3	-0.3
North America	3.1	3.5	3.1	2.5	2.3	2.3	2.7	2.8	3.1	3.2
Oceania	0.3	0.3	0.4	0.4	0.4	0.2	0.4	0.4	0.4	0.4
Africa	5.1	6.1	7.3	8.6	9.9	12.2	14.4	16.1	16.8	18.0
Asia	28.3	31.9	39.6	48.7	50.9	46.8	50.9	55.8	51.8	49.8
Latin America/Caribbean	4.7	5.5	6.4	6.9	7.4	7.9	7.9	7.9	7.9	7.8

Source: Adapted from *World Population Prospects: The 2000 Revision*, Volume III, United Nations Population Division.

natural increase is third to Africa and Latin America. Europe and North America have low rates of natural increase and the percentage of their population over the age of 64 is correspondingly high. They also have the highest life expectancy at birth and the highest percent urban population. Per capita gross national product is highest in North America, Oceania, and Europe, while the crude death rate is lowest in Oceania, followed by North America, Latin America, Europe, and the former Soviet Union.

United States and Canada

In both the United States and Canada, the most striking recent demographic trend is the aging of the population. As far back as 1980, the median age of the U.S. population was 30.2 years, whereas Canada's was slightly below this at 29.9 years. This median age was the same as in 1950, before the postwar baby boom. By the year 2000 the median age of the United States increased to 35.3 years while that of Canada climbed to 36.8 years. The increase in median ages across these two countries can be attributed to the general decline in fertility, which is more pronounced in Canada than in the United States, and the general increase in average life span witnessed during the later part of the twentieth century. The baby boom cohort, which was 20 to 34 years in 1980, became 40 to 54 years in 2000. This is the age group that has shown the largest relative increase in population within this period.[50]

The Depression cohort (babies born in the Depression years of low birth rates) is now 60 and over, so this group decreased between 1970 and 1980 with even further decreases in 1990 and 2000. Table 8-9 shows the 1990 and 2000 distribution of the population by age group in the United States.

The changing age structure in both the United States and Canada is a result of the change in fertility behavior. Both the crude birth rate and the general fertility rate decreased dramatically between 1950 and 1995 but increased slightly thereafter (Table 8-10). These changes in fertility can be observed at every age (Figure 8-4).

The fertility rate in Canada has continued to drop relative to that of the United States since the mid-1990s. The birth rate in Canada was 1.52 children per woman in 1999 compared with 2.08 per woman in the United States for the same period. It is projected that given the current trend in Canada's birth rate, the natural increase will become negative within the next twenty years. The situation in the United States is not expected to be as acute within this period. The aging of the U.S. population is less rapid than in Canada because of its higher fertility rate. In 1990, 12.6 percent of the U.S. population was 65 and over, compared with 11.6 percent in Canada

TABLE 8-9   United States Population by Age Group, 1990 and 2000

Age Group	Percentage 1990	2000
Under 5	7.4	6.8
5–9	7.3	7.3
10–14	6.9	7.3
15–19	7.1	7.2
20–24	7.6	6.7
25–34	8.6	14.2
35–44	15.1	16.0
45–54	10.2	13.4
55–59	4.2	4.8
60–64	4.3	3.8
65 and over	12.6	12.4

Source: Adapted from *Demographic Trends in the Twentieth Century and Census 2000, Summary File 1*, United States Census Bureau, 2000.

TABLE 8-10   Crude Birth Rates and General Fertility Rates; United States, 1950 to 2000

Year	Crude Birth Rate per 1,000 Population	General Fertility Rate per 1,000 women (15–44)
1950	24.1	106.2
1960	23.7	118.0
1970	18.4	87.9
1980	15.9	68.4
1990	16.7	70.9
1995	14.8	65.6
2000	14.7	67.5

Source: U.S. Department of Health and Human Resources, "National Center for Health Statistics," *Health, United States,* 2002. Hyattsville, MD (2003):83.

by 1991. By 2000, 12.4 percent of the U.S. population was 65 and over, whereas Canada's was 13.0 percent in 2001.

The total fertility rate in the United States in the early 1980s was about 1.8 births per woman, in contrast to nearly 3.7 in the late 1950s. The average family size declined correspondingly, from a high of 3.67 in 1960 to 3.28 in 1980. The marriage rate decreased from 90.2 marriages per year per 1,000 unmarried women age 15 and older in 1950 to 64.6 in 1981.[51]

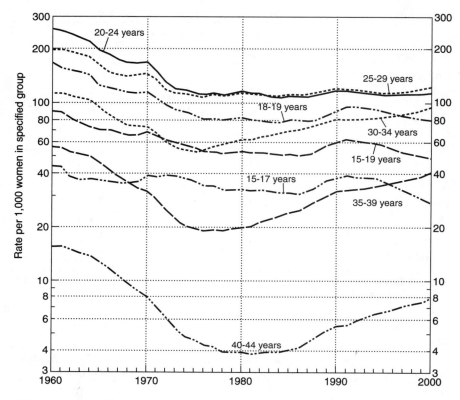

FIGURE 8-4   Age-Specific Fertility Rates, United States, 1960 to 2000.
Source: National Center for Health Statistics, *National Vital Statistics Report* 50, no. 5 (2002): 5.

The divorce rate appeared to be leveling off at around 22.8 divorces per 1,000 married women ages 15 and older, after having more than doubled since 1967 and almost tripled since 1940.[52] The proportion of nonfamily households (individuals living alone or sharing living quarters with unrelated persons) increased from 18.8 percent in 1970 to 26.6 percent in 1980.

Although fertility rates in the United States are low, teenage rates are very high as compared to other industrialized countries (Table 8-11). There were 54.26 births per 1,000 women under 20 years of age in the United States from 1995 to 2000, compared to 20.11 in Canada, 9.83 in France, 7.22 in Israel, and only 5.21 in The Netherlands.

TABLE 8-11 Fertility Rates and Percentage of All Births for Women under 20 Years of Age (Selected Countries, 1995–2000)

Country	Births per 1,000 Women under 20 Years	Percentage of All Births (year 2000)
Brazil	74.07	16
Canada	20.11	8
Denmark	8.02	3
France	9.83	3
Germany	12.78	4
Israel	7.22	4
Mexico	69.52	13
Russia	35.63	17
Sierra Leone	211.90	17
Sweden	7.25	2
Thailand	50.31	20
The Netherlands	5.21	1
Uganda	211.30	13
United States	54.26	15

Source: Generated from *The World Youth, 2000,* Population Reference Bureau (PRB).

However, as shown in Table 8-12, teenage fertility in the United States decreased slightly after 1995, and even though the decline was more rapid for blacks than for whites, the fertility rates in 2000 remained almost twice as high for black teenagers than for whites.

Impact of Demographic Trends on Utilization

As noted extensively throughout this book, many demographic characteristics of the population are related to health, disease, and service utilization. Therefore, it is obvious that demographic trends have definite health policy implications. This section briefly examines, for illustrative purposes, the impact on the health care system of three important demographic trends: (1) the post–World War II baby boom, (2) the aging of the population, and (3) the millennial generation.

TABLE 8-12   Race-Specific Teenage Fertility Rates: United States, 1980 to 2000

	TOTAL			WHITE			BLACK		
				Age Groups					
Year	*10–14*	*15–17*	*18–19*	*10–14*	*15–17*	*18–19*	*10–14*	*15–17*	*18–19*
1980	1.1	32.5	82.1	0.6	25.5	73.2	4.3	72.5	135.1
1983	1.1	31.8	77.4	0.6	25.0	68.8	4.1	69.6	127.1
1985	1.2	31.0	79.6	0.6	24.4	70.4	4.5	69.3	132.4
1988	1.3	33.6	79.9	0.6	26.0	69.6	4.9	75.7	142.7
1990	1.4	37.5	88.6	0.7	29.5	78.0	4.9	82.3	152.9
1993	1.4	37.8	92.1	0.8	30.3	82.1	4.6	79.8	151.9
1995	1.3	36.0	89.1	0.8	30.0	81.2	4.2	69.7	137.1
1998	1.0	30.4	82.0	0.6	25.9	74.6	2.9	56.8	126.9
2000	0.9	27.4	79.2	0.6	23.6	72.7	2.4	50.4	121.3

Source: National Center for Health Statistics, *National Vital Statistics Report* 50, no. 5 (2002).

*The sum of white and black fertility rates do not equal total since the numerators and denominators of the calculated rates are different. For example, white (10–14) births = 8, population is 890, therefore, rate is 8.9. For black (10–14) births = 18, population is 1245, therefore, rate is 14.5. Total (10–14) births = 26, population is 2,135, therefore, rate is 12.2.

The Baby Boom

Between 1946 and 1964, 76.4 million babies were born in the United States, one-third of the total population in 1980 and one-quarter of the population today. The postwar increase in the fertility rate occurred in many countries, including Canada, New Zealand, Australia, and the former Soviet Union. The baby boom created unusually large cohorts of births compared to those of the 1930s and early 1940s and compared to the baby bust years of the 1960s and 1970s.[53] As one author put it, the boom generation can be thought of as a "moving bulge in the population that, like a pig swallowed by a python, causes stretch marks and discomfort along the way."[54]

The moving through time of the baby boom cohort (Figure 8-5) by the early 1980s was mostly between ages 20 and 30. The small proportion of the population ages 45 to 49 at that time (65 to 69 in 2000) reflects the depression cohort, while the drop in fertility in more recent years is shown in the baby bust cohort under 40 (year 2000). The population distribution over 50 resembles a pyramid as older age groups are thinned by death.

The fact that there was a great upsurge in fertility between 1945 and 1960 affects all aspects of people's daily lives. Contrary to the Depression or the "good times" cohort, which "by virtue of this smaller number, upon encountering each inpatient lifecycle event [has] experienced relative abundance,"[55] the baby boom cohort has been experiencing, and can expect, problems and frustrations as it passes through the lifecycle.[56] Problems of overcrowded classrooms and shortages of teachers through the 1960s and 1970s and school closings and unemployment problems in the 1980s are all related directly to the baby boom phenomenon.

The recent increase in the number of births and in the crude birth rate during the 1970s and the early 1980s was also caused by the baby boom of

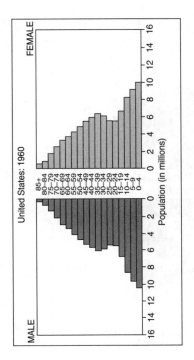

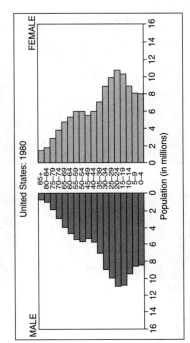

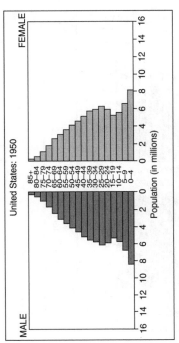

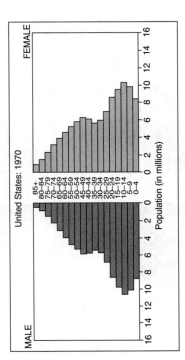

FIGURE 8-5 Population Age-Sex Pyramids, United States, 1950 to 2050. *Source:* Printed from U.S. Census Bureau, Population Division, International Programs Center Branch, August 2003, *http://www.census.gov.*

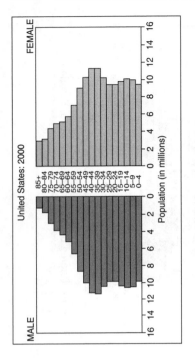

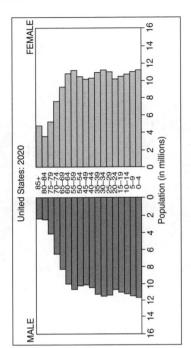

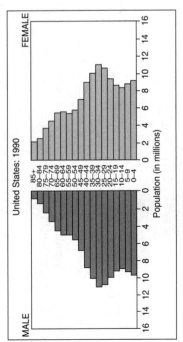

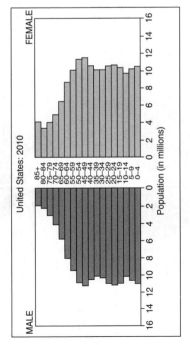

FIGURE 8-5 (continued)

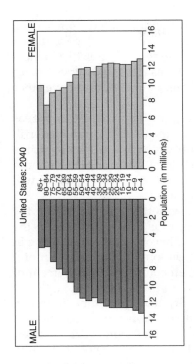

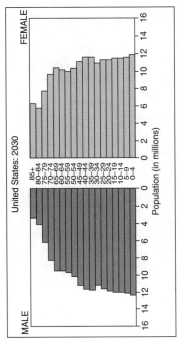

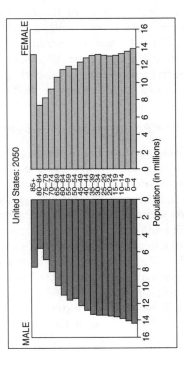

FIGURE 8-5 (continued)

the 1950s. The so-called echo effect of the baby boom resulted from several factors including the baby boom generation postponing marriage and children.[57] Thereafter the total fertility rate (TFR) rose slowly (after 1986) reaching 2.08 by 1990. Although the total fertility rate has remained above 2 since the late 1980s, the total births peaked at 4.2 million in 1990 and have since declined slightly to about 3.9 million.

The number of births remained fairly high in the early 1990s but, as Figure 8-5 projects, they should continue to decline (even though the fertility rate remains constant) because the baby bust cohort is now in its prime childbearing ages (1995 to 2005). Thereafter the number of births should remain constant at the level of the 1990s because the age-sex pyramid will assume a somewhat stationary, rectangular profile.

As the baby boom generation ages and as fertility remains low, the median age of the population is pushed up, thus artificially raising the crude death rate.[58] When the baby boom cohort becomes elderly, starting in 2020, crude death rates will go up even more, as some 15 percent (or more) of the population then will be 65 or older when compared to 11 percent of the same age group in 1980.

Meanwhile, using the age-specific mortality and morbidity figures in Chapter 5, it can be projected that if rates for these factors remain constant, or nearly constant, the number of motor vehicle accidents, homicides, suicides, and cases of depression and heart disease will continue to increase through the early and middle parts of the twenty-first century. This projection is because the baby boom cohort will have entered the age 65 and over category by the year 2012 or thereabout. Similarly, if morbidity rates remain constant, the prevalence of cancers, heart diseases, stroke, and respiratory conditions will continue to increase during the early 2000s, using age as the major determinant. Obviously other factors operate to change the disease patterns.

Aging of the Population: The Senior Boom

In the year 2000, the number of Americans age 65 and older reached an estimated 35 million, an average of 13 percent of the total population. With declining birth rates and a progressively aging population, people 65 and older (especially those 75 and older) are the fastest growing group in America.[59] As shown in Table 8-13, the proportion of the United States population age 65 and older rose from 4.1 percent in 1900 to 12.8 percent in the year 2000. As a result of low birth rates and greater life expectancy, the proportion of the elderly (age 65 and older) has gone up from 4 percent in 1900 to about 13 percent in the year 2000. If this trend continues, this proportion is expected to rise to 20 percent by the year 2030 (meaning 1 in every 5 Americans will be age 65 or older).

Because of the effects of the small Depression cohorts, this growth slowed in the 1990s and is expected to remain slow in the first decade of the

TABLE 8-13   Percentage of Population 65 and Older: United States, 1900 to 2050

Year	% of Total Population Ages 65 and Older	Median Age of Total Population
1900	4.1	22.9
1910	4.3	24.1
1920	4.7	25.3
1930	5.5	26.5
1940	6.8	29.0
1950	8.1	30.2
1960	9.2	29.5
1970	9.8	28.1
1980	11.2	30.2
1990	12.5	32.9
2000	12.8	35.3
PROJECTIONS:		
2010	13.3	36.9
2020	16.4	38.0
2030	20.1	39.0
2040	20.7	39.1
2050	20.4	39.1

Source: Adapted from *Older Population by Age: 1900–2050*, based on U.S. Census Bureau data, United States Administration on Aging, February 2003.

2000s. Thereafter, however, the baby boom (1946 to 1965) cohort will become a senior boom and the proportion of the population over age 65 will grow rapidly to about 20 percent by the year 2030. Again, after 2030, the population of this group probably will fall sharply as the baby bust cohorts of the 1960s and 1970s become age 65 and over.[60]

In the United States in 2002, life expectancy at age 65 is more than 16.6 years for men and 19.5 years for women. Age-specific death rates for males 65 to 74 years declined by almost 40 percent between 1950 and 2000; for females, approximately 42 percent.[61]

The leading causes of death in the elderly were the same in 2000 as in the 1950s, with heart disease, cancer, and stroke accounting for over 75 percent of all causes.[62] Mortality trends from heart disease parallel the decline for all other causes combined. Death rates from stroke have been falling even more rapidly than the death rates from heart disease. However, death rates from cancer have been rising, with rapid increases in recent years resulting primarily from cancer of the lung. Older people generally require more health and social services than the general population, especially after age 75. Arthritis and rheumatism, followed closely by heart conditions, are the most common causes of activity limitation at age 65 and over.[63] A study conducted as early as 1982 reported that 39 percent of more than 4,200 individuals age 65 and over had some form of hypertension with about 25 percent of these either untreated or poorly controlled.[64] Hearing impairment affects 21 percent of the elderly population.[65]

These problems are important factors because they often lead to withdrawal, isolation, depression, further disability, and dependence.[66] Finally, approximately half the elderly individuals have no teeth, or dentures that fit poorly or do not wear,[67] predisposing them to malnutrition and increasing their already high susceptibility to disease and disability.[68] Health services utilization is higher among the elderly population. In 1980 in the United States, persons aged 65 and over averaged 6.4 physician visits during the year as compared to 5.1 for those 45 to 64, and 4.4 for those under the age of 45.[69] There is every indication that these differences are widening especially with the advancing medical technology and efforts to increase longevity. Rates of hospital utilization also are much higher for the elderly, who occupy more than 30 percent of acute care beds while comprising only 1.6 percent of the total population.[70]

The impact of aging on health care utilization is, of course, highly dependent on this group's health. However, it is not easy to determine what changes are related to age and occur in everyone and which ones are pathologic and represent the development of disease.[71] Death, disease, and disability in the older population stem mostly from chronic conditions. These tend to originate early in life and develop gradually.

This does not mean, however, that the elderly population in the years to come will be a sicker population.[72] Fries predicts a continued decline in premature deaths resulting from chronic conditions and the emergence of a pattern of natural death at the end of a natural life span.[73] As he points out, some chronic illnesses definitely can be stopped. Elimination of cigarette smoking greatly delays the date of emphysema onset and reduces the risk of lung cancer.

The decline in mortality rates, which is caused principally by a drop in arteriosclerosis and cerebrovascular disease, is the first demonstration of a national decrease in mortality rates from a major chronic disease. It is attributed by most observers to changes in lifestyle (primary prevention) and to better treatment of hypertension (secondary prevention).[74] Fries suggests that through further lifestyle changes, chronic illnesses can be postponed and morbidity can be compressed until near the end of life span (which he calculates as ideally 85 years).

The impact aging of the population will have on the health care system thus is dependent on present health policy. An effective health care policy for the elderly should stress health maintenance and promotion, disease prevention, comprehensive and integrated health and social services, and personal autonomy and social interaction.

Millennial Generation

The new generation—the millennial generation—was born according to various demographers sometime between 1977 and 2002 and is currently in the age range of 2 to 25. In the year 2000, the millennial generation totaled up to 77–79 million in population and represents the single highest generation in the past one hundred years—even slightly larger than the huge years of the baby boomers. They follow Generation X where there was a significant decline in the annual marker of births between 1965 and 1980–82. This new millennium generation will have a dramatic impact on business and health care institutions for the pre-teen, adolescent, and young adult groups. Their impact on school systems has been overwhelming and, further, they will have an impact on the labor markets and housing environment. As this generation matures, they will make a significant impact on the health care system, more specifically, if they begin to produce children at a rate equal to or greater than that which was produced during the baby boom generation, there will be an unprecedented high birth rate that could quite easily outpace any previous birth rate in the past century. This generation is reinvigorating the youth market—with more emphasis placed on civic, service, and teamwork aspects of life. This generation could quite easily establish a new consciousness in an era of uncertainty in world affairs.[75]

Summary

Demography is one of the disciplines necessary for the use of epidemiology in health services management. It supplies the tools for the analysis of population composition and distribution, of changes in its components, and for the estimation and projection of health care's future.

All of these are essential for an epidemiologic approach to health services management because health, disease, and utilization are all related to population characteristics. Furthermore, demographers supply health services managers with some of the tools, including methods for estimating and projecting population, needed to relate the delivery of health services to the population. Accompanying any trend in population, demographics is a health care management implication.

References

1. Population Reference Bureau Staff, "Transitions in World Population," *Population Bulletin* 59, no. 1 (Washington, D.C.: Population Reference Bureau, 2004).
2. H. S. Shryock et al., *The Methods and Materials of Demography*, condensed ed., ed. E. G. Stockwell (San Diego: Academic Press, 1976), 91.
3. United Nations, Population Division of the Department of Economics and Social Affairs, *World Population Prospects, 2000* (2002 revision) New York, NY.

4. United Nations, *World Population Prospects*.
5. U.S. Census Bureau, International Data Base, *http://www.census.gov/ipc/www/idbnew.html*.
6. C. W. Tyler, Jr. and C. W. Warren, "Public Health and Population," in *Maxcy-Rosenau-Last Public Health and Preventive Medicine*, 14th ed., ed. R. B. Wallace, 45–57 (Stamford, Conn.: Appleton and Lange, 1998).
7. Tyler and Warren, "Public Health and Population," 45–57.
8. J. A. McFalls, "Population: A Lively Introduction," 4th ed., *Population Bulletin* 58, no. 4 (Washington, D.C.: Population Reference Bureau, 2003).
9. United Nations, *Demographic Yearbook 2000* (New York, NY Sales Section, United Nations: 2003).
10. United Nations, Department of Economic and Social Affairs Statistics Division, *Principles and Recommendations for Population and Housing Censuses*, Revision 1 (New York, NY Sales Section, United Nations: 1997).
11. United Nations, *Principles and Recommendations for Population and Housing Censuses*.
12. A. Haupt and T. T. Kane, *The Population Reference Bureau's Population Handbook*, 4th ed. (Washington, D.C.: Population Reference Bureau, Inc., 1997), 63.
13. Population Reference Bureau, *2002 World Population Data Sheet of the Population Reference Bureau* (Washington, D.C.: Population Reference Bureau, 2002).
14. A. Haupt and T. Kane, *Population Handbook, International Edition*, 4th ed. (Washington, D.C.: Population Reference Bureau, 1998), 51.
15. U.S. Office of Management and Budget, *Final Report and Recommendations from the Metropolitan Area Standards Review Committee to the Office of Management and Budget Concerning Changes to the Standards for Defining Metropolitan Areas* (Washington, D.C.: 2000, U.S. OMB), *http://www.whitehouse.gov/omb/inforeg/metro2000.pdf*.
16. T. C. Ricketts et al., *Using Geographic Methods to Understand Health Issues* (Rockville, Md.: Agency for Health Care Policy and Research, 1997), 3.
17. Population Reference Bureau, *2002 World Population Data Sheet of the Population Reference Bureau*.
18. M. R. Lavin, *Understanding the Census: A Guide for Marketers, Planners, Grant Writers and Other Data Users* (Kennore, N.Y.: Epoch Books, Inc., 1996), 156.
19. D. J. Jolley and P. Elliott, "Socio-economic Confounding," in *Geographical and Environmental Epidemiology: Methods for Small-Area Studies*, eds. P. Elliott et al., 115–124 (Oxford: Oxford University Press, 1996).
20. A. B. Bernstein et al., *Health Care in America: Trends in Utilization* (Hyattsville, Md.: National Center for Health Statistics, 2003), 7.
21. Tyler and Warren, "Public Health and Population," 45–57.
22. Haupt and Kane, *The Population Reference Bureau's Population Handbook*, 14.
23. H. S. Shryock and J. S. Siegel, *The Methods and Materials of Demography*, (NY, NY: Academic Press, 1976), 278.
24. Haupt and Kane, *The Population Reference Bureau's Population Handbook*, 14–15.
25. Haupt and Kane, *The Population Reference Bureau's Population Handbook*, 16–18.
26. Haupt and Kane, *The Population Reference Bureau's Population Handbook*, 16–18.

27. Statistics Canada, CANSIM, Table 051-0004 and Catalogue No. 91-213-XIB, *http://www.statcan.ca/english/Pgdb/demo04a.htm*; Statistics Canada, CANSIM II, Table 051-0001, *http://www.statcan.ca/english/Pgdb/ demo10a.htm*.
28. Haupt and Kane, *The Population Reference Bureau's Population Handbook*, 20–21.
29. Shryock, *The Methods and Materials of Demography*, 283–284.
30. Shryock, *The Methods and Materials of Demography*, 349.
31. Shryock, *The Methods and Materials of Demography*, 349–406.
32. Haupt and Kane, *The Population Reference Bureau's Population Handbook*, 35–37.
33. Haupt and Kane, *The Population Reference Bureau's Population Handbook*, 36.
34. CIA—*The World Factbook—United States, http://www.cia.gov/cia/publications/factbook/geos/us.html*.
35. *Quick Reference Guides on Canada—People: Net Migration Rate (Facts about Canada), http://www.reference-guides.com/cia_world_factbook/Canada/People/ Net_migration_rate/*.
36. Population Reference Bureau, *2002 World Population Data Sheet of the Population Reference Bureau*.
37. D. A. Swanson and J. S. Siegel, *The Methods and Materials of Demography* (San Diego, Calif.: Elsevier Academic Press, 2004).
38. J. P. McManus, ed., *American Demographics* (March 2004):c2, c4, 3, 5, 7, 9, 14, 16, 18, 23, 33.
39. M. J. Batutis, "Estimating Population II," *American Demographics* (May 1982):38–40.
40. M. J. Batutis, "Estimating Population I," *American Demographics* (April 1982):3–5.
41. Shryock, *The Methods and Materials of Demography*, 426–428.
42. Haupt and Kane, *The Population Reference Bureau's Population Handbook*, 45–53.
43. Shryock, *The Methods and Materials of Demography*, 439.
44. Shryock, *The Methods and Materials of Demography*, 439–482.
45. J. Saunders, *Basic Demographic Measures* (Lanham, Md.: University Press of America, 1988), 63–75.
46. R. Arwin, "Methods on Data Sources for Population Projections of Small Areas," in *Population Forecasting for Small Areas*, P. M. Hauser, ed. 15–26 (Oak Ridge, Tenn.: Associated Universities, 1977).
47. Statistics Canada, *How Communities Can Use Statistics* (Ottawa: Minister of Studies and Services, 1981), 53.
48. Statistics Canada, *How Communities Can Use Statistics*, 53.
49. Lavin, *Understanding the Census*, 41.
50. C. Russell, *Demographics of the U.S.: Trends and Projections* (Ithaca, N.Y.: New Strategist Publications, Inc., 2003), 308–309.
51. A. P. Sanoff, "As Americans Cope with a Changing Population," *U.S. News and World Report* 9 (1982):27.
52. J. A. Weed, "Divorce: Americans' Style," *American Demographics* (March 1982):12–17.
53. Haupt and Kane, *The Population Reference Bureau's Population Handbook*, 5–12.
54. L. Y. Jones, *Great Expectations: America and the Baby Boom Generation* (New York: Ballantine Books, 1982), 512.
55. C. L. Harter, "The Good Times' Cohort of the 1930s," *Population Reference Bureau Report* 3, no. 3 (1977):4.

56. Haupt and Kane, *The Population Reference Bureau's Population Handbook*, 12.
57. M. M. Kent and M. Mather, "What Drives U.S. Population Growth?" *Population Bulletin* 57, no. 4 (2002):7.
58. Haupt and Kane, *The Population Reference Bureau's Population Handbook*, 12.
59. B. J. Soldo, "America's Elderly in the 1980s," *Population Bulletin* 35, no. 4 (1980):3.
60. Soldo, "America's Elderly in the 1980s," 7.
61. National Center for Health Statistics, *Health, United States, 2004* (Hyattsville, MD: National Center for Health Statistics, 2004).
62. National Center for Health Statistics, *Health, United States, 2004* (Hyattsville, MD: National Center for Health Statistics, 2004).
63. Metropolitan Life Insurance Company, "Health of the Elderly," *Statistical Bulletin* 63, no. 1 (1982):3.
64. W. E. Hale et al., "Screening for Hypertension in an Elderly Population: Report from the Dunedin Program," *Journal of the American Geriatrics Society* 29 (1981):123–125.
65. A. R. Somers, "The High Cost of Care for the Elderly: Diagnosis, Prognosis, and Some Suggestions for Therapy," *Journal of Health Politics and Law* 3 (1978):163–180.
66. J. G. Ouslander and J. C. Beck, "Defining the Health Problems of the Elderly," *Annual Review of Public Health* 3 (1982):55–83.
67. M. G. Kover, "Health of the Elderly and the Use of Health Services," *Public Health Reports* 1 (1977):9–19.
68. Ouslander and Beck, "Defining the Health Problems of the Elderly," 55–83.
69. Kover, "Health of the Elderly and the Use of Health Services," 5.
70. Soldo, "America's Elderly in the 1980s," 18.
71. Ouslander and Beck, "Defining the Health Problems of the Elderly," 60.
72. National Center for Health Statistics, *Health, United States, 2003* (Hyattsville, Md.: National Center for Health Statistics, 2003), 46.
73. J. F. Fries, "Aging, Natural Death, and the Compression of Morbidity," *New England Journal of Medicine* 303, no. 3 (1980):130–135.
74. M. P. Stern, "The Recent Decline in Ischemic Heart Disease Mortality," *Annals of Internal Medicine* 91 (1979):630–640.
75. S. Mitchell, *American Generations*, 3d ed. (Ithaca, N.Y.: New Strategist Publications, Inc., 2000), 8–12.

9

Evidence-Based Health Services Management— A Practice Approach

In the previous chapters, the focus was on basic health and epidemiological measurement. Specifically, efforts to create a healthy public and models to perform public health and epidemiological practice assessments were outlined and presented. Further, a basic understanding of rates and their role in many health services from an epidemiological perspective was discussed based on concepts of statistical and analytical/empirical thinking. A recurring message throughout this material was that public health managers must make sound scientific decisions based on evidence and must not base decisions on anecdotes, rhetoric, or generalities that reflect unsound nonscientific thought or policies. Thus, this chapter furthers these concepts of promoting evidence-based public health and health services management and presents some very basic strategies for moving public health practice into the assessment, policy development, and assurance activities using evidence for making such decisions.

Public health must reframe, reconstruct, and quit believing the past will create the future. There have been recent accounts by individuals who still believe and espouse the ideas and thoughts that defend the tradition of public health.[1,2,3]

The following thoughts have been expressed "many of our services— WIC, prenatal, health education, for example—are seen as unnecessary and unproductive benefits for undeserving populations,"[4] because Evans believes that, "part of the problem we face is a hardened America, with a mean-spirited, begrudging attitude toward social justice, affirmative action, equity and compassion."[5] Koop suggested that the public must grumble, advocate for programs and offices, stand tall, articulate, and become confrontational.[6] These thoughts will not create a public health practice in the twenty-first century that will be a leader in providing population-based services to communities by implementing the core functions of public health assessment, policy development, and assurance. Public health services are not seen as unnecessary or unproductive because of a hardened attitude toward social justice or equity, but because of the inability to provide evidence that these programs have been necessary or productive. Public health must shelve the rhetoric, reframe the system, and act on evidence-based epidemiological policies. This chapter provides some approaches and directions to take public health into the twenty-first century by using evidence-based tools for the practice of public health and the management and utilization of health services.

Assessing Public Health Evidence

The Institute of Medicine (IOM) Report suggests that public health lacks the infrastructure to successfully complete the core public health functions of assessment, policy development, and assurance. Further, in a recent edition of the *American Journal of Preventive Medicine*, the focus on research and measurement in public health practice is an indication of the need to provide the tools for effective measurement in public health practice. In fact, the main objective of this issue of the *Journal* was how to best measure the effectiveness of public health practice.[7] Attempts to develop a strategy for measuring local public health practice and methods to assess the public health core functions have been demonstrated by several authors.[8,9,10,11]

The great attention to this topic indicates the need for public health practitioners to take notice and recognize that the abilities of the health services sector must be expanded to create public health scientists and health services managers with epidemiologic, behavioral, statistical, and demographics measurement skills.

Richards surveyed local health departments (370) to assess performance of the core functions by asking twenty-six questions related to assessment, policy development, and assurance (Table 9-1). The results clearly indicate public health is weakly positioned to implement evidence-based decisions because only 46 percent of the surveyed health departments do assessment functions. Within this function, the indicators on immunization (No. 7) received the highest response (79 percent) and the hospital indicator (No. 5) received the lowest (18 percent). Of further importance is that the functions of policy development recorded 53 percent and assurance was 68 percent. Within these functions, the indicators scoring the highest were meetings (95 percent), officials (91 percent), media (95 percent), and standards (87 percent). These results indicate that the practitioners of public health in local, state, and federal agencies must expand their capabilities beyond the levels that have been identified and promote population-based health (i.e., public health practice) from an evidenced-based perspective. Public health is failing with a grade of 56 percent. Note the indicators in Table 9-1 that receive a score of 90 percent or better (meetings, officials, and media). The ability to promote the practice of pubic health is excellent, but it is not based on evidence because most evidence-based indicators all reflect values of less than 60 percent.

TABLE 9-1   Assessing Public Health Practices—Core Functions: Assessment, Policy Development, Assurance

Indicator	Question	% Yes*
Assessment		**46**
1. Needs	In the past three years in your jurisdiction, has there been a health needs assessment that included using morbidity, mortality, and vital statistics data?	51
2. Age-specific	In the past three years in your jurisdiction, have there been any age-specific surveys to assess participation in preventive and screening services?	32
3. Behavioral	In the past three years in your jurisdiction, has the population been surveyed for behavioral risk factors?	43
4. Investigation	In the past three years in your jurisdiction, has there been timely investigation of any unusual adverse health events?	65
5. Hospital	In the past three years in your jurisdiction, has there been a review of hospital discharge data to determine age-specific leading causes of hospitalization?	18
6. Work-related	In the past three years in your jurisdiction, has there been a review of work-related morbidity and mortality?	38
7. Immunized	In the past three years in your jurisdiction, has there been an analysis of data on children two years of age who have been immunized with the basic series?	79
8. High-risk	In the past three years in your jurisdiction, has there been an analysis of health services needed by high-risk population groups?	47
Policy Development		**53**
9. Review	In the past three years, has there been a public review of the public health mission for your agency's jurisdiction?	24
10. Meetings	In the past year, as a part of the job, have you and your senior staff members regularly participated in meetings with other community health organizations?	95

TABLE 9-1   (continued)

Indicator	Question	% Yes*
Policy Development (continued)		
11. Officials	In the past year in your jurisdiction, has there been a formal attempt to inform elected officials about the potential public health impact of actions under their consideration?	91
12. Advocates	In the past year in your jurisdiction, have elected or other government officials been strong advocates for public health?	65
13. Prioritized	In the past three years in your jurisdiction, have community health initiatives been prioritized on the basis of established problems and resources?	56
14. Policy	In the past three years, has your health department published an explicit policy agenda for the department?	25
15. Candidates	In the past year, has there been a formal attempt to inform candidates for elective office about health priorities for your jurisdiction?	56
16. Plan developed	In the past year in your jurisdiction, has a community health action plan developed with shared input from local, regional, and state levels been used?	31
17. Plan used	In the past year in your jurisdiction, has a community health action plan, developed with public participation, been used?	19
18. Agreements	In the past three years, has your health department entered into any written agreements with key health care providers or funding sources to define service roles?	63
Assurance		**68**
19. Codes	In the past three years in your jurisdiction, have local health codes been reviewed to ensure they were up to date?	53
20. Standards	In the past three years in your jurisdiction, have public health services been reviewed to ensure they comply with applicable professional and regulatory standards?	87
21. Safety	In the past year in your jurisdiction, has there been a program to ensure environmental safety?	66
22. Access	In the past year in your jurisdiction, has there been a program to ensure access to basic personal health services for those unable to afford them?	69

TABLE 9-1 (continued)

Indicator	Question	% Yes*
Assurance (continued)		
23. Effect	In the past year in your jurisdiction, has there been any evaluation of the effect that public health services have on community health?	37
24. Budget	In the past year in your jurisdiction, has there been any evaluation of the effect that budget changes for your health department would have on public health problems?	55
25. Informing	In the past year in your jurisdiction, has there been a formal attempt to inform the public about health problems?	86
26. Media	In the past year in your jurisdiction, have reports on public health problems been provided to the local media?	95
Overall Total		**56**

*n = 370

Source: Adapted with permission from T. B. Richards et al., "Assessing Public Health Practice: Application of Ten Core Function Measures of Community Health in Six States," in *American Journal of Preventive Medicine*, Vol. 11, No. 6, Supplement, pp. 36–40, ©1995, Oxford University Press.

A study in the state of Washington that evaluated the local health department's capacity using APEX reported similar results.[12] They noted that "the strengths reported by the local health departments in Washington reflect the historical strengths of the public health systems in the United States." [13] That is, they do a good job carrying out the traditional public health functions. However, the weaknesses noted clearly reemphasize the fact that public health is not well positioned to promote evidence-based decisions. They identified four broad areas that reflect significant weaknesses. They are as follows:

1. Inadequate health department access to legal counsel, particularly among smaller health departments
2. Lack of clarity about their mission and role
3. Lack of expertise in data collection and analysis, program evaluation, and community health assessment
4. Inability to use data effectively to guide established community public health priorities and program planning policy[14]

As a result of these identified weaknesses, they call for an increased capacity to collect, analyze, and interpret health data and to use the data to guide policy. The suggestion to place epidemiologists, statisticians, health services managers, and planning and policy officers in local health departments, or alternatively request technical assistance and training for present staff, is a clear signal that the ability to promote evidence-based decisions for planning and policy is greatly needed. Pratt and associates conclude that the changing nature of public health and the management of health services from the individual focus on clinical-based service to the population-based focus on community services is resulting in confusion and difficulty in adjusting to the new role.[15] They note that "addressing the health problems of the community as a whole is a very different mission from that of providing limited clinical services for the needy."[16]

Evidence-Based Public Health Practice

This book is an attempt to promote evidence-based decision making, planning, policy, and analysis using the traditional measures of statistics, epidemiology, demography, and methods for assessing healthy communities as well as new applications using marketing and small-area analysis measurement tools to work with ideas and numbers. As evidenced by the previous discussion, public health community epidemiological investigation is not practicing its discipline effectively. The discipline has been in jeopardy recently by not being able to demonstrate that public health programs have been efficient and/or effective in demonstrating improvement in outcome measures or indicators. Lamarche notes that the public health model is in peril due to limitless spending without health, difficulty adapting to emerging problems, and a diminishing impact on health.[17] The new public health paradigm must shift in focus from individuals to populations; use health as a starting point; rethink resource allocations from curative and hospital care to ambulatory care, primary care, home care; and to substitute nonclinical personnel for physicians.[18] These thoughts clearly point to the new role for public health; this is the opportunity to reframe the discipline. However, there is a caution: Evidence is lacking to support this role for public health, and public health practitioners cannot continue to rely on intuition as the basis for making decisions or assessing outcomes. For example, Fox notes:

> Despite progress, we continue to encounter barriers in the struggle to determine effective interventions for troublesome public health problems. The dilemma of where to spend our money only can worsen as we face greater demands on limited local, State, and Federal resources. We cannot

ignore the importance of research- [evidence-] based successful interventions. [We must:]

1. Ensure that the research surrounding our interventions is sound and that the data are valid and reliable. This will require vigilant attention to data collection.
2. Assure early buy-in from agency officials, community providers and, most importantly, recipients [customers].
3. Adopt an ongoing epidemiologic approach to program management for continuous evaluation and quality improvement.[19]

Evidence-Based Framework for Health Services Management

To promote evidence-based public health and health services management by using evidence-based tools, public health personnel and managers must borrow from the work that has been done in clinical medicine that reflects clinical practice guidelines and clinical pathways. There are five basic elements that can provide the framework for providing evidence-based public health community assessment, including policy development and assurance. These five elements and how they relate to public health practice are embodied in the principles of lifelong learning, which will be discussed in subsequent sections.

The elements that provide this evidence-based framework can be thought of as a cycle that begins with *setting priorities* by using assessment tools to determine the importance of the problem being investigated (i.e., What is the evidence or methods used for prioritizing the problem?). Once priorities are determined, it is important to establish public health practice or management *guidelines* by using epidemiological tools and to answer the question, "How should the problem be managed?" (i.e., What protocols should be followed to ensure a positive outcome?). *Measuring performance* typically uses epidemiological measurement tools to determine how the problem is being managed and to report on the process and variation in the outcomes that have been defined for the community. To complete the cycle of setting priorities, setting guidelines, and measuring performance, it is necessary to focus on *improving performance*. Typically, to improve performance the tools for epidemiological measurement are applied to the problem to determine areas where improvement in outcomes can take place so that public health professionals are better able to manage the problem. The results from this final step lead again to a new determination of setting priorities based on an analysis of how performance might be improved.

This cycle of setting priorities, setting guidelines, measuring performance, and improving performance, which is dependent on lifelong learning, is continuous and, therefore, moves the process of evidence-based public health always to the next level of outcome improvement defined by decisions based on evidence. The application these five evidence-based strategies (lifelong learning, setting priorities, setting guidelines, measuring performance, and improving performance) to a population-based problem has been attempted by Ellrodt and Cho.[20]

Table 9-2 outlines eleven steps to follow for adapting the five evidence-based strategies for a community and/or a population in public health practice or health services management setting.

TABLE 9-2 Evidence-Based Strategies for Population-Based Health

Evidence-Based Strategies	*Evidence-Based Activities*
Lifelong Learning	▪ Develop and articulate a succinct problem statement ▪ Implement a thorough literature search ▪ Assess the quality of the article(s)
Setting Priorities	▪ Public health and management evaluation teams determine the significance of the expected outcomes of the interventions
Setting Guidelines	▪ Develop Public Health Practice Guideline(s) for each important element of assessment, policy development, and assurance ▪ Utilize guidelines for program community function (e.g., assessment)
Measuring Performance	▪ Develop a systematic approach to process measurement and reporting—epidemiological measurement ▪ Develop a systematic approach to outcomes measurement and reporting—epidemiological measurement ▪ Implement guidelines
Improving Performance*	▪ Measure and report process variation and community outcomes ▪ Use process and outcomes measures with updated literature searches and appraisals to continually improve population health status in the community

*At this point, based on level of performance, new priorities are set and the cycle is continuous.

Evidence-Based Assessment—Setting Priorities

In public health practice, several tools and/or methods for setting priorities [Model Standards, Assessment Protocol for Excellence in Public Health (*APEXPH*), Planned Approach to Community Health (PATCH), Plan-Do-Check-Act (PDCA) cycle] have been discussed elsewhere. In addition to these methods, a public health practitioner must use epidemiologic and statistical skills along with quality improvement measurement and community readiness (Civic Index) to establish population-based priorities.[21] By using these methods of priority setting, various agencies have developed criteria for determining priorities. The criteria range from the potential to change health outcomes, potential to change costs, prevalence of the condition (morbidity, mortality), and the burden of illness. Further, a generic priority-setting process to develop public health practice guidelines and manage health services has been create by Hayward and Laupacis.[22] This process includes the following steps:

1. Select priority-setting criteria and assign a weight to each.
2. Solicit nominations for topics for guidelines development.
3. Reduce list of topics to a number for which data about criteria can be gathered.
4. Obtain data for priority ranking.
5. For each topic, assign a score for each criterion.
6. Calculate summary priority score and rank topics by this score.
7. Review priority list and schedule guidelines development projects.[23]

These steps address the basic question of the importance of this problem. The answer using this process and the priority-setting tools and methods noted here focuses the decision to be based on evidence rather than intuition or hope. For example, the Hanlon method for setting priorities is an attempt to use an evidence-based approach to identify the important problems to be addressed.[24,25]

A Method for Setting Priorities* The method described here is a modification of a method developed by J. J. Hanlon.

Health problems are prioritized on the basis of size, seriousness, and effectiveness of available interventions. This formula assesses the relative importance of a problem.

$$D = (A + 2B)\ C$$

---

*Abridged with permission from *APEXPH: Assessment Protocol for Excellence in Public Health,* ©1991, the National Association of County Health Officials.

where

A = size of problem

B = seriousness

C = effectiveness of interventions

D = program priority score

This model implies that the seriousness of a health problem is twice as important as its size and the most important determinant of opportunity is the effectiveness of available interventions.

Alternatively, the "Size of the Problem" ratings can be established by giving the health problem with the highest frequency a rating of 10, the problems with the lowest frequency a rating of 0 or 1, and the other problems ratings according to where they are relative to the most common or least common problems.

Size of the Health Problems   Give each health problem being considered a numeric rating on a scale of 0 to 10 that reflects the percentage of the local population affected by the particular problem—the higher the percentage affected, the larger the numeric rating.

Table 9-3 is an example of how the numeric rating can be established. The scale shown is for illustrative purposes only and is not based on scientific or epidemiologic data; a community establishing priorities should establish a scale appropriate to the level of the health problems in that community and utilize the best available evidence for establishing the priorities.

Seriousness of the Health Problems   To score the seriousness of a health problem, use a scale of 1 to 10. The more serious the problem, the higher the number. In the priority-setting process, the seriousness of a health problem is considered to have a greater impact than its size; for this reason, in the final calculation, the "Seriousness Rating" given will be multiplied by a factor of 2.

Every community must establish its own criteria for rating the seriousness of health problems. Once criteria for rating the seriousness of health

TABLE 9-3   Size of Problem Rating Scale

Percentage of Population with the Health Problem	"Size of Problem" Rating
25% or more	9 or 10
10% through 24.9%	7 or 8
1% through 9.9%	5 or 6
0.1% through 0.9%	3 or 4
0.01% through 0.09%	1 or 2
less than 0.01% (1/10,000)	0

TABLE 9-4 Seriousness of Problem Rating Scale

How Serious a Health Problem Is Considered	*"Seriousness" Rating*
Very serious (e.g., very high death rate; premature mortality; great impact on others) (below estimated objectives 2010)	9 or 10
Serious	6, 7, or 8
Moderately Serious	3, 4, or 5
Not Serious (above estimated objectives 2010)	0, 1, or 2

problems are decided on, the seriousness of every health problem must be judged against the same criteria.

The following questions are helpful in setting criteria for rating the seriousness of health problems.

- What is the emergent nature of the health problem? Is there an urgency to intervene? Is there public concern? Is the problem a health problem?

- What is the severity of the problem? Does the problem have a high death rate or high hospitalization rate? Does the problem cause premature morbidity or mortality?

- Is there actual or potential economic loss associated with the health problem? Does the health problem cause long-term illness? Will the community have to bear the economic burden?

- What is the potential or actual impact on others in the community (e.g., measles spread in susceptible population)?

An example of criteria for scoring for seriousness is shown in Table 9-4.

Effectiveness of Available Interventions for Health Problems The effectiveness of interventions to reduce the health problem is an important component in priority setting. However, precise estimates are usually not available for specific health problems. It is helpful to define upper and lower limits of effectiveness and assess each intervention relative to these limits. For example, vaccines are a highly effective intervention for many diseases; those diseases receive a high "Effectiveness of Intervention Rating." At the other end of the scale are diseases such as arthritis, for which interventions now available are mainly ineffective. With this in mind, each health problem is scored for the effectiveness of available interventions according to the table (Table 9-5). The best real-world expectations of available interventions, based on evidence of successful intervention programs, should guide this strategy. Three questions are suggested:

1. How effective is the actual intervention (tools, methodology, devices, drugs, vaccines, etc.)?

TABLE 9-5   Effectiveness of Available Interventions Rating Scale

Effectiveness	Degree of Effectiveness	"Effectiveness" Rating
Very effective	80% to 100% effective	9 or 10
Relatively effective	60% to 80% effective	7 or 8
Effective	40% to 60% effective	5 or 6
Moderately effective	20% to 40% effective	3 or 4
Relatively ineffective	5% to 20% effective	1 or 2
Almost entirely ineffective	Less than 5% effective	0

    2. How effective is the application of the intervention (what percentage of the population can be reached? Affected?)?

    3. What is the potential of the intervention (fully funded, staffed, state-of-the-art)?

Calculate Priority Scores for the Health Problems   Calculate priority scores using the Health Problem Priority Setting Worksheet (Figure 9-1). Priority scores are calculated from the scores recorded in columns A, B, and C for each health problem and are recorded in column D. The formula used for this calculation is:

$$D = (A + 2B) \, C$$

Once priority scores are recorded for all health problems, assign a priority rank for each problem, based on the size of its priority scores, and record it in column E. For example, the health problem with the highest priority score is given a rank of 1, the problem with the next highest priority score,

Health Problem	A Size	B Serious	C Effectiveness of Intervention	D Priority Score (A + 2B) C	E Rank

List the health problems as determined through data collection, community perceptions, or other means.

FIGURE 9-1   Health Problem Priority Setting Worksheet

a rank of 2, and so on. Health problems with the same priority score are given the same priority rank.

Evidence-based Management—Setting Guidelines

All too often after priorities are determined, health care practitioners are reluctant to establish guidelines to manage or implement the program identified as a priority. To manage a community program or problem, four steps should be followed.

1. Formulate questions related to the priority that may be answered.
2. Critically review the best available evidence for managing the problem (i.e., locate and synthesize the evidence needed to answer the questions).
3. Evaluate the benefits, risks, and costs for options related to implementing the program.
4. Determine the relative level of the expected outcome to conclude whether benefits outweigh risks and costs.[26]

By assessing effectively these four steps, a health services manager and/or a public health analyst will be able to base a decision on evidence as to the development of a guideline for the identified priority. If the evidence suggests that public health professionals are unable to set guidelines because they do not have evidence, then they should alter their course or review their priorities.

To obtain evidence to develop community guidelines, the literature must be reviewed to determine the most likely articles to provide valid results. There are several issues to assess at this point, but two of the most important are the grades of recommendation supported by evidence and the type of the community problem to be developing guidelines based on the relevance of the article.

The grades of evidence are based on several approaches as to the quality of evidence supporting a particular recommendation. Table 9-6 lists the designs for a study to determine the quality of evidence they support. For instance, a randomized clinical trial is of the highest quality, whereas a single case report is considered poor quality evidence. Health analysts must base their programmatic and community-based guidelines on evidence-based studies. The level or grade of evidence based on research designs is just an initial step to develop evidence for the creation of community or public health practice guidelines.

In addition to the research design issue, Oxman and others developed guides for selecting articles most likely to provide valid results based on purpose of investigation (therapy or prevention, diagnosis, harm, prognosis) and integration of studies (e.g., overview articles, practice guidelines,

TABLE 9-6   Quality of Evidence Grades by Research for Assessing Community
Practice Guidelines

Grade	Quality of Evidence—Research Designs
A	Randomized, prospective, community, and/or clinical trial with low false-positive and low false-negative errors
B	Randomized, prospective, community, and/or clinical trial with high false-positive and/or high false-negative errors
C	Nonrandomized prospective, community, and/or clinical trials
D	Cohort studies (incidence studies)
E	Case-control studies
F	Prevalence studies (cross-sectional studies)
G	Descriptive/ecologic studies
H	Case series/case reports
I	Individual evidence (personal experience/expert opinion)
J	One meta-analysis
K	One cost-effectiveness or decision-analysis study
L	One summary study that pools data from other studies

decision analysis, and economic analysis).[27] (See Table 9-7.) By combining
the grades of evidence for the types of study with the guides for selecting
articles, a public health analyst or health services manager will be able to
base the development of the community practice guideline on significant
levels of evidence.

Evidence-based Programs—Measuring Performance

The Evidence-Based Medicine Working Group notes that they have

> frequently been surprised by discrepancies between what they perceived
> they were doing and what they found when they audited their . . . records.
> Because these discrepancies are common it is important to measure physi-
> cian [and community] performance to ensure that effective care is being
> provided."[28]

In public health, the same issues occur. However, public health practitioners are more concerned with the performance of community health programs provided by public health agencies than doing community health
assessments to measure performance. For public health to practice the core
functions of assessment, policy development, and assurance, there must be
a link and/or a direct connection to the environment of the managed care
network that already produces a data set of performance measures. These
performance measures are called Health Plan Employer Data and
Information Set (HEDIS) and were updated in 1995, with a set of Medicaid

TABLE 9-7 Guides for Selecting Articles That Are Most Likely to Provide Valid Results

Primary Studies	
Therapy	Was the assignment of patients to treatments randomized?
	Were all the patients who entered the trial properly accounted for and attributed at its conclusion?
Diagnosis	Was there an independent blind comparison with a reference standard?
	Did the patient sample include an appropriate spectrum of the sort of patients to whom the diagnostic test will be applied in clinical practice?
Harm	Were there clearly identified comparison groups that were similar with respect to important determinants of outcome (other than the one of interest)?
	Were outcomes and exposures measured in the same way in the groups being compared?
Prognosis	Was there a representative patient sample at a well-defined point in the course of disease?
	Was follow-up sufficiently long and complete?

Integrative Studies	
Overview	Did the review address a clearly focused question?
	Were the criteria used to select the articles for inclusion appropriate?*
Practice guidelines	Were the options and outcomes clearly specified?
	Did the guideline use an explicit process to identify, select, and combine evidence?*
Decision analysis	Did the analysis faithfully model a clinically/community important decision?
	Was valid evidence used to develop the baseline probabilities and utilities?*
Economic analysis	Were two or more clearly described alternatives compared?
	Were the expected consequences of each alternative based on valid evidence?*

*Each of these guides makes an implicit or explicit reference to investigators' need to evaluate the validity of the studies that they are reviewing to produce their integrative article. The validity criteria to use in making this evaluation depends on the area being addressed (therapy, diagnosis, harm, or prognosis) and on whether those that are presented as the part of the table are dealing with primary studies.

Source: Adapted with permission from A. D. Oxman et al., "Users' Guide to the Medical Literature: I. How to Get Started," in *Journal of the American Medical Association*, Vol. 270, No. 17, p. 2094, ©1993, American Medical Association.

HEDIS measurements currently being produced.[29] HEDIS, as used by some managed care health professionals, has been recommended to be proxy measures for public health measurements as a sort of a backing into population-based health measurement.[30]

Most think the fit of HEDIS measurement to population-based health measurement is not exact; in fact, the National Commission for Quality Assurance does not see HEDIS as interchangeable with public health performance targets but as a convergence of interest.[31] Public health benchmarks are detailed in *Healthy People 2000* and *2010*[32,33] and are used by public health practitioners and health services managers as targets to continuously monitor improvement of the stated outcome indicators.[33] A major problem with the promulgated Year 2000 standards is that they are "implicit rather than explicit"[34] (i.e., they are not based on evidence). An implicit standard or target, such as the Year 2000 objectives, is traditionally based on asking experts what they think, either as individuals or as groups (e.g., consensus panel—such as the Year 2000 objectives). This approach requires processing all information by each individual, and whoever uses the standard must accept the experts' opinion on faith. The presumption is that experts are reasoning in an analytical fashion rather than arriving at their answers intuitively.

The Year 2010 objectives have shown modest improvement in their targets by basing some of their objectives on evidence. In a later section on lifelong learning and the learning cube, it is shown that intuitive knowledge is the weakest form of evidence. Thus, implicit evidence means not formally described or written down.

The alternative approach to the establishment of standards, practice guidelines, performance measures, and so on is the "explicit approach." This approach is characterized by a systematic analysis of evidence (see Tables 9-2 and 9-6), estimation of outcomes and costs, and assessment of preferences. Eddy notes that *"explicit* means formally described and written down. Whereas the implicit approach accepts the beliefs of experts—without requiring any explicit descriptions of the evidence considered, the consequences of different options, or the value judgments behind the chosen option—the explicit approach holds that these descriptions are essential to the accurate assessment of a [community], and to the intelligent design and use of a [community–public health practice] guideline."[35]

The need for "explicit evidence" changes the demands on the practice of public health management of health services and the practitioners who set standards, targets, or guidelines. They must change their approach from simple intuition and belief statements to reasoning through a public health program or problem step by step and justifying the conclusions. This change has several consequences:

1. *Setting standard or practice guidelines will be considerably more difficult, take longer, and cost more than the traditional approach of simply*

asking experts what they think. Compared with the implicit approach, public health personnel will have to lower their sights on the speed and volume with which guidelines can be designed and raise their sights on the level of investment required.

2. *Most public health experts and health services managers are not trained to do all the tasks required to understand the consequences of a health practice, to design a guideline for its use, or to develop a standard as an objective outcome measurement.* Although public health knowledge is critical and indispensable, knowledge of statistics, quantitative analysis, epidemiology, quality improvement measurement, economics, and other disciplines is also required. The appropriate model is a team (a grand rounds approach).

3. *Participating as a member of a team requires sharing control.* Experts accustomed to providing all the answers and having their recommendations adopted without challenge must understand that their knowledge and insights, although still indispensable, paint only a part of the picture. Their beliefs must be merged with other factors to determine the proper use of a program.[36]

For the measurement of public health services and management performance, a set of guidelines must be established, which, given the gap between perception (implicit evidence) and reality (explicit evidence), appears to be essential for further advancement of evidence-based public health. Five steps are suggested for measuring clinical performances that may be used for public health performance measurement.

1. What is to be measured?
2. Is the needed information available?
3. How is an appropriate sample of community and/or patients identified?
4. How large should the sample be?
5. How will the information be interpreted?[37]

Much of this book has dealt with the statistical questions, and it is not the intent to detail the issues related to each of these questions. However, it is critical for the health services manager to realize that these are steps to be followed for developing evidence-based public health performance measures. There are several reports, in addition to the Year 2000/2010 *Healthy People* objectives, that provide lists of potential performance indicators.[38,39,40] Each of the lists is primarily a result of implicit-based evidence; however, it is clear that there is much movement toward developing more explicit definitions of performance measurement.

Performance Measurement—How Will the Information Be Collected?   There is considerable debate concerning the issue of how the information will be collected for measuring performance in health management situations. Much of the controversy centers around the proposed functions of an information network or system to collect the data. It has been reported there are three functions: (1) to support patient care—a disappearing responsibility in public health, that is, decline in the process of clinical services, (2) to support administrative and business transactions, and (3) to support outcomes management and performance reporting—including the health status of a community.[41] To respond to these efforts or at least provide a partial response, there has been the development of Community Health Information Networks (CHIN), Community Health Management Information Systems (CHMIS), and Information Network for Public Health Officials (INPHO), including several independent hospital, community-based systems.[42,43]

Each of these information systems faces the reality of implementing a system that is difficult, time-consuming, and expensive. A recent report notes that "you don't have to have a network or electronic superhighway to do community health assessments. But you do have to have agreement on data elements, definitions, how data is reported, and what's meaningful. Getting agreement on this is much harder than accomplishing network building."[44]

Recently, it has been noted that some high-profile CHIN and CHMIS initiatives that damaged the reputation of community networks have proponents who believe integrated delivery systems and the Internet will aid the cause of community population-based information systems.[45]

As public health searches to find its niche on the information superhighway, it must focus its efforts more on responding to the core public health functions of assessment, policy development, and assurance and not on patient management (a disappearing function) or clinical services from professional providers—these functions will be serviced by the managed care networks. The opportunity for public health in performance measurement is to link with managed care networks to provide population-based health information and measurement—a significant need of the managed care providers. Of course, public health must meet its own objectives related to the core functions.

There also has been debate over the nature of these systems (CHIN, CHMIS, INPHO). CHMIS, for example, was envisioned as a centralized data repository. Collected information from other systems in the community is sent to the CHMIS database. Databases include health plans, physician groups, and institutional providers (hospitals, nursing homes, business coalitions). CHIN, on the other hand, does not require a central data repository but supports an integrated set of applications that connect systems and networks, allowing users to access the other systems and download data they need.[46] It appears the CDC/INPHO system is a cross between these two approaches (e.g., the centralized data repository of the federal government and the attempted connecting of primary care services as proposed by CHMIS).[47]

Certainly, the idea and the importance of a public health information system to meet the core functions are appealing. A major trend that is having an effect on the evolution of population-based health information systems for evaluating the performance of public health is the need for evidence-based public health practice. This is not the only factor related to this need of public health and health services utilization systems development. Other trends include the following:

1. Growth and spread of managed care plans; however, in 2000 those plans have become less important in the provision of health services

2. Increasing consumer/community demand for accountability by hospitals, physicians, and health plans during the 1980s

3. Growing interest in clinical practice and public health practice focusing on quality improvement, disease management, and population-based assessment, including continuous quality improvement, epidemiologic measurements, and outcome measures; these efforts require increased and more targeted data collection and data analysis (the major premise of this book)

4. More consumer/community customer demand for and more health plan focus on performance measurement, and reporting, including pressure on health plans to demonstrate their ability to manage the care of defined populations (evidence-based population health care)

5. Development of HEDIS and other performance data sets (CHIN, CHMIS) and report cards

6. Increasing interest on the part of public health specialists and health services managers in taking these basic evidence-based epidemiological tools and using work already being done by health plans and providers to assess the health of entire communities, not just employer groups[48]

Evidence-based Programs—Improving Performance

The objective of developing evidence-based performance and/or outcomes measures is to evaluate public health programs and be able to show improvement. The use of quality improvement measurement in public health has been detailed in this book for the purpose of managing, analyzing, and improving performance by using quality improvement tools and traditional statistical/epidemiologic methods. The data systems for performance measurement should be designed toward this end of improving outcomes. Table 9-8 suggests the levels of development in a quality

TABLE 9-8 A Quality Improvement Process for Improving Performance and Outcomes in Public Health Practice

Improvement Performance Level	Definition	Behavioral Objective	Behavior	Measurement
1. Business as usual	No attempt to allow public health organizations to expand or change	—	A. Programs do not actively support quality improvement measurement	None
			B. Inspection and record review is primarily the quality improvement tool	
			C. Quality is only for industrial processes	
			D. Training is provided on an exception basis	
			E. CQI/TQM infrastructure incomplete	
2. Initiation	Beginning planning and initial actions designed to create a desirable cultural change	■ Recognition of the horizontal multifunctional process vs. vertical	A. Organization's mission defined in terms of the primary processes	A. List of macro/key processes
			B. Workplace input solicited to identify subprocesses of key process	B. Subprocess list
			C. Responsibility is determined and accepted for identified processes	C. List of process owners

TABLE 9-8 (continued)

Improvement Performance Level	Definition	Behavioral Objective	Behavior	Measurement
2. Initiation		■ Workforce involvement in organizational processes	A. Teams have been formed around selected subprocesses rather than categorical programs	A. Process team charter
		■ Organizational performance measures focus on customer needs	A. Primary external customer is identified	A. List of customers
			B. Customer needs/requirements are identified	B. Customer feedback
			C. Indicators are identified based on customer requirements	C. List of indicators
3. Implementation	A higher degree of action than has been exhibited in initiation level	■ Document baseline organizational subprocesses: assessment, policy, and assurance	A. Document selected processes	A. Use of quality improvement tools (flowchart, cause and effect, etc.)
			B. Performance data has been expressed in terms of its central tendency and variability	B. Mean, median, range, and standard deviation as applicable

TABLE 9-8 (continued)

Improvement Performance Level	Definition	Behavioral Objective	Behavior	Measurement
3. Implementation		▪ Assess program capabilities	A. An operational definition of the customer requirement has been established	A. Customer-defined limits
			B. Program performance is described	B. Use of quality control charts
			C. Customer requirement is compared with the process performance	C. Process performance model
		▪ Select program processes to review interorganizationally (e.g., immunization program)	A. Processes have been selected	A. List of interorganizational processes
			B. An assessment has been completed on selected processes	B. Use quality improvement tools (Pareto, cause-and-effect diagrams, etc.)
		▪ Increase workforce involvement with organizational processes	A. Teams are identified around all subprocesses	A. Process team charter
		▪ Start to identify "best-in-class"	A. Survey most likely candidates for leaders	A. Survey of the process

TABLE 9-8 (continued)

Improvement Performance Level	Definition	Behavioral Objective	Behavior	Measurement
4. Expansion	A wider range of quality improvement efforts and an increasing degree of activity in executing planned strategies	▪ Document baseline processes and data availability	A. Document selected processes	A. Use of quality improvement tools (flowchart, cause-and-effect diagrams, etc.)
			B. Identify customers (internal/external)	B. List of customers (internal/external)
			C. Teams gather pertinent data	C. Data
			D. Performance data expressed in terms of central tendency and variability	D. Mean, median, range, and standard deviation as applicable
		▪ Make program process changes	A. Assess variation by using comparison analysis to measure special vs. common cause variation	A. Percentage assignable
			B. Process control charts are used to monitor performance	B. Control chart interpretation
			C. Process teams use analytical tools to determine root cause of conditions	C. Cause-and-effect/scatter diagrams

TABLE 9-8 (continued)

Improvement Performance Level	Definition	Behavioral Objective	Behavior	Measurement
4. Expansion		▪ Make program process changes	D. Effects of corrective action are monitored to verify the results	D. Control chart
5. Integration	Quality improvement is embodied in the way public health does business	▪ Process capability achieved for customer requirements	A. Process capability studies are processed	A. Completed capability studies
			B. Process teams determine the type and amount of improvement needed	B. Improvement plan
			C. Fundamental changes to process design are implemented	C. Process documentation
		▪ Participation of communities in continuous process improvement	A. Community performance meets or exceeds requirements	A. Program/service criteria data
			B. Community participation in periodic reviews	B. Process team leaders
			C. Community input is solicited in design/changes	C. Community feedback

TABLE 9-8 (continued)

Improvement Performance Level	Definition	Behavioral Objective	Behavior	Measurement
5. Integration		■ Establish benchmarks for performance (best-in-class)	A. Measurement criteria are established for performance B. Benchmark assessment instrument is used by public health to develop strategy for continuous quality improvement	A. List of criteria/benchmark matrix B. Benchmark matrix (best-in-class)

Source: Reprinted from *Journal for Healthcare Quality*, 14(1), 8–13, with permission of the National Association for Healthcare Quality, 4700 W. Lake Avenue, Glenview, IL 60025–1485. Copyright ©1992 National Association for Healthcare Quality.

improvement process for performance in public health practice. The five levels assess the total participation by the organization in the actual improvement of the critical process through the application of tools and methodology. Key concepts are worker involvement, methodology, and use of tools.[49] A public health agency can evaluate the current state of continuous quality improvement (CQI) in its organization by using this benchmarking process and can aid in moving the agency forward to develop standards and/or practice guidelines for evidence-based performance for improving the outcomes in public health programs.[50]

In addition to using these benchmarks, the Evidence-Based Medicine Working Group has developed strategies for clinical action to improve performance and outcome measurement.[51] Figure 9-2, adapted from the Evidence-Based Medicine Working Group, outlines the strategies or determinants for community public health action to improve performance using evidence-based guidelines. Thus, the practice environment (community), prevailing opinion, public health attitudes, and evidence-based practice guidelines all contribute to community public health action for improving performance. Through this process measurement, it is possible to determine compliance with guideline recommendations. Compliance with evidence-based practice guidelines by measuring outcomes is the only means by which public health practitioners are able to demonstrate programs and patient care improvement. Thus, in public health practice the goal must be to link the quality improvement process to outcome measurement in order to provide the

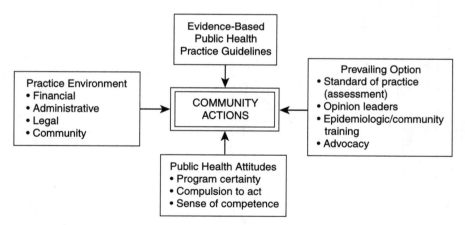

FIGURE 9-2 Community Action Strategies for Improving Performance. *Source:* Adapted from "Evidence-Based Care: 4. Improving Performance: How Can We Improve the Way We Manage This Problem?" by the Evidence-Based Care Resource Group, by permission of the publisher, *Canadian Medical Association Journal* 150, no. 11 (1994).

opportunity to optimize community and patient health status. Reinertsen outlined the useful and complementary roles of outcome measurement and quality improvement measurement.[52] In essence, quality improvement focuses on existing variation and complexity in processes to continually improve the process and thereby the outcome. Outcome measurement focuses more on the reported outcomes and not the process that created the outcomes.[53]

The public health organization, by adopting these quality improvement strategies, sets the stage for implementing changes and modifications in current public health practice guidelines. Many of the current practices in public health are not based on evidence, and it is hoped that by adopting the strategies outlined here the public health practitioner will promote the practice of evidence-based public health practice focusing on the process and the outcome.

Evidence-based Learning—Learning to Be More Effective

To promote the evidence-based public health epidemiological practice model, a new approach for learning is advocated: lifelong learning. To ensure the use of the evidence-based framework as proposed, it is critical for health officials to base their future decision on evidence. To practice evidence-based learning and how to be a more effective learner, it is necessary to be able to critically appraise the public health and medical literature. Further, this learning must occur in an environment in which the health officials and managers have opportunities to listen, to present, and to evaluate the medical/public health literature. There are at least three ways that health professionals may learn to be more effective and prepare for lifelong learning so they can base their decisions on evidence. They are as follows:

1. The public health epidemiologic learning cube
2. Public health grand rounds
3. Critical appraisal of the public health/medical literature

The Public Health and Health Services Management Learning Cube   This cube was created by Sackett and others who promoted the acquisition of critical appraisal skills for advanced lifelong learning in the medical field, specifically by using the materials and methods of clinical epidemiology.[54] To further the notion of lifelong learning for evidence-based public health and/or population-based medicine, the cube can also be a model for learning. The basic cube for public health and health services learning is based on clinical/community evidence, clinical/community problem, and critical appraisal skills (Figure 9-3).

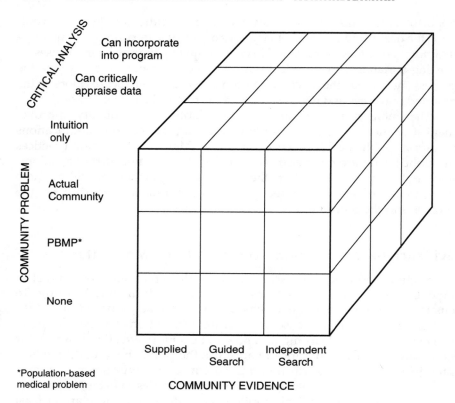

FIGURE 9-3   The Public Health/Health Services Management Learning Cube.
Source: Adapted with permission from *Clinical Epidemiology: A Basic Science for Clinical Medicine*, D. L. Sackett, ©1985, published by Little, Brown and Company.

The weakest form of learning occurs where there is no clinical/community problem, the community/clinical evidence is supplied, and the critical appraisal level is by intuition only (the lower left cell of the cube). This is considered the "core knowledge" approach and is the least effective way to learn and is based on the weakest form of evidence.

This learning cube generates twenty-seven different learning situations. The most advanced learning situation is when the clinical/community problem is an actual program, the level of clinical evidence is an independent and/or guided search, and the critical appraisal level is such that it can be incorporated into the program. This level of learning is highly self-directed and produces an effective public health practitioner. Table 9-9 gives the strengths of public health and management learning based on the cube elements. In addition to this health learning cube, the Evidence-Based Care Resource Group devised a set of guidelines for teaching and learning evidence-based medicine that is valuable for the field of public health practice and health services management. They suggest the following:

TABLE 9-9 Relationship of Lifelong Learning Concepts to Level of Evidence in Public Health Practice and Health Services Management

	Evidence		
Concepts	*Weak*	*Moderate*	*Strong*
Community evidence	Supplied	Guided search	Independent search
Community problem	None	PBMP*	Actual program
Critical appraisal	Intuition only	Can critically appraise data	Can incorporate into program

*Population-based medical problems

1. Learning should be applied and participatory.
2. Learning should be self-directed.
3. Learning should be practice based and practical.
4. Learning should focus on high-priority problems.
5. Efficiency should be emphasized.
6. Expectations should be reasonable.[55]

By applying these guidelines and focusing on the learning cube, the individuals in public health practice and health services management can become more effective learners and base their decisions on evidence and not on intuition, rhetoric, or anecdotal information.

Table 9-10 gives the reader an evaluation form to determine where his or her agency is in the learning cycle. The health practitioner can substantiate program additions, deletions, or modifications based on the learning levels within the evidence-based model. Obviously, there are situations that are unsatisfactory, and program decisions must not be based on such levels.

A final note on the proof to support evidence-based medicine or management of health practice is to see whether patients and/or communities show improved health status. The authors of evidence-based medicine state:

> Our advocating evidence-based medicine in the absence of definitive evidence of its superiority in improving patient outcomes may appear to be an internal contradiction. As has been pointed out, however, evidence-based medicine does not advocate a rejection of all innovations in the absence of definitive evidence . . . and on biologic rationale. The rationale in this case is that physicians [public health practitioners] who are up-to-date as a function of their ability to read the current literature critically, and are able to distinguish strong from weaker evidence, are likely to be more judicious in the . . . [programs] they recommend. Physicians who understand the properties of diagnostic tests are able to use a quantitative approach to those tests and are likely to make more accurate diagnoses. (Similarly, public health practitioners who understand the programs and are able to use the quality improvement tools are more likely to base outcome measurement on evidence.) While this rationale appears compelling to us, compelling rationale has often

TABLE 9-10 Evaluation Form for Assessing Lifelong Learning Skills for Evidence-Based Health Services Utilization and Public Health Practice

	Health Practice Learning Domain	
Evidence-Based Rating	Role Model of Practice of Evidence-Based Population Health/Medicine	Leads Practice of Evidence-Based Population Health/Medicine
Unsatisfactory	Seldom cites evidence to support community decisions	Never assigns problems to be resolved through literature
Needs improvement	Often fails to substantiate decisions with evidence	Produces suboptimal volume or follow-through of problem resolution through literature
Satisfactory	Usually substantiates decisions with evidence	Assigns problems and follows through with discussion, including methodology
Good	Substantiates decisions; is aware of methodologic issues	Discusses literature retrieval, methodology of papers, application to individual patient and community program
Excellent	Always substantiates decisions or acknowledges limitations of evidence	Discusses literature retrieval, methodology of papers, application to individual patient and community program

Source: Adapted with permission from "Evidence-Based Medicine: A New Approach to Teaching the Practice of Medicine" by the Evidence-Based Medicine Working Group, *Journal of American Medical Association*, Vol. 268, No. 17, p. 2422, ©1992, American Medical Association.

proved misleading. Until more definitive evidence is adduced, adoption of evidence-based [public health and health services management] medicine should appropriately be restricted to two groups. One group comprises those who find the rationale compelling, and thus believe that use of the evidence-based [public health] medicine approach is likely to improve clinical [program and community] care. A second group comprises those who, while skeptical of improvements in patient [community] outcome, believe it is very unlikely that deterioration in care results from the evidence-based approach and who find that the practice of [public health] medicine in the new paradigm is more exciting and fun.[56]

Grand Rounds—Tutorial Style

Grand rounds are traditionally conducted in medicine in the southwest cell of the cube, where clinical evidence is supplied, there is no clinical problem, and critical appraisal is based on intuition (Figure 9-3). In public health practice and health services management, grand rounds must be introduced first to pursue evidence for programs and to meet the core functions of assessment, policy development, and assurance. In addition, the grand rounds should become tutorial, where a population-based medical problem (PBMP) is supplied as the community evidence and the critical appraisal of the problem is based on management's ability to apply the rules or guides to critically assess the evidence as proposed in the PBMP.

Initially, a major goal of the grand rounds was to review the literature, in a PBMP format, on the issues of how to effectively evaluate the literature from an evidence-based perspective. Thus, articles on causation, therapy, assessment, prognoses of disease, quality of care, and the economic evaluation of a program should all be read to understand the guidelines for evaluating these topics.

When this step is accomplished (there are agencies doing this using a similar format to promote evidence-based population health and/or medicine), the next step is to begin, using epidemiologic tools, to establish a process by which health programs are systematically reviewed for evidence-based assessments, policies, and assurances. This approach can be local or at the state/federal level and the results should be reported and distributed to other agency personnel. Public health officials and health services managers must survive the onslaught of attack by legislators and consumers who say that health practitioners are unable to show in a valid statistical format that the programs improve outcomes; the response must show that "our results must be based on evidence." The evidence-based learning framework of grand rounds for public health must be adopted and become commonplace in the agency.

Critical Appraisal of the Public Health/Medical Literature

Several articles over a period of the past fifteen years have received the attention of the health and medical advocates who see critical appraisal skills as a required subject for medical students and other clinicians. There is no such movement in public health practice. The skills, methods, and knowledge outlined here are to help the public health practitioners report on the health of the public and to ensure that decisions are based on evidence and the use of critical appraisal skills. Certainly, agencies can base their recommendations related to the implementation of various community programs on practice guidelines from clinical studies; but the ability to determine if the program worked or had an impact has not been accomplished. Outcomes that have not been based on evidence and recommendations that have not been driven by the evaluation of programs are subject to modification or termination. The critical appraisal skills outlined here and the evidence-based public health model proposed are offered in the spirit of articulating public health as a major force in the development, planning, and evaluation of population-based medicine in the twenty-first century.

Figure 9-4 shows the critical appraisal skills for evaluating the literature related to four goals: (1) use of a diagnostic test, (2) learning the clinical course and prognosis of a disorder, (3) determining etiology or causation, and (4) distinguishing useful from useless or even harmful therapy. Other types of studies and their critical appraisal skills were noted in Table 9-7. Depending on the type of study evaluated, there are three questions to determine the strengths and weaknesses of the research.

1. Are the study results valid?
2. What were the results?
3. Will the results help in improving the health status of the patients/communities?

Practical answers to these three questions are shown in Table 9-7 and Figure 9-4.

Specifically, primary care strategies concerning therapy/prevention, diagnostic tests, harm/benefits, and prognosis are presented. For integrative studies that respond to these questions, see Table 9-7 and, in addition, see the Users' Guides to the Medical Literature series by the Evidence-Based Medicine Working Group.[57,58,59,60,61,62,63] It is suggested that the public health agency, when implementing the tutorial-based grand rounds, begin with these user guides and the basics of critical appraisal as noted in Table 9-7. Although the focus of most of these guides is from a clinical perspective, it takes very little creativity to note how these critical appraisals can be adapted to acquire lifelong learning skills in order to practice public health from an evidence-based perspective.

Critical Appraisal Guides for Public Health and Health Services Management

In addition to the critical appraisal guides in Table 9-7 and Figure 9-4, appraisal guides have been developed to evaluate literature based on assessment, planning, and policy issues in public health practice.[64] Specifically, three guides are presented for evaluating the public health literature.

1. Articles based on rates and ratios—used in assessment and policy analysis
2. Articles based on numbers and percentage—used in health status and resource allocation problems
3. Articles based on measures of central tendency—used for assessing program performance and improvement

The appraisal guides are shown in Figures 9-5 to 9-7.

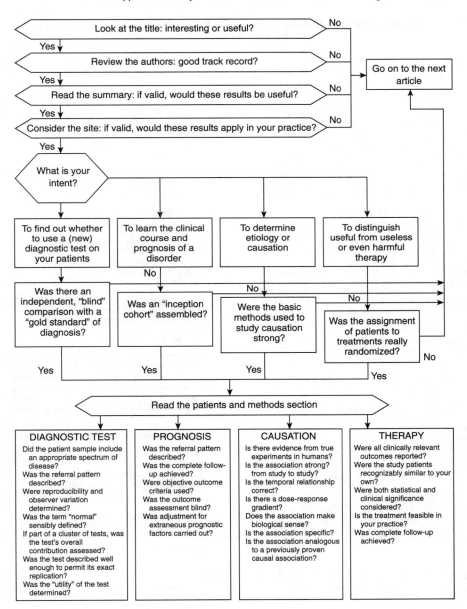

FIGURE 9-4 Readers' Guide for the Critical Appraisal of the Clinical Literature. *Source:* Reprinted with permission from R. B. Haynes et al., "Problems in Handling of Clinical and Research Evidence by Medical Practitioners," in *Archives of Internal Medicine*, Vol. 143, p. 1971, © 1983, American Medical Association.

CRITICAL APPRAISAL GUIDES EVALUATING THE PUBLIC HEALTH LITERATURE MEASURES BASED ON RATES AND RATIOS

Citation:

1. Purpose of investigation (What is the research question? What is measured?)
   _____
   _____
   _____
   _____
   _____

2. Community research designs (evidence-based policy and planning):
   ☐ Randomized community trial
   ☐ Cohort study (community)
   ☐ Control community vs study community
   ☐ Cross-sectional (prevalence survey)
   ☐ Ecological (comparison analysis)
   ☐ Community series
   ☐ Descriptive profile (county, state, national)

3. Evidence-based evaluation—does this study represent or report problems related to:
   ☐ Ecological fallacy
   ☐ Variations in the base (i.e., per 100; 1,000; 10,000)
   ☐ False associations
   ☐ Small denominator and variation of rates
   ☐ Advantages and disadvantages of the rate

4. Is this study about rates and/or ratios?
   ☐ Yes   ☐ No

5. Do you understand the type of frequency measure being used (rate/ratio/proportion)?
   ☐ Yes   ☐ No

6. What is the data source used in this study?
   ☐ Vital statistics   ☐ Program data
   ☐ Census data—U.S.   ☐ Clinical data
   ☐ Survey data   ☐ Unable to tell

7. Do the data for the study represent:
   ☐ Residence data   ☐ Other (i.e., workplace)
   ☐ Occurrence data   ☐ Region
   ☐ Census tract   ☐ National
   ☐ ZIP code
   ☐ County

8. The analysis involves:
   ☐ Counts   ☐ Ratios
   ☐ Rates   ☐ Indexes
   ☐ Proportions

9. Determine the specific rate being used.
   ☐ Mortality (death)   ☐ Natality (births)
   ☐ Morbidity (illness)

10. What type of rate is being used?
    ☐ Crude   ☐ Specific
    ☐ Adjusted
    ☐ Standardized Mortality Ratio (SMR)
    ☐ Proportionate Mortality Ratio (PMR)
    ☐ Risk or rate ratio
    ☐ Incidence/prevalence
    ☐ Other

11. What is the constant (k) used to calculate the rate/ratio/proportion? Determine what could be used. Is there a standard? What is that standard for this type of rate?
    Type of rate_____

Constant (k)	Used	Standard
100		
1,000		
10,000		
100,000		

What constants are used in this study?

12. Are the numbers and rates both provided in the study?
    ☐ Yes   ☐ No

13. Has the proper conversion of rates to numbers and numbers to rates been presented?
    ☐ Yes   ☐ No

14. What is the geographic level of the data?
    ☐ Household   ☐ District
    ☐ Block   ☐ State
    ☐ Region

FIGURE 9-5   Appraisal Guide: Rates and Ratios

15. What time period does this study cover?
   - ☐ < 1 year   ☐ 4–5 years
   - ☐ 1 year   ☐ > 5 years
   - ☐ 2–3 years   ☐ Specified period

16. What does the numerator represent (i.e., the type of event)?
   - ☐ Birth
   - ☐ Death
   - ☐ Marriage
   - ☐ Divorce
   - ☐ Abortion
   - ☐ Death by cause
   - ☐ Other
   - ☐ Demographic variables
   - ☐ Social variables
   - ☐ Hospital discharge
   - ☐ Hospital admission
   - ☐ Cases

17. What is the source of the numerator?
   _____
   _____
   _____

   Is this information reliable?
   - ☐ Yes   ☐ No

18. What time period is considered for the numerator?
   - ☐ < 1 year   ☐ 4–5 years
   - ☐ 1 year   ☐ > 5 years
   - ☐ 2–3 years   ☐ Specified period

19. How was the denominator (i.e., population-at-risk) derived in this study?
   - ☐ Estimate   ☐ Total count (U.S. census)
   - ☐ Projection   ☐ Other

20. What is the source of the population-at-risk (denominator) data?
   - ☐ Census data   ☐ Program/clinic
   - ☐ State documents   ☐ Records
   - ☐ Other

   Is this information reliable?
   - ☐ Yes   ☐ No

21. Is the numerator data from the same time period as the denominator data?
   - ☐ Yes   ☐ No

22. What is the standard or basis for comparison to determine if the rate is high or low?
   - ☐ District   ☐ National
   - ☐ State   ☐ 2000 objective

23. Is the rate high or low?*
   - ☐ Yes   ☐ No

24. Has statistical significance been determined for the rate?
   - ☐ Yes   ☐ No

   Is it necessary to determine significance?
   - ☐ Yes   ☐ No

25. Determine the significance of the rate using the following formula:

$$SE = \frac{R}{\sqrt{d}}$$

   where SE = standard error
   R = rate per population
   $\sqrt{}$ = square root
   d = number of events on which rate is based

26. Are the confidence intervals for the rates given? If not, calculate using the following formula:

$$CI = R \pm 1.96 \frac{R}{\sqrt{d}}$$

   where CI = confidence interval
   R = rate
   $\sqrt{}$ = square root
   d = number of events on which rate is based
   1.96 = two standard errors

27. Has statistical significance been determined for the count (event)?
   - ☐ Yes   ☐ No

   Is it necessary to determine significance?
   - ☐ Yes   ☐ No

28. Determine the significance of the event using the following formula:

$$SE_d = \sqrt{d}$$

   where SE = standard error
   $\sqrt{}$ = square root
   d = number of events on which rate is based

---

*The rate must be compared with a standard (i.e., above or below the selected standard).

FIGURE 9-5 (continued)

29. The results from this evaluation analysis suggest program:
    ☐ Change ☐ Contraction
    ☐ Expansion ☐ No change

30. What program change or modification would be a practical application of this analysis?
    _____
    _____
    _____

31. Is there strong evidence as indicated by the results to influence policy?
    ☐ Yes ☐ No

32. Is there evidence to warrant further investigation?
    ☐ Yes ☐ No

33. What programs in community/public health could be influenced by the results of this study?
    1. _____
    2. _____
    3. _____
    4. _____
    5. _____
    6. _____

FIGURE 9-5 (continued)

CRITICAL APPRAISAL GUIDES EVALUATING THE PUBLIC HEALTH LITERATURE MEASURES BASED ON NUMBERS AND PERCENTAGES

Citation: _____

1. Purpose of investigation (Why are the data presented? What is measured?)
   _____
   _____
   _____
   _____
   _____

2. Is this study about numbers and/or percents?
   ☐ Yes   ☐ No

3. Do the data for the study represent (i.e., data source):
   ☐ Clinical data   ☐ Program data
   ☐ Census data   ☐ Unable to tell

4. Evidence-Based Evaluation does this study represent:
   ☐ Arithmetic errors
   ☐ Percentage errors
   ☐ Improbable precision
   ☐ Misleading presentation
   ☐ Incomplete data
   ☐ Improper or faulty comparisons
   ☐ Improper sampling
   ☐ Failure to allow for the effect of chance

5. Are the data:
   ☐ Qualitative   ☐ Quantitative

6. What type of variable is being measured?
   ☐ Discrete   ☐ Continuous

7. Arithmetic error evaluation.
   Did you accept the value because it appears in print?
   ☐ Yes   ☐ No
   Is the subject matter important to you?
   ☐ Yes   ☐ No
   Did you check the author s calculations before accepting them?
   ☐ Yes   ☐ No

Did you find mistakes?
☐ Yes   ☐ No
If yes, list problems. If no, proceed with appraisal.
_____
_____
_____
_____
_____
_____
_____
_____

8. Percentage error evaluation.
   What type of percentage was determined?
   ☐ Simple percent
   ☐ Percentage change
   ☐ Percentages point of change (relative change)
   Were percentages computed correctly?
   ☐ Yes   ☐ No
   Were percentages based on levels rather than based on change in the level?
   ☐ Yes   ☐ No
   Was adding or subtracting of percentages calculated?
   ☐ Yes   ☐ No

9. Selection of base value for percentage calculations.
   How is the base value selected?
   Is the base value small?
   ☐ Yes   ☐ No
   Is the base value representative of the period of comparison?
   ☐ Yes   ☐ No

10. False percentages.
    Were the percentages added (beware of adding percentages)?
    ☐ Yes   ☐ No

FIGURE 9-6   Appraisal Guide: Numbers and Percentages

Do results show decreasing percentages (beware of decreasing percentages)?
☐ Yes   ☐ No
Do numbers accompany percentages (beware of percentages unaccompanied by the actual numbers)?
☐ Yes   ☐ No
Do percentages show huge differences (beware of huge percentages)?
☐ Yes   ☐ No

11. Precision.
Is the result (number or percentage) presented to several decimal points (if not, be skeptical)?
☐ Yes   ☐ No
Is the degree of precision warranted by the evidence?
☐ Yes   ☐ No
Did you ask how could anyone have found that out?
☐ Yes   ☐ No
Did you approach results with a healthy skepticism?
☐ Yes   ☐ No

12. Misleading presentation.
Are accompanying numbers presented?
☐ Yes   ☐ No
Are percentages calculated appropriately?
☐ Yes   ☐ No
Are there attempts to misinform the audience?
☐ Yes   ☐ No

13. Incomplete data.
Are all data provided to make an accurate evaluation?
☐ Yes   ☐ No

Are you able to check the original measurement and make appropriate calculations?
☐ Yes   ☐ No

14. Faulty comparisons.
Were the proper comparisons made?
☐ Yes   ☐ No
Did the two groups being compared represent like characteristics?
☐ Yes   ☐ No
Is chance an effect that was not properly assessed?
☐ Yes   ☐ No

15. You used your Statistical Guides to:
☐ Calculate the error of the number
☐ Calculate the significance of the number
☐ Calculate the error of the percentage
☐ Calculate the significance of the percentage

16. The results for this critical thinking evaluation suggest?
☐ Information   ☐ Contraction
☐ Change   ☐ No change
☐ Expansion

17. Is program change or modification a potential application of this analysis?
☐ Yes   ☐ No

18. Is there strong evidence as indicated by the results to influence policy?
☐ Yes   ☐ No

19. Is there evidence to warrant further investigation?
☐ Yes   ☐ No

FIGURE 9-6   (continued)

CRITICAL APPRAISAL GUIDES EVALUATING THE PUBLIC HEALTH LITERATURE MEASURES
BASED ON CENTRAL TENDENCY

Citation: _____

1. Purpose of investigation (What is the research question? What is measured?)
   _____
   _____
   _____
   _____
   _____

2. What type of community research design is being prepared? (Evidence-based policy and planning):
   ☐ Randomized community trial
   ☐ Cohort study (community)
   ☐ Control community vs. study community
   ☐ Cross-sectional (prevalence survey)
   ☐ Ecological (comparison analysis)
   ☐ Community series
   ☐ Descriptive profile (county, state, national)

3. Evidence-based evaluation—does this study represent or report problems related to:
   ☐ Ecological fallacy
   ☐ Variations in the base (i.e., per 100;1,000; 10,000)
   ☐ False associations
   ☐ Small denominators
   ☐ Advantages/disadvantages of the measures (mean, median, mode, range, variance, standard deviation)

4. Is this study or report about averages and/or dispersions?
   ☐ Yes   ☐ No

5. Do you understand the type of measure being used (mean, median, mode, range, variance, standard deviation)?
   ☐ Yes   ☐ No

6. What is the data source used in this study?
   ☐ Vital statistics   ☐ Program data
   ☐ Census data—U.S.   ☐ Clinical data
   ☐ Survey data   ☐ Unable to tell

7. Do the data for the study represent:
   ☐ Residence data
   ☐ Other (e.g., workplace)
   ☐ Occurrence data

8. Does the analysis involve:
   ☐ Means   ☐ Ranges
   ☐ Medians   ☐ Variances
   ☐ Modes   ☐ Standard deviations

9. Is the level of measurement appropriate for the statistic?

	Yes	No
Normal...mode	☐	☐
Ordinal...median	☐	☐
Interval...mean standard deviation	☐	☐
Ratio......mean standard deviation	☐	☐

10. Does this study commit any statistical sins?

	Yes	No
The mean of the means	☐	☐
Skewed distributions (used appropriate statistics)	☐	☐
Level of measurement	☐	☐
Data distortion problem— mean	☐	☐

11. Are the numbers (counts) and the measurements (statistics) both provided in the study?
    ☐ Yes   ☐ No

12. What is the geographic level of the data?
    ☐ Household   ☐ District
    ☐ Block   ☐ State
    ☐ Census tract   ☐ Region
    ☐ Zip code   ☐ National
    ☐ County

13. What time period does this study cover?
    ☐ < 1 year   ☐ 4–5 years
    ☐ 1 year   ☐ > 5 years
    ☐ 2–3 years   ☐ Specified period

FIGURE 9-7 Appraisal Guide: Measures of Central Tendency

14. What does the numerator represent (i.e., the type of event)?
    □ Birth
    □ Death
    □ Marriage
    □ Divorce
    □ Abortion
    □ Death by cause
    □ Other

    □ Demographic variables
    □ Social variables
    □ Hospital discharge
    □ Hospital admission
    □ Cases

15. What is the source of the numerator data?

    _____
    _____
    _____
    _____
    _____

    Is this information reliable?
    □ Yes   □ No

16. What time period is considered for the numerator?
    □ < 1 year   □ 4–5 years
    □ 1 year   □ > 5 years
    □ 2–3 years   □ Specified period

17. With what are the computed measures being compared?
    □ Program/clinic   □ National
    □ District   □ 2000 objective
    □ State

18. The results from this "evaluation analysis" suggest program
    □ Change   □ Further study
    □ Expansion   □ No change
    □ Contraction

19. What program or modification would be a practical application of this analysis?

    _____
    _____
    _____
    _____
    _____
    _____

20. Is there strong evidence as indicated by the results to influence policy?
    □ Yes   □ No

21. Is there evidence to warrant further investigation?
    □ Yes   □ No

FIGURE 9-7   (continued)

Summary

Evidence-based public health practice and health services management are essential to meet the challenges being faced by the health industry in terms of scarce resources, government downsizing, improved performance, improved health outcomes, and decisions based on evidence and not intuition, opinion, or anecdotal information. This chapter has provided a framework for arriving at evidence-based decisions. A case was made for public health and health services management to refocus its approach in areas of assessment (setting priorities), management (setting guidelines), programs (measuring and improving performance), and lifelong learning (grand rounds, the cube, and critical appraisal) and to develop these areas by promoting evidence-based health practice.

Several assessment tools were outlined that can be used to critically appraise the medical and public health literature. By wisdom and not convention, public health practitioners and health services managers will begin to make progress toward creating healthy communities. This will take shape as they adopt the health practice guidelines for basing decisions on evidence.

In the previous chapters, the focus was on the tools for measurement and improvement to bring the rhetoric of evidence-based public health practice and management into the mainstream of epidemiology, statistics, and measurement. Thus, the analytic tools for problem identification and problem analysis were detailed. The basis for these tools is predicated on sound epidemiologic and statistical methods, which are also highlighted as appropriate for the application of the improvement tools. Next, a chapter on small-area analysis is presented to further develop quality measurement for application by problem solvers.

References

1. "Koop Urges Public Health to 'Take the High Road,'" *Nation's Health* (December 1995):1, 8.
2. E. R. Brown, "President's Column: Advocacy and Public Health," *Nation's Health* (December 1995):2.
3. "'Marketing Our Value' Is Public Health's Challenge, Says Evans," *Nation's Health* (December 1995):8.
4. Ibid.
5. Ibid.
6. "Koop Urges Public Health to 'Take the High Road,'" *Nation's Health*, 8.
7. G. M. Christenson and S. Dandoy, eds., "Research and Measurement in Public Health Practice," *American Journal of Preventive Medicine* 11, no. 6 Supplement (1995).
8. A. S. Handler et al., "A Strategy for Measuring Local Public Health Practice," *American Journal of Preventive Medicine* 11, no. 6 Supplement (1995):29–35.
9. T. B. Richards et al., "Assessing Public Health Practice: Application of Ten Core Function Measures of Community Health in Six States," *American Journal of Preventive Medicine* 11, no. 6 Supplement (1995):36–40.
10. C. A. Miller et al., "A Screening Survey to Assess Local Public Health Performance," *Public Health Reports* 109 (1994):659–664.
11. C. A. Miller et al., "A Proposed Method for Assessing the Performance of Local Public Health Functions and Practices," *American Journal of Public Health*, 84 (1994):1743–1749.
12. M. Pratt et al., "Local Health Departments in Washington State Use APEX to Assess Capacity," *Public Health Reports* 111, no. 1 (1996):8–91.
13. Ibid., 88.
14. Ibid., 90.
15. Ibid., 91.
16. Ibid.
17. P. A. Lamarche, "Our Health Paradigm in Peril," *Public Health Reports* 110, no. 5 (1995):556–560.
18. Ibid.
19. C. E. Fox, "Why We Fail to Replicate Pilot Results: Adopting Realistic Expectations," *Public Health Reports* 110, no. 5 (1995):562.
20. A. G. Ellrodt and M. Cho, "Introduction to Evidence-Based Practice," in *Patient-Focused Care in the Hospital: Restructuring and Redesign Methods to Achieve Better Outcomes*, vol. 4, ed. C. E. Aydin et al. (New York: Faulkner & Gray, 1995), 301–328.

21. M. E. Lara and C. Goodman, eds., *National Priorities for the Assessment of Clinical Conditions and Medical Technologies: Report of a Pilot Study* (Washington, D.C.: National Academy Press, 1990), 77–81.
22. R. S. A. Hayward and A. Laupacis, "Initiating, Conducting and Maintaining Guidelines Development Programs," *Canadian Medical Association Journal* 148, no. 4 (1993):507–512.
23. Ibid., 508.
24. J. J. Hanlon, "The Design of Public Health Programs for Underdeveloped Countries," *Public Health Reports* 69 (1954):1028–1033.
25. G. E. Pickett and J. J. Hanlon, *Public Health Administration and Practice*, 9th ed. (St. Louis, Mo.: CV Mosby, 1990), 226–227.
26. Evidence-Based Care Resource Group, "Evidence-Based Care: 2. Setting Guidelines: How Should We Manage This Problem?" *Canadian Medical Association Journal* 150, no. 9 (1994):1417–1423.
27. A. D. Oxman et al., "Users' Guide to the Medical Literature: I. How to Get Started," *JAMA* 270, no. 17 (1993):2093–2095.
28. Evidence-Based Medicine Working Group, G. Guyatt and D. Rennie, eds., *Users' Guides to the Medical Literature: Essentials of Evidence-Based Clinical Practice* (Chicago: American Medical Association, 2002).
29. D. L. Sackett et al., *Evidence-Based Medicine: How to Practice and Teach EBM*, 2d ed. (Edinburgh: Churchill Livingstone, 2000).
30. Ibid., 67.
31. Ibid.
32. U.S. Department of Health and Human Services, *Healthy People 2010, 2d ed., with Understanding and Improving Health*, 2 vols. (Washington, D.C.: Government Printing Office, 2000).
33. U.S. Department of Health and Human Services, Healthy People 2000: National Health Promotion and Disease Prevention Objectives, DHHS Pub. (PHS) 91-50212 (Washington, D.C.: Government Printing Office, 1991), GPO Stock No. 017-001-0474-0.
34. M. R. Traska, *Managed Care Strategies 1996: An Annual Report on the Latest Practice and Policies in the New Managed Care Environment* (New York: Faulkner & Gray, Inc., 1996), 67.
35. D. M. Eddy, "Practice Guidelines: What Are They, and How Are They Designed?," 138.
36. Ibid., 140.
37. Evidence-Based Care Resource Group, "Evidence-Based Care: 3," 1576.
38. D. R. Nerenz and B. M. Zajac, *Ray Woodham Visiting Fellowship Program Project Summary Report* (Chicago: Hospital Research and Educational Trust, 1991).
39. "Measuring the Quality of Health Care," *Employee Benefit Research Institute (EBRI) Issue Brief* 159 (1995):15.
40. B. M. Zajac et al., "Health Status of Populations as a Measure of Health System Performance," *Managed Care Quarterly* 3, no. 1 (1995):29–38.
41. Traska, *Managed Care Strategies 1996*, 174.
42. Ibid.
43. E. L. Baker et al., "CDC's Information Network for Public Health Officials (INPHO): A Framework for Integrated Public Health Information and Practice," *Journal of Public Health Management Practice* 1, no. 1 (1995):43–47.

44. Traska, *Managed Care Strategies 1996*, 181.
45. F. Bazzoli, "Restoring the Image of Networks," *Health Data Management* 4, no. 11 (1996): 38–50.
46. Traska, *Managed Care Strategies 1996*, 174.
47. Baker et al., "CDC's Information Network for Public Health Officials (INPHO)," 43–47.
48. Traska, *Managed Care Strategies 1996*, 169–170.
49. Headquarters Air Force Logistics Command, "Benchmark Matrix and Guide: Part III," *Journal for Healthcare Quality* 14, no. 1 (1992):8–13.
50. Ibid., 8.
51. Evidence-Based Care Resource Group, "Evidence-Based Care: 4. Improving Performance: How Can We Improve the Way We Manage This Problem?" *Canadian Medical Association Journal* 150, no. 11 (1994):1793–1796.
52. J. L. Reinertsen, "Outcomes Management and Continuous Quality Improvement: The Compass and the Rudder," *Quality Review Bulletin* (January 1993):5–7.
53. Ibid., 6.
54. D. L. Sackett et al., *Clinical Epidemiology: A Basic Science for Clinical Medicine* (Boston: Little, Brown and Company, 1985).
55. Evidence-Based Care Resource Group, "Evidence-Based Care: 5. Lifelong Learning: How Can We Learn to Be More Effective?" *Canadian Medical Association Journal* 150, no. 12 (1994):1971–1973.
56. Evidence-Based Medicine Working Group, "Evdence-Based Medicine: A New Approach to Teaching the Practice of Medicine," *JAMA* 268, no. 17 (1992): 2420–2425.
57. J. A. M. Gray, *Evidence-Based Healthcare: How to Make Health Policy and Management Decisions* (Edinburgh: Churchill Livingstone, 2001).
58. Evidence-Based Medicine Working Group, "Users' Guides to the Medical Literature: III. How to Use an Article about a Diagnostic Test, A. Are the Results of the Study Valid?" *JAMA* 271, no. 5 (1994):389–391.
59. Evidence-Based Medicine Working Group, "Users' Guides to the Medical Literature: IV. How to Use an Article about Harm," *JAMA* 271, no. 20 (1994): 1615–1619.
60. Evidence-Based Medicine Working Group, "Users' Guides to the Medical Literature: V. How to Use an Article about Prognosis," *JAMA* 272, no. 3 (1994):234–237.
61. Evidence-Based Medicine Working Group, "Users' Guides to the Medical Literature: VI. How to Use an Overview," *JAMA* 272, no. 17 (1994):1367–1371.
62. Evidence-Based Medicine Working Group, "Users' Guides to the Medical Literature: VII. How to Use a Clinical Decision, Analysis, B. What Are the Results and Will They Help Me in Caring for My Patients?" *JAMA* 273, no. 20 (1995):1610–1613.
63. Evidence-Based Medicine Working Group, "Users' Guides to the Medical Literature: VIII. How to Use Clinical Practice Guidelines, A. Are the Recommendations Valid?" *JAMA* 274, no. 7 (1995):570–574.
64. G. E. A. Dever, *Creating Critical Thinkers* (Atlanta: Georgia Department of Human Resources, 1993).

10

Epidemiologic Assessment: Small Area Analysis

In public health practice, there is a high demand for assessment—a core function—of the needs of a community from an epidemiologic perspective. Traditionally, there has been a keen interest in using small area analysis, mainly in response to the pressure from federal agencies to monitor the progress of a community toward the Year 2000 and 2010 objectives. Further, and a more recent development, is the need to develop data systems that will allow effective outcome assessment and epidemiological measurement of a program, community, county, or a customer. Associated with this type of measurement in public health practice is the need to analyze information effectively that represents small areas. To do this, public health practitioners and health service managers need to understand epidemiologic measurement as discussed in Chapter 5 and additionally understand how to analyze communities from a epidemiological perspective using small area analysis (SAA).

A review of the literature reveals two major, almost parallel, uses of small area analysis:

1. Small area analysis of epidemiologic data in performing widespread needs assessments
2. Small area analysis of community-level variations in hospital admissions for various medical and surgical conditions (i.e., variation in hospital utilization statistics)

The *epidemiologic needs assessment approach* using small area analysis dates back to the time of Hippocrates but is probably best recognized with the 1854 analysis of cholera deaths by John Snow in the Soho district of London, England.[1] Of course, this approach of epidemiologic needs assessment is prevalent and very popular in the SAA of health planning, disease investigation, demographic analysis, and indicator profiling providing quality of life reports. All approaches tend to rely heavily on mapping and other geographic methods to display the small area data.

The *hospitalization utilization approach* using small area analysis was reported as early as 1856 by a physician in London (William A. Guy). He noted that annual rates for hospitalization varied from 325 per 1,000 population to one per 1,000 population. He hypothesized that the explanation for the variation in use rates between the two areas was related to behavioral characteristics of the populations, specifically to "acts of self indulgence."[2] In the modern era, the study by Coger in 1938 on tonsillectomy is recognized as the landmark report. Of course, now the issues of costs, quality improvement, medical outcomes, and consumer demands have propelled this type of analysis forward.[3]

What Is Small Area Analysis?

Small area analysis is a method of measuring variations and comparing rates of mortality, morbidity, and the cost of health care use among defined populations.[4] Because considerable variation in mortality, morbidity, and hospital use has been found to exist among small communities, which is often masked when analyzing larger geographic areas, a need to have appropriate statistical/epidemiologic/quality measurement tools is important for the proper assessment of public health practices and utilization of health services. These tools can be used to address these variations and to determine the significance of the differences and further to monitor these areas over periods of time for variation. Thus, small area analysis identifies variations (differences) in the use (rate) of inpatient hospital services, mortality data, and social, economic, demographic, and psychographic factors, showing those rates in defined small areas (market areas). Each service area (county, city, ZIP code, census tract, or health market area) rate can be compared with other small areas or the state rate, providing information that could be lost or hidden if only state rates were analyzed.

The data usually has been age and sex adjusted, meaning that any differences cannot be attributed to age or sex. Sometimes such adjustments can obscure age/sex variations when small areas are compared. To use the methods and techniques for small area analysis effectively, there are some simple yet important concepts to learn.

Simple Concepts Important to Know for Small Area Analysis

Table 10-1 presents several concepts that must be evaluated by the health practitioner or analyst who takes on the task of epidemiologic measurement and outcome assessment for small area analysis. Although these concepts are simplistic, they are essential to performing a valid analysis of small areas.

TABLE 10-1 Simple Concepts Important to Know for Epidemiologic Measurement for Small Area Analysis

Numerator	*vs.*	*Denominator*
■ Cases (morbidity) ■ Deaths (mortality) ■ Visits (utilization)		■ Population-at-risk ■ Service area
Numbers	*vs.*	*Rates*
■ Allocation of resources		■ Assessment of health status
Small Numbers	*vs.*	*Large Numbers*

■ Large error, statistically unreliable aggregate:
  ■ Space (geographics)
  ■ Time (years, months, etc.)
  ■ Groups (ages, socioeconomic)
■ Identify trends
		■ Statistically reliable trends
		■ Area comparisons

Significant	*vs.*	*Nonsignificant*
■ Clinical vs. statistical ■ Programmatic vs. statistical		■ Sample size too small
Service Area	*vs.*	*Market Area*
■ Where *do* patients come from?		■ Where *should* patients come from?
Community Health Status	*vs.*	*Individual Health Status*
■ Populations in communities ■ Community diagnosis		■ Individuals in clinics ■ Clinical diagnosis
*Program Impact-Evaluation**	*vs.*	*Community Impact-Evaluation**
Must determine the difference between:		
1. Program-based evaluation 2. Service-based evaluation	*vs.*	1. Community-based evaluation 2. Population-based evaluation

*Cannot infer that the program was responsible for improvement in community indicators.

■ The numerator/denominator concept

The numerator/denominator concept is of paramount importance to population-based analysis for small areas. Obviously, the numerator provides counts that can be translated into rates using the appropriate denominator (population-at-risk). Epidemiologic measurement in public health practice must understand the nature of a program service-oriented denominator (all patients in the program or clinic) versus a community-based population-oriented denominator (total population in a service area or population-at-risk). When making decisions for improvement in an indicator, health practitioners must be responsible and report results based on the appropriate target population and use the correct denominator.

■ Numbers versus rates

The relationships of numbers to rates at first glance seem rather obvious as to their differences in terms of use. However, public health analysts need to be aware that there is a place for both of these values. Specifically, if the analyst is most concerned with resource allocation, then the actual number of events to be addressed must be known because each event requires a certain dollar amount, amount of space, or personnel time. However, if the concern is about the relative health status of one community compared with another, the rates are essential to standardize the comparison for further evaluation. Recall in a previous chapter that there were occasions for using the counts and occasions for using the rates, depending on the specifics of the analysis required—person, place, or time.

■ Small numbers versus large numbers

Small numbers versus large numbers, of course, is the primary issue concerning the analysis of small areas. Notably, small numbers produce large errors and are usually statistically unreliable compared with large numbers, which generally produce statistically reliable trends. The methods described in this chapter based on the binomial and Poisson distributions are presented to deal with the issue of small numbers (counts) in epidemiologic measurement. Further, assessments make use of the binomial and Poisson distributions to evaluate small areas from an outcome and improvement perspective. To avoid or compensate for the small number problems, it is customary to aggregate the data by geography (i.e., combining two or more small areas), time (analyzing several time periods or using a three- or five-year moving average), or groups (e.g., age or socio-economic status can be combined to produce a larger number).

■ Significance versus nonsignificance

A result, if significant or nonsignificant, is usually evaluated by statistical tests. Several tests can determine the significance of numbers for small geographic areas. However, the real issue is the importance of this statistically significant difference in terms of clinical and programmatic policy. The evaluations of all statistical tests must be further evaluated for policy implications—clinically and programmatically. In small area analysis, this is especially true because small numbers can produce significant results but the confidence limits provide the range or interval, which in the case of small numbers can be so wide as to be of no practical value except to alert the analyst to a potential invalid evaluation.

■ Service areas versus market areas

The concept of a service area versus a market area is seldom considered as an issue by the public health analyst. In the era of managed care and quality improvement, these terms take on a significant meaning. As public health analysts apply the public health core functions of assessment, policy development, and assurance within their agencies, they must understand that a service area (where patients come from) and a market area (where patients should come from) are different from a population-based area, which includes both a service area and a market area. In other words, public health is concerned primarily with the population-at-risk for defining needs of a program; however, hospitals have almost always been concerned with service areas and market areas. The future for public health is in the understanding of all these areas because managed care providers are most interested in population-based analysis and public health agencies at present control much of the data for developing population-based indicators. Health service providers desperately seek to get a handle on this type of information.

■ Individual focus versus community (population-based) focus

As discussed in an earlier chapter, there has been a shift away from the individual focus of clients in clinics to the community- or population-based focus of populations in communities. Public health practice has been responsible for assessing the community health status by completing a community diagnosis (population-in-communities) report on the health status of areas. However, as public health shifted into clinical programs (individuals-in-clinics), the health status measurement of individuals was attempted. The result was that very feeble efforts were attempted to evaluate the status of individuals in programs and certainly can be considered as one of the factors contributing to the present disarray of public health evaluations. However, public health in the future is well positioned to focus on the population-based assessments and fulfill the core functions of public health.

■ Program impact versus community impact

Finally, program impact evaluation as opposed to community impact evaluation has been used inappropriately to suggest impact at both ends of the spectrum—program and community. Traditionally, health programs have made the inference that if community indicators have improved, then the program was responsible. However, there is not always proof available to document this situation. Assessment must, however, begin to evaluate the program that is service-based using proper numerators and denominators to determine if the program has had any influence on improving outcomes. This is not to say the program has not had an effect, but assuming credit for improvement is not based on evidence. Future endeavors, if public health stays in the program business, must be evaluated from the program perspective using program cases (numerators) and program denominators. Of course, public health must continue to evaluate communities and assess change and improvement. The purpose of this book is to bring the appropriate tools to the practice of public health and health services management so that quality measurement can become part of the skills advanced and applied by the public health practitioner and the health services manager.

The understanding of the concepts discussed in the bullet list here allows for a more realistic use and application of the statistical tests for small area analysis. In epidemiology, the traditional tools are used to understand the variation of a process; and the small area analysis concepts and tools are used to also understand the variation of the characteristic being evaluated but further to determine the significance of the variation based on confidence limits of a count, rate, proportion, ratio, or index. Obviously, the two approaches are almost identical. If the assessment is more concerned with the process over time, the traditional epidemiologic tools as discussed in Chapters 7 and 8 are used, and if one is mostly concerned with variation in space or geography, then using small area analysis is another tool for epidemiologic measurement. No matter the viewpoint, the intent or purpose must be to continuously monitor the situation, hold the gains, and improve the outcomes or process. Using small area analysis as an analytical tool must likewise become the skill of the new public health scientist; evaluating small areas (e.g., census tracts, ZIP codes, blocks, counties) is crucial to quality measurement. Obviously, the spatial pattern over time will exhibit characteristics that can be high risk or low risk and, therefore, must be monitored to demonstrate improvement either based on a Year 2010 standard or an objective (such as used in quality assurance) or based on a continuous quality improvement (CQI) model in which it does not matter if certain geographic areas have met the objective, there is always room for continuous improvement in the indicator. A first step toward this process is to know what is expected based on a standard or a predetermined value identified from a specific process. For example, if it is known for infant mortality the Year 2000 objective was seven infant deaths per 1,000 live births—that is a standard; however, an analysis of fifteen small areas revealed an infant mortality of sixteen infant deaths per 1,000 live births, which is a value based on the process. In both instances, the small area analysis methods are applied to determine the pattern of variation and to see if any of the areas can be determined to be at high and low risk and, thereby, represent a special situation that must be investigated. Initially, however, the evaluation of small areas must determine the number of expected events (e.g., deaths, cases, utilization) to occur in the area investigated. This concept of determining the number of expected events can also be used in the evaluation of programs if the process is evaluated against a standard. However, in quality improvement, control charts generally evaluate the outcome indicator based on the process and therefore focus on the continuous quality improvement (CQI) of the outcome that continues to evaluate levels beyond a standard.

Determining the Number of Expected Events

Each of the following two methodologies is statistically valid for small area analysis and should produce the same results. The selection of one methodology over the other, therefore, depends solely on the availability of data and personal preference. The examples provided here are based on determining the number of expected deaths; however, for detecting the number of expected cases for use related to utilization rates, the same methods may apply.

Using the Actual Number of Deaths (Events)

The expected number of deaths can be calculated using the following formula:

$$E = \frac{P_1}{P_2} \times D$$

where

> E = expected deaths
> P_1 = population being investigated
> P_2 = standard population
> D = actual deaths in standard population

The ratio, P_1/P_2, should be age-sex-race specific. If the subject is deaths among white men ages 55 to 64, both P_1 and P_2 should refer to the number of white men of these ages; however, if deaths among the overall population are being studied, P_1 and P_2 should refer to the total population.

For example, in a state between 2000 and 2004 there were fifty-two deaths from fires and flames among men ages 60 to 64. There were 113,128 men of this age in the state; 4,055 were in the city being investigated. Assuming that the risk of dying in a fire was the same in the city as in the state as a whole, the expected number of deaths in the city was calculated as follows:

$$E = \frac{P_1}{P_2} \times D$$

$$E = \frac{4,055}{113,128} \times 52$$

$$E = 1.9 \text{ deaths}$$

Thus, 1.9 (rounded to 2) is the expected number of such deaths in the city among men ages 60 to 64. There were three actual deaths because of fires and flames in the city being investigated, a difference of one death.

Using Death Rates

If, instead of the actual number of deaths (events), death rates are available for the standard population, the expected number of deaths is given by

$$E = P_1 \times M_2$$

where

> P_1 = population being investigated
> M_2 = specific death rate in the standard population

Because $M_2 = \dfrac{D}{P_2}$, it can be shown that this is algebraically equivalent to the previous method.

Using Death Rates—An Example

Situation: In Burke County, Georgia (small area), the acute myocardial infarction (AMI) rate for 1994 through 2003 is 147.0 per 100,000 population, representing 306 deaths. The rate in the standard population (in Georgia from 1994 to 2003) is 107.9 per 100,000 population.

Solution: $E = P_1 \times M_2$

$$E = 208{,}224 \times \left(\frac{107.9}{100{,}000} \right)$$

$$E = 208{,}224 \times 0.001079$$

$$E = 224.7$$

where

E = expected deaths

P_1 = 208,224 (1994–2003 population for Burke County)

M_2 = 107.9 (AMI rate of Georgia)

Thus, 224.7 deaths can be expected in Burke County for 1994 through 2003 for AMI, and in actuality 306 deaths had been observed during 1994 through 2003.

Significance of "Excess Deaths" or "Excess Events"

A problem can also be defined by an excess of morbidity or mortality (i.e., use rate problems or epidemiology/needs assessment problems). In an analysis of "excess deaths," for example, there are two major steps. Initially, it must be determined whether there is a difference between the number of deaths expected and the number that actually occurred (observed). If so, it must be determined whether the excess deaths result merely from chance or are actually significant statistically. This analysis can require the following data on both the population being investigated and the standard population:

- Demographic data categorized by age, sex, race, occupation, or other specifics
- Mortality data categorized by cause of death, either in actual number observed or in death rates

As already noted, if death rates are available for the selected standard population, the expected number of deaths can be derived for the population being investigated.

Testing the Significance of Results (Excess Deaths/Events)

Once the difference between the expected and the observed (actual) deaths has been determined, a statistical test must be applied to determine whether the difference has any significance. If so, a greater than expected number of deaths is not likely to be the result of chance alone; however, there is always a possibility that a certain number of events in 100 could have occurred solely on the basis of chance.

The significance of a difference can be tested by means of standardized mortality ratios (SMRs), which are developed and tested using the standard error and confidence intervals, or the chi-square "goodness-of-fit" test. Although each of these methods is statistically sound for this purpose, public health analysts with limited statistical backgrounds generally find the SMR easier to use. It requires more subjective judgment to interpret the results, whereas the chi-square test is somewhat more complex and can require some statistical expertise.

Standardized Mortality Ratio   SMR is calculated as follows:

$$SMR = \frac{Observed\ deaths}{Expected\ deaths} \times 100$$

A ratio of 100 indicates that the observed number of deaths equals the expected number of deaths. A ratio of 130, for example, indicates that there were 30 percent more deaths than expected; a ratio of 90 indicates 10 percent fewer deaths than expected.

The next step is to calculate the confidence interval of the SMR. The calculation of a 95 percent confidence interval of an SMR is obtained by

$$CI = SMR \pm (1.96 \times SE)$$

where

SE = standard error

$$SE = \frac{SMR}{\sqrt{d}}$$

d = number of observed deaths

Data on observed and expected deaths in a county, as compared with a state, is presented in Table 10-2. The SMR is 89.97 or rounded to 90 and the SE is 5.58. The resulting confidence interval is 79 to 101. To interpret the confidence interval of an SMR, the following is suggested:

- If the lower confidence limit is below 100 and the upper limit is above 100, there is no significant difference between the number of observed and the number of expected deaths.
- If the lower confidence limit is above 100, then the number of observed deaths is significantly higher than expected, and it is unlikely that the excess is merely a chance occurrence.
- If the upper confidence limit is below 100, the number of observed deaths is significantly fewer than expected.
- If a confidence interval is quite wide, regardless of what the limits are, more data is required or the data should be grouped before any conclusion can be reached. Although no clear-cut rules specify what constitutes a "wide" range, a range of fifty or more is excessive.

In the following example (Table 10-2), it is somewhat difficult to decide whether the result is significant, because the upper confidence limit is barely above 100. It can be concluded that the SMR seems moderately,

TABLE 10-2 Observed and Expected Deaths from Heart Disease for County A, by Age Group, 2000–2004

Age Group	Observed Deaths	Expected Deaths
20–29	16	16
30–39	18	20
40–49	22	18
50–59	51	56
60–69	55	72
70–79	62	64
80–89	22	28
90+	14	15
TOTAL	260	289

$$SMR = \frac{260}{289} \times 100 = 89.97$$

$$SE = \frac{SMR}{\sqrt{d}} = \frac{89.97}{\sqrt{260}} = 5.58$$

95 percent confidence interval

$$CI_{95\%} = 89.97 \pm (1.96 \times 5.58)$$

Upper limit $= 89.97 + 10.94 = 100.91$

Lower limit $= 89.97 - 10.94 = 79.03$

$$CI = 79 \text{ to } 101$$

although not significantly, low at the 95 percent confidence level. A strict interpretation is that it is not significant.

Chi-Square Test   The chi-square or "goodness-of-fit" test makes it possible to compare an observed frequency with an expected frequency distribution. The formula for chi-square is

$$\chi^2 = \Sigma \frac{(O - E)^2}{E}$$

where

O = observed deaths

E = expected deaths

Table 10-3 presents the calculation of chi-square for the data presented in Table 10-2. The computed chi-square value of 6.97 is compared with a tabular value of chi-square with $(k - r)$ degrees of freedom, where k equals the number of categories that can be calculated for $(O - E)^2 / E$ (i.e., the number of age groups in this example), and r equals the number of restrictions (quantities) that were determined from observed data and used in calculating the expected frequencies.

In most cases in which the expected frequencies are determined by using the chi-square test (or the SMR), the only observed quantity involved in calculating the expected frequencies is the population (P_1). Under these circumstances, the degree of freedom is $(k - 1)$. However, in the example in

TABLE 10-3   Calculations of Chi-Square for Observed and Expected Deaths from Heart Disease for County A, 2000–2004

Age Group	Observed Deaths	Expected Deaths	$\frac{(O - E)^2}{E}$
20–29	16	16	0.00
30–39	18	20	0.20
40–49	22	18	0.89
50–59	51	56	0.45
60–69	55	72	4.01
70–79	62	64	0.06
80–89	22	28	1.29
90+	14	15	0.07
TOTAL	260	289	6.97

$\chi^2 = 0.00 + 0.20 + 0.89 + 0.45 + 4.01 + 0.06 + 1.29 + 0.07$
$\chi^2 = 6.97$

Table 10-3 there are no restrictions, as the expected frequencies were not calculated from the observed data but from a standard.

There are eight degrees of freedom (eight age groups). The value of chi-square for eight degrees of freedom at the 95 percent level is 15.507.[*] If the calculated value (6.97) is less than the tabular value, as is the case here, then it can be said that there is no significant difference between the observed and the expected deaths. If the calculated value were greater than the tabular value, the difference would be significant. Both methods (i.e., the SMR and the X^2) provide the same result.

Epidemiologic Measurement and Small Area Analysis

When analyzing small areas, especially for epidemiology/needs assessment type problems and quality measurement, there are specific methods to be used when the analysis involves any of the following:[5,6,7,8]

- Counts
- Rates
- Proportions
- Ratios
- Indexes

Depending on the assumptions related to the use of the statistical tests and the nature of the data used, it is possible that some of the tests can be appropriate to analyze hospital utilization statistics (i.e., use rates). If the assumptions are met, then there is a "green light" for analysis.

Small Area Analysis—Hypothesis Testing

To compare one geographic area, time period, or age group with a standard, there are specific tests based on counts, rates, and proportions to use to test the hypotheses of no difference between the two categories. Listed in Table 10-4 is a summary of these statistics for counts, rates, and proportions. Using these tests, it is shown how they can be applied to the analysis of small areas. Additionally, the use of confidence intervals is demonstrated as a method for assessing the significance of small area variations. The formulas for determining confidence limits for counts, rates, and proportions are also shown in Table 10-4.

---

[*]A value obtained by looking at the χ^2 probability distribution.

TABLE 10-4   Small Area Analysis: Area/Standard Comparisons (One-Sample Tests)[*]

Hypothesis Test On	Test Statistic	Confidence Interval[†]
One count	$z = \dfrac{x - \mu_0}{\sqrt{\mu_0}}$	$x \pm 1.96\sqrt{x}$
One rate	$z = \dfrac{r - \theta_0}{\sqrt{\theta_0/\text{PYRS}}}$ [**]	$r \pm 1.96\sqrt{\dfrac{r}{\text{PYRS}}}$ [**]
Alternative rate[‡]		$\dfrac{1000}{n}(d \pm 1.96\sqrt{d})$
		$\text{SE} = \dfrac{r}{\sqrt{d}}$
One proportion	$z = \dfrac{p - \pi_0}{\sqrt{\dfrac{\pi_0(1 - \pi_0)}{n}}}$	$p \pm 1.96\sqrt{\dfrac{p(1 - p)}{n}}$
Many proportions[§]	$\chi^2 = \sum \dfrac{(O - E)^2}{E}$	

[*]H_0 (Null Hypothesis) = no difference between the observed area (sample) and the expected (population) standard.

[**]PYRS = person-years-at-risk (population-at-risk)

[†]The confidence interval is a range that is expected to contain the population parameter being estimated. The level of probability can be 0.05, 0.01, or 0.001.

[‡]There are several alternatives to calculating confidence intervals for a rate; each is applicable. The choice to use one over the other is a personal preference.

[§]The X^2 can be used to compare one proportion or many proportions. Because this is the only test presented in this book for measuring variations in many proportions, it is, therefore, included here.

Small Area Analysis—Confidence Interval Estimation

Assessing confidence intervals for a single parameter for a small area is an acceptable alternative to significance testing if small proportions or low counts bring into question the approximation model used (i.e., binomial, Poisson, normal), specifically the assumptions concerning the sampling distribution of proportions and counts that are approximated by the binomial and Poisson distributions, respectively.

To use these distributions, some facts are essential to an appropriate evaluation of the results.

- For *small proportions or low counts*, an acceptable alternative is to perform the significant test using the confidence interval approach.

- If the *null value* is included in the confidence interval, the result is equivalent to nonsignificance.

- If the *null value* is not included in the confidence interval, the result is equivalent to significance.

- For *small sample sizes*, the tests for the normal approximation to the binomial or Poisson distribution for proportions and counts, respectively, as outlined in this book might not hold; however, tables for the binomial and Poisson can be used to determine the exact limits.

- Assessing significance using confidence intervals is a perfectly acceptable procedure and is recommended for small sample sizes (i.e., data representing small areas).

It is always necessary to construct a confidence interval when presenting data derived from a sample of a population or when presenting rates for a population. Such calculations are often based on relatively low numbers of values, and the width of the confidence interval will take this into account. If few values are used, the confidence interval will be quite wide. With a great many values, however, the confidence interval is narrower, indicating that the estimates are more accurate.

The confidence interval can be particularly illuminating for the presentation of nonsignificant results. If the sample size is too small, the width of the confidence interval shows clearly the large range of values compatible with the observed result and thus allows one to see the possibly important effects that would be glossed over by giving only the negative result of the significance test. If the sample size is adequate for nonsignificant results, the range covered by the confidence interval should be narrow enough to exclude the possibility of medically important effects.[9]

The probability that the true population rate is contained within the confidence interval is called the degree of confidence. The value most commonly used for the degree of confidence is 0.95, or 95 percent. This indicates that users of the data can be 95 percent confident that the true value lies within the calculated confidence interval. In other words, there is a 95 percent probability that the confidence interval includes the true value and a 5 percent probability that it does not. When a 5 percent chance of error is not acceptable, a 99 percent confidence interval is commonly used.

Statistical Guides for Outcome Assessment and Epidemiological Measurement in Analyzing Small Areas

This section outlines several statistical guides to be used for evaluating small areas from an epidemiologic perspective and assessing outcomes in public health practice. The guides focus on the typical tests of hypotheses and the use of confidence intervals for assessing patterns based on defined limits from a spatial perspective. These guides are presented for counts, rates, and proportions.

Statistical Guide 1: Counts (Hypothesis Test)

A Single Count (Comparing a Small Area with a Standard)*

- Analyzing a single count
- Hypothesis test for a count
- Problem: Is the number of infant deaths observed in a small area from an expected number based on a standard (state, region, or national objective—Year 2010 objective may also be used)?
- Null hypothesis (H_0)

  H_0: observed count = standard count (i.e., no difference in the two counts)
- Test statistic† (normal approximation to the Poisson)

  z test

$$z = \frac{x(\text{observed count}) - x_1(\text{standard count})}{\sqrt{x_1(\text{standard count})}}$$

  or

$$z = \frac{x - \mu_0}{\sqrt{\mu_0}}$$

  where

  z = normal approximation to the Poisson

  x = observed count in the area

  μ_0 = standard count to be compared (expected count)
- Data: infant deaths in:

  Burke County, Georgia (1994–2003) = 62 infant deaths

  Georgia (1994–2003) = 12,854 infant deaths

  Expected based on standard = 50.9 infant deaths

---

*The comparison can be a geographic area, a time period, or an age group.

†Assumptions/requirements: that the count is based on independent events and that, for the z test, the count is more than ten. Also the normal approximation can be used when it is reasonable to assume that cases (events) are occurring independently and randomly in time and space. This is less likely to be true for infectious diseases and for diseases in which there is strong evidence of clustering.

■ Analysis

$$z = \frac{62 - 50.9}{\sqrt{50.9}}$$

$$z = \frac{11.1}{7.1}$$

$$z = 1.56$$

■ Determining the expected count (standard)*

1. Infant mortality is based on the number of live births.
2. Burke County had 3,912 live births; Georgia had 988,147.
3. Burke County has 0.00396 proportion of the state births.
4. It would be expected that Burke County would have 0.00396 of the state infant deaths.
5. The state had 12,854 infant deaths. Therefore,

    Expected deaths = 0.00396 × 12,854 = 50.9

■ Results

Compare the z value of 1.56 to the standard normal distribution (critical value) at the 0.05 significance level. The critical value at this level is 1.96.

■ Interpretation

Because 1.56 is less than 1.96, there is no significant difference between the number of infant deaths in Burke County compared with the expected number based on the state standard. That is, this one county shows no variation from the standard, so the county is within the limits established by the test using the standard as the expected.

Statistical Guide 2: Counts (Confidence Intervals)

A Single Count (Confidence Intervals for a County Representing a Small Area)

■ Analyzing a single count using confidence intervals.

■ Confidence intervals for a count draws attention to results actually obtained rather than concentrating on the decision to reject or not to reject; confidence intervals give a range of values that

---

*The method used here is "using the actual number of deaths."

$$E = \frac{P_1}{P_2} \times D$$

at a given probability level is likely to contain the true count; thus, the confidence interval presents the result and conveys the inherent variability in the estimate of that result.

■ Problem: at the 95 percent confidence level, what is the range in the number of infant deaths that can be expected? That is, if the number of infant deaths in an area is assumed to be a sample in time and space, what is the confidence level that the sample count is reflective of the true count for that area or time period?

■ Confidence intervals do not require the predetermination or specifications of a null value.

■ Test statistic

1. For $n \leq 100$, use tables based on Poisson distribution (see Table 10-5).

2. For $n > 100$, a normal approximation to the Poisson distribution is used:

$$x \pm 1.96\sqrt{x}$$

where

$x = \text{count}$

$1.96 = \text{critical value at the 95 percent significance level}$

■ Data: infant mortality (1994–2003)

Burke County = 62 infant deaths

■ Analysis

1. Exact confidence limits per Poisson distribution table (Table 10-5)

Lower Limit	Actual	Upper Limit
47.5	62	79.5

2. Confidence limits per normal approximation formula:

$$x \pm 1.96\sqrt{x}$$

$$62 \pm 1.96(7.9)$$

$$62 \pm 15.5$$

or

Lower Limit	Actual	Upper Limit
46.5	62	79.5

TABLE 10-5   Exact Confidence Limits for Poisson Count[*]

	95% Confidence Level	
x	x_l	x_u
56	42.302	72.721
57	43.171	73.850
58	44.042	74.978
59	44.914	76.106
60	45.786	77.232
61	46.660	78.357
62	47.535	79.481
63	48.411	80.604
64	49.288	81.727
65	50.166	82.848

[*]x is an observed Poisson count, x_l and x_u are the lower and upper limits for the population count.

■ Results

There is a 95 percent confident level that the actual number of infant deaths could be as low as 47.5 (46.5) and as high as 79.5 (77.5). Thus, if another sample is taken for a 10-year period from the same small area, it can be expected that 95 percent of the time the count of infant deaths would fall between these lower and upper limits. Of course, 5 percent of the time, just by chance, the count could be outside these limits.

■ Interpretation

Remembering that the expected count (50.9) calculated from the previous guide on counts was the *null value*, it can then be determined if the confidence level limits include the value. That is, is 50.9 located between the lower limit (47.5) and the upper limit (79.5)? If they do (and they do in this example), then the result is equivalent to nonsignificance. If the null value was not included, then the result could be considered significant. The results obtained here verify earlier results that there is no significant difference, plus there is now a range of possible values the actual count could have fallen in and still be representative of the true count.

Statistical Guide 3: Rates (Hypothesis Test)

A Single Rate (Comparing a Small Area with a Standard)*

- Analyzing a single rate
- Hypothesis test for a rate
- Problem: Is the infant mortality rate observed in a small area different from an expected rate based on a standard (state, region, or national objective—Year 2010 objective can be used)?
- Null hypothesis

    H_0: observed rate = standard rate (i.e., no difference between the two rates)

- Test statistic[†] (normal approximation to the Poisson)

z test

$$z = \frac{r(\text{observed count}) - r_1(\text{standard count})}{\sqrt{r_1(\text{standard count}) / \text{population-at-risk}}}$$

or

$$z = \frac{r - \theta_0}{\sqrt{\theta_0 / \text{PYRS}}}$$

where

z = normal approximation to the Poisson

r = observed rate in the area

θ_0 = standard rate to be compared

PYRS = person-years-at-risk (population-at-risk), the denominator for the observed rate

- Data: infant mortality rate

    1. Observed rate

        Burke County, Georgia (1994–2003) = 15.8 per 1,000 live births

        = 62 infant deaths

        = 3,912 live births

---

*The comparison can be a geographic area, a time period, or an age group.

[†]Assumptions/requirements: that the count is based on independent events and that, for the z test, the count is more than ten. Also the normal approximation can be used when it is reasonable to assume that cases (events) are occurring independently and randomly in time and space. This is less likely to be true for infectious diseases and for diseases in which there is strong evidence of clustering.

2. Standard rate

   Burke County, Georgia (1994–2003) = 13.0 per 1,000 live births
   = 12,854 infant deaths
   = 988,147 live births

■ Analysis

$$z = \frac{15.8 - 13.0}{\sqrt{13.0 / 3.912}}$$

$$z = \frac{2.8}{\sqrt{3.323}}$$

$$z = \frac{2.8}{1.82}$$

$$z = 1.54$$

Note: The population at risk must be expressed in 1,000s because the rate is expressed per 1,000. Thus,

   $3,912/1,000 = 3.912$

■ Results

Compare the z value of 1.54 to the standard normal distribution (critical value) at the 0.05 significance level. The critical value at this level is 1.96.

■ Interpretation

Because 1.54 is less than 1.96, there is no significant difference between the rate of infant mortality in Burke County compared with the standard rate for the state of Georgia.

Note: The results obtained here for the rate are similar to that obtained for the counts: no significant difference. Most times, the results will be identical.

Statistical Guide 4: Rates (Confidence Intervals)

A Single Rate (Confidence Intervals for a County Representing a Small Area)

■ Analyzing a single rate using confidence intervals.

■ Confidence intervals for a rate draw attention to results actually obtained rather than concentrating on the decision to reject or not to reject; confidence intervals give a range of values that at a given probability level are likely to contain the true rate; thus, the confidence interval presents the result and conveys the inherent variability in the estimate of that result.

■ Problem: At the 95 percent confidence level, what is the range in the infant mortality rate that can be expected? That is, if the rate in an area is assumed to be a sample in time and space, what is the confidence level that the sample rate is reflective of the true rate for that area or time period?

■ Confidence intervals do not require the predetermination or specification of a null value.

■ Test statistic

1. For $n \leq 100$ (i.e., if numerator of rate is based on fewer than 100 events), use tables based on Poisson distribution.
2. For $n \geq 100$, a normal approximation to the Poisson distribution is used.

$$r \pm 1.96 \frac{r}{\text{PYRS}}$$

where

r = observed rate in the area

1.96 = critical value at the 95 percent significance level

PYRS = person-years-at-risk (population-at-risk—the denominator on which the observed rate is based).

■ Data: infant mortality rate (1994–2003)

1. Observed rate
   Burke County, Georgia = 15.8 per 1,000 live births
   = 62 infant deaths
   = 3,912 live births

2. Standard rate
   Georgia = 13.0 per 1,000 live births
   = 12,854 infant deaths
   = 988,147 live births

■ Analysis
Exact confidence limits per Poisson distribution table (see Table 10-5):

Lower Limit	Actual	Upper Limit
47.5/15.8 = 3.01	15.8 (62 deaths)	70.5/15.8 = 5.03
12.8		20.8

■ Confidence limits per normal approximation formula[*]

$$r \pm 1.96 \sqrt{\frac{r}{\text{PYRS}}}$$

$$15.8 \pm 1.96 \sqrt{\frac{15.8}{3.912}}$$

$$15.8 \pm 1.96(2.0097)$$

$$15.8 \pm 3.94$$

Lower Limit	Actual	Upper Limit
11.86	15.8	19.74

■ Results

A 95 percent confident level is that the actual rate of infant mortality could be as low as 11.86 (12.8—exact) and as high as 19.74 (20.8—exact). Thus, if another time period is sampled from the same small area, it can be expected that 95 percent of the time the rate would fall between these upper and lower limits. Of course, 5 percent of the time, just by chance, the rate could be outside these limits.

■ Interpretation

Remembering that the expected rate (13.0) noted in the previous guide on rates was or could be on the *null value*, it can then be determined that confidence limits include the value. If they do (and they do in this example), then the result is equivalent to nonsignificance. If the *null value* was not included, then the result could be considered significant. The results obtained here verify the earlier results of no significant difference, plus there is now a range of possible values that the actual rate could have been and could still be representative of the true rate. *This is an important aspect to the evaluation of variation of events in small area analysis.*

Statistical Guide 5

When Rates Are Not Independent The two previous guides were based on the fact that the two rates were independent. However, in public health practice and in health services management there are situations in which the rates are not independent. Because this is the case, the method for calculating differences in rates when they are not independent must be altered.

---

[*]The population-at-risk (PYRS) must be expressed in 1,000s because the rate is expressed per 1,000. Thus, 3,912/1,000 = 3.912.

■ High frequency events (≥100)

When comparing an observed rate with another rate or a standard rate that may not be independent, a slightly modified formula is needed:

$$\mu = (r - s)\sqrt{\frac{n}{s - s^2}}$$

where

> r = the observed rate or rate to be compared
>
> s = the standard rate (e.g., in the state, region, nation)
>
> n = the denominator (population on which the rate is based)

The formula is calculated as follows:

1. Square the standard rate s. Change all rates to a per-person basis by dividing by the rate's denominator.
2. Subtract the square of s from s: $s - s^2$.
3. Divide the denominator on which the rate is based, n, by the difference of $s - s^2$: $\sqrt{\dfrac{n}{s - s^2}}$
4. Find the square root of the quotient from the last step: $\sqrt{\dfrac{n}{s - s^2}}$
5. Subtract the standard rate s from the observed rate, r: $r - s$.
6. Multiply the square root in the fourth step by the difference in the fifth step: $\mu = (r - s)\sqrt{\dfrac{n}{s - s^2}}$

If μ exceeds 1.96, it can be concluded that the rate differs significantly at the 95 percent confidence level from the standard rate with which it is compared. If it exceeds 2.58, it is significantly different at the 99 percent level.

If, for example, a county has a population of 16,400 persons and a death rate of 20.9 per 1,000, the objective can be to find out whether the county rate is significantly different from the state rate of 16.8 per 1,000. These rates are not independent because the events that were used to calculate the observed rate are also included in the calculation of the standard rate (i.e., the county is a subset of the state). Thus,

Observed rate: $r = 20.9$ per 1,000

Standard rate: $s = 16.8$ per 1,000

Population (denominator n on which the observed rate is based) = 16,400. By applying the previous formula

$$\mu = (r - s)\sqrt{\frac{n}{s - s^2}}$$

we set the following six steps:

1. $(0.0168)^2 = 0.0168 \times 0.0168 = 0.000282$
2. $0.0168 - 0.000282 = 0.016518$
3. $\dfrac{16,400}{.016518} = 992,856.27$
4. $\sqrt{992,856.27} = 996.42173$
5. $0.0209 - 0.0168 = 0.0041$
6. $0.0041 \times 996.42173 = 4.09\ (\mu)$.

Because the value of 4.09 (μ) is greater than 2.58, it can be concluded that the difference between the rates is significant at the 99 percent level. In other words, there is 99 percent confidence that the county death rate is higher than the state death rate.

■ Low frequency events (at least one rate is based on less than 100 events)

When rates are based on a very low number of events (e.g., births, deaths, cases), the actual number of events is used instead of the rate:

$$\mu = \frac{(o - e)}{\sqrt{e}}$$

where

o = the observed number(s) to be compared

e = the standard number (e.g., state, region, nation)

This formula is calculated as follows:

1. Find the square root of the standard number e: $\sqrt{e}$.
2. Subtract the standard number e from the observed number o: $o - e$.

3. Divide the difference between the observed and standard numbers (step 2) by the square root of e: $\dfrac{(o-e)}{\sqrt{e}}$

Thus, to determine whether a county infant mortality rate is significantly higher than the state infant mortality rate,

$$\mu = \frac{(o-e)}{\sqrt{e}}$$

where

$o = 20.2$ per 1,000 (65 deaths)

$e = 17.5$ per 1,000 (56 deaths)

Thus,

$$\sqrt{56} = 7.48$$
$$65 - 56 = 9$$
$$\frac{9}{7.48} = 1.20$$

Because the value 1.20 is less than 2.58, it can be concluded that the two rates are not significantly different at the 99 percent confidence level.

Summary—Analyzing Small Areas (One Sample)

A summary of methods for analyzing small areas is provided for (1) counts, (2) rates, and (3) proportions.

Figure 10-1 gives a guide for selecting the appropriate method to use for analyzing one small area or time period or group when counts, rates, or proportions are involved. Further, Figure 10-2 gives the actual formulas used for performing the analysis using counts, rates, and proportions for small areas. Not all methods were discussed in this section; however, in the subsequent section those methods not discussed for one sample are presented for the two or more sample situations.

Comparing Two Small Areas

In epidemiologic/needs assessment studies focusing on quality improvement and outcomes measurement, a comparison of two areas is common. A health agency might wish to determine if the geographic area is statistically different from another area. To analyze this type of problem, it usually involves counts (cases), rates, proportions, and the ratio of the two rates. This section provides statistical guides for the purpose of analyzing data

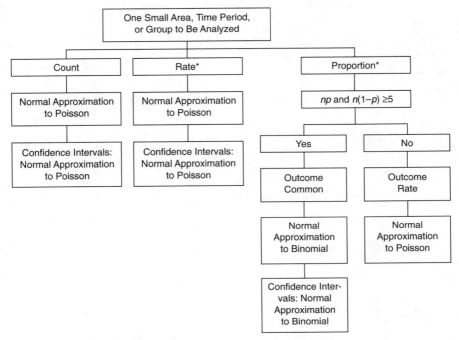

*When rates are not independent, see Statistical Guide 5 for appropriate methods.

FIGURE 10-1   Selection Guide for Epidemiological Measurement and Small Area Analysis—A Reference Chart for One Sample Situation

from two small areas. Table 10-6 provides an overview of the statistical tests by which to test the null hypothesis that the two areas are not different. Further, Table 10-6 provides the formulas for computing the confidence intervals when data from the two areas is being compared.

Statistical Guide 6

Counts: Comparing Two Small Areas*

- Analyzing two counts (comparing one group or area with another)
- Hypothesis test for the difference between two counts

---

*If two counts are to be compared directly, then the counts must be based on the same time period or same underlying distribution in space or time. If this is not the case, then the counts must be converted to rates to correct for the different periods of observation, and it is the rates that must be compared. For the methods presented here, the two counts should be more than ten.

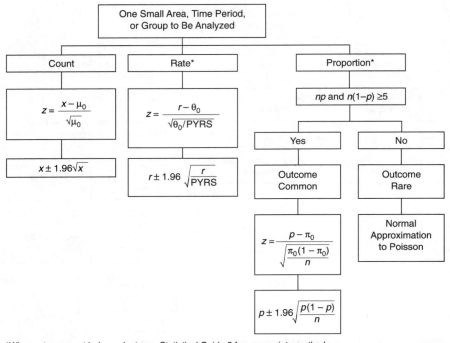

*When rates are not independent, see Statistical Guide 5 for appropriate methods.

FIGURE 10-2   Selection Guide for Epidemiological Measurement and Small Area Analysis—Formulas for One Sample Situation

- Problem: Is the number of AMI deaths observed in Burke County different from the total cancer deaths observed in Burke County during 1994–2003?
- Null hypothesis

  H_0: Observed number (AMI) = Observed number (total cancer) (i.e., no difference in the number of deaths between the two classifications)
- Test statistic (normal approximation to Poisson)

  z test

$$z = \frac{x_1(\text{observed count}) - x_2(\text{observed count})}{\sqrt{x_1(\text{observed count}) + x_2(\text{observed count})}}$$

or

$$z = \frac{x_1 - x_2}{\sqrt{x_1 + x_2}}$$

TABLE 10-6 Small Area Analysis: Comparing Two Small Areas (Two-Sample Tests)

Comparison Of	Hypothesis Test*	Confidence Interval†
Independent counts (z test)	$z = \dfrac{x_1 - x_2}{\sqrt{x_1 + x_2}}$	$(x_1 - x_2) \pm 1.96\sqrt{x_1 - x_2}$
Independent rates (z test)	$z = \dfrac{r_1 - r_2}{\sqrt{\dfrac{r}{\text{PYRS}_1} + \dfrac{r}{\text{PYRS}_2}}}$ $r = \dfrac{\text{PYRS}_1(r_1) + \text{PYRS}_2(r_2)}{\text{PYRS}_1 + \text{PYRS}_2}$	$(r_1 - r_2) \pm 1.96\sqrt{\dfrac{r_1}{\text{PYRS}_1} + \dfrac{r_2}{\text{PYRS}_2}}$
Independent proportions (z test)	$z = \dfrac{p_1 - p_2}{\sqrt{\dfrac{pq}{n_1} + \dfrac{pq}{n_2}}}$ $p = \dfrac{n_1 p_1 + n_2 p_2}{n_1 + n_2}$	$(p_1 - p_2) \pm 1.96\sqrt{\dfrac{p_1 q_1}{n_1} + \dfrac{p_2 q_2}{n_2}}$
(χ² test)	$\chi^2 = \sum \dfrac{(O - E)^2}{E}$	

*H_0 (null hypothesis): no difference in the two populations from which the samples are selected.

†The confidence interval is a range that is expected to contain a low to high range comparing one sample (region) with another sample (region).

where

z = normal approximation to the Poisson

x_1 = observed count for area 1 or time period 1

x_2 = observed count for area 2 or time period 2

■ Data

AMI: Burke County, Georgia (1994–2003) = 306 deaths (x_1)

Total cancer: Burke County, Georgia (1994–2003) = 344 deaths (x_2)

■ Analysis

$$z = \frac{306 - 344}{\sqrt{306 + 344}}$$

$$z = \frac{-38}{\sqrt{25.5}}$$

$$z = -1.49$$

■ Results

Compare the z value of -1.49 to the standard normal distribution (critical value) at the 0.05 significance level. The critical value at this level is ± 1.96.

■ Interpretation

Because -1.49 is more than -1.96, there is no significant difference between the AMI deaths for Burke County and total cancer deaths for Burke County.

Statistical Guide 7

Rates: Comparing Rates between Two Small Areas

■ Analyzing two rates (comparing one small area with another)
■ Hypothesis test for the difference between rates for two areas
■ Problem: Is the infant mortality rate observed in one small area different from the observed mortality rate from another area?
■ Null hypothesis

H_0: Observed rate (area 1) = Observed rate (area 2) (i.e., no difference in the two rates)

■ Test statistic (normal approximation to Poisson)

z test

$$z = \frac{\text{Rate (area 1)} - \text{Rate (area 2)}}{\sqrt{\dfrac{\text{Pooled rate}}{\text{Population-at-risk (area 1)}} + \dfrac{\text{Pooled rate}}{\text{Population-at-risk (area 2)}}}}$$

or

$$z = \frac{r_1 - r_2}{\sqrt{\dfrac{r}{\text{PYRS}_1} + \dfrac{r}{\text{PYRS}_2}}}$$

where

z = normal approximation to Poisson

r_1 = rate for area 1

r_2 = rate for area 2

r = pooled rate (is equivalent to a weighted average of the two observed rates weighted by person-years or population-at-risk [see Figure 10-3 to calculate])

PYRS_1 = person-years-at-risk (population-at-risk for area 1)

PYRS_2 = person-years-at-risk (population-at-risk for area 2)

- Data: infant mortality rates
  - Area 1

    Burke County, Georgia (1993–2003) = 15.8 per 1,000 live births

    = 62 infant deaths

    = 3,912 live births

Note: The pooled rate is calculated using

$$r = \frac{\text{PYRS}_1(r_1) + \text{PYRS}_2(r_2)}{\text{PYRS}_1 + \text{PYRS}_2}$$

$$r = \frac{13,912(15.8) + 66,067(13.6)}{3,912 + 66,067}$$

$$r = 13.7$$

FIGURE 10-3 How to Calculate the Pooled Rate

■ Area 2

Augusta District, Georgia (1993–2003) = 13.6 per 1,000 live births

= 900 infant deaths

= 66,067 live births

■ Analysis

$$z = \frac{15.8 - 13.6}{\sqrt{\dfrac{13.7}{3.912} + \dfrac{13.7}{66.1}}}$$

$$z = \frac{2.2}{\sqrt{3.5 + 0.21}}$$

$$z = \frac{2.2}{1.9}$$

$$z = 1.15$$

■ Results

Compare the z value of 1.15 to the standard normal distribution (critical value) at the 0.05 significance level. The critical value at this level is 1.96.

■ Interpretation

Because 1.15 is less than 1.96, there is no significant difference between the two areas.

■ Determining confidence intervals for rates in this example:

Test statistic: normal approximation to Poisson

$$CI = (r_1 - r_2) \pm 1.96 \sqrt{\frac{r_1}{PYRS_1} + \frac{r_2}{PYRS_2}}$$

$$CI = (15.8 - 13.6) \pm 1.96 \sqrt{\frac{r_1}{PYRS_1} + \frac{r_2}{PYRS_2}}$$

$$CI = 2.2 \pm 1.96\sqrt{4.04 + 0.206}$$

$$CI = 2.2 \pm 1.96(2.06)$$

$$CI = 2.2 \pm 4.04$$

$$CI = -1.84 \text{ to } 6.24$$

■ Interpretation

At the 95 percent level of confidence, Burke County, Georgia, could have an infant mortality rate ranging from a figure of 1.84 per 1,000 lower than Augusta to 6.24 per 1,000 higher.

Statistical Guide 8

Ratio of Two Rates—Using Confidence Intervals to Determine Significance
When comparing an observed rate with an arbitrarily set standard, goal, or
target value, the confidence interval for the observed rate provides the significance of the difference. If the standard is included in the confidence
interval of the observed rate, there is no significant difference at the level of
confidence chosen. The situation is somewhat more complex, however,
when comparing rates of two different areas or of two different times for the
same area. This requires a direct extension of the concept of a confidence
interval. The objective is to determine whether a difference between the
rates is significant or whether it is caused solely by random effects. Different
methods must be used, depending on whether the rates are independent.

Two rates are independent when they do not include any of the same
observations of events (e.g., births, deaths) in their numerator. Thus, rates
from overlapping time periods or areas are not independent. For example,
rates from a county and the state that the county is in are not independent;
rates from two different counties are independent.

To determine whether there is a significant difference between two
independent rates, the confidence interval for the ratio between the two
rates or the difference between the two independent rates is used.

■ Ratio of two rates. The ratio is defined as

$$R = \frac{r_1}{r_2}$$

where

R = ratio

r_1 = rate for area 1 or period 1

r_2 = rate for area 2 or period 2

The 95 percent confidence interval for the ratio is defined as

$$R = 1.96 \sqrt{\frac{1}{d_1} + \frac{1}{d_2}}$$

where

d_1 = number of events for area 1 or period 1 (i.e., the rate
   numerator)

d_2 = number of events for area 2 or period 2

To establish a significant difference, it must be determined
whether the confidence interval contains the number 1. If it does
not, it can be stated that the two rates are significantly different.
If the interval does contain the number 1, it cannot be concluded

TABLE 10-7 Data for Calculating the Ratio of Two Rates

Years	Number of Infant Deaths	Infant Mortality Number of Live Births	Rate per 1,000 Live Births
1961–1965	200	5,000	40
1966–1970	100	4,000	25

Source: Reprinted from J. C. Kleinman, "Infant Mortality," *Statistical Notes for Health Planners,* vol. 2. (Washington, D.C.: National Center for Health Statistics, 1976).

that there is a significant difference. Kleinman provided the example in Table 10-7.[10]

$$R = \frac{40}{25} = 1.6$$

The 95 percent confidence interval is

$$CI = R \pm 1.96 \sqrt{\frac{1}{d_1} + \frac{1}{d_2}}$$

$$CI = 1.6 \pm 1.96(1.6) \sqrt{\frac{1}{200} + \frac{1}{100}}$$

$$CI = 1.6 \pm 1.96(1.6)\sqrt{0.015}$$

$$CI = 1.6 \pm 0.384$$

$$CI = 1.216 \text{ to } 1.984$$

Thus, the infant mortality rate for 1961 through 1965 can be said, with 95 percent confidence, to be from 1.22 to 1.98 times the rate for 1966 through 1970. Because the interval does not contain 1, there is a statistically significant difference in the area's infant mortality rate between the two time periods. If the interval did contain 1, there would not be a statistically significant difference.

A Selection Guide for Analyzing Small Areas (Two Samples)

Test selection to evaluate variation in small areas can be a difficult task. Statistical guides (Figures 10-4 and 10-5) are offered to ease the decisions in selecting appropriate tests when analyzing counts, rates, proportions, or ratios for two or more groups or small areas. The cornerstone of small area analysis is variation. Thus, the significance of the variation must be assessed.

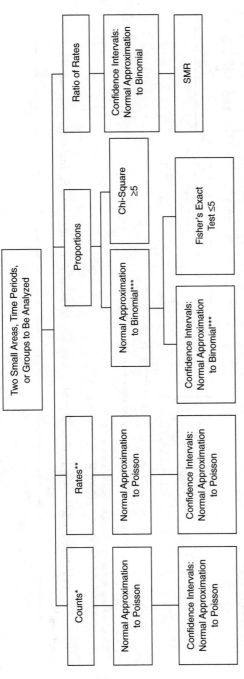

Two Small Areas, Time Periods, or Groups to Be Analyzed

Counts*
— Normal Approximation to Poisson
— Confidence Intervals: Normal Approximation to Poisson

Rates**
— Normal Approximation to Poisson
— Confidence Intervals: Normal Approximation to Poisson

Proportions
— Normal Approximation to Binomial***
  — Chi-Square ≥5
  — Fisher's Exact Test ≤5
— Confidence Intervals: Normal Approximation to Binomial***

Ratio of Rates
— Confidence Intervals: Normal Approximation to Binomial
— SMR

*Two counts should be > 10

** When rates are not independent, see Statistical Guide 8 for approiate methods.

*** 1. Total sample size > 20
2. $n_1 p$, $n_2 p$, $n_1 q$, $n_2 q$ all >5 for sample sizes between 20 and 40.
3. Valid for total sample size that is in both groups ≥40.

FIGURE 10-4 Selection Guide for Epidemiological Measurement and Small Area Analysis—A Reference Chart for Two Sample Selections

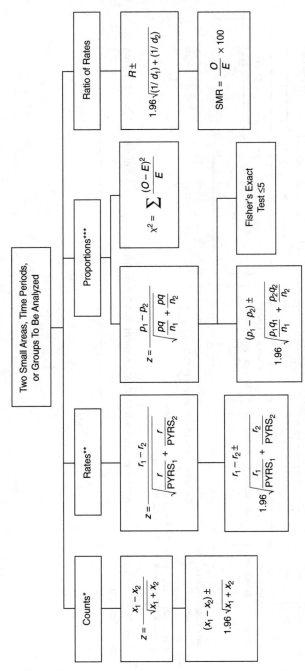

*Two counts should be > 10

** When rates are not independent, see Statistical Guide 8 for appropriate methods.

*** 1. Total sample size > 20

2. n_1p, n_2p, n_1q, n_2q all >5 for sample sizes between 20 and 40.

3. Valid for total sample size that is in both groups ≥40.

FIGURE 10-5 Selection Guide for Epidemiological Measurement and Small Area Analysis—Formulas for Two Sample Selections

Summary

The analysis of small areas is of paramount importance in the assessment of outcomes in the quality improvement process. As managed care expands, the need for program-based outcome evaluations and the analysis of small areas in the quality improvement environment are critical. This chapter provides these statistical tools for the public health analyst to provide valid and reliable measurement for small areas. Further, public health analysts and health services managers can use many of the small area analysis techniques and measurements presented in this chapter to focus on the core public health problems. The concept of a rate and population-at-risk are central to the analysis of problems related to the management of health services, the understanding of small area variation, and the analysis of communities to monitor the improvement of outcomes. This chapter provides the tools and methods for epidemiologic investigation of small areas and the quality improvement measurement to monitor the effective delivery of health services and improving the process.

The epidemiologic analysis of small areas and the measurement of rates and their significance allow administrators to determine the magnitude of a problem; what warrants further analysis; how to monitor a process to hold the gains; and how to identify potential special causes to focus for improvement. Certainly, a much more practical use for these statistical and epidemiologic methods is to monitor current conditions and establish where improvement can occur in the future. Finally, determining the significance of the results obtained from small area analysis and quality improvement measurement may be more of a practical decision than a statistical one.[*]

References

1. L. D. Stamp, *Some Aspects of Medical Geography* (Oxford: Oxford University Press, 1964), 16.
2. J. D. Clark, "Variations in Michigan Hospital Use Rates: Do Physicians and Hospital Characteristics Provide the Explanation," *Social Science and Medicine* 30, no. 1 (1990):67–82.
3. Center for Evaluative Clinical Sciences, Dartmouth Medical School, *The Dartmouth Atlas of Health Care* (Chicago: American Hospital Publishing, 1996).
4. M. Spitzer and P. Caper, "Quality Measurement through Small Area Analysis Techniques," in *Innovations in Health Care Quality Measurement*, ed. P. L. Spath (Chicago: American Hospital Publishing, 1989), 11–21.
5. D. G. Altman, *Practical Statistics for Medical Research* (London: Chapman and Hall, 1991).

---

[*]The data utilized in this chapter is presented for illustrative purposes only. Not all values reflect actual places or times.

6. D. G. Altman et al., eds., *Statistics with Confidence*, 2d ed. (London: BMJ Publishing Group, 2000).

7. L. E. Daly and G. J. Bourke, *Interpretation and Uses of Medical Statistics*, 5th ed. (Oxford: Blackwell Science Ltd., 2000).

8. H. Motulsky, *Intuitive Biostatistics*. (New York: Oxford University Press, 1995).

9. L. E. Daly et al., *Interpretation and Uses of Medical Statistics*, 4th ed. (Oxford: Blackwell Scientific Publications, 1991).

10. J. C. Kleinman, "Infant Mortality," *Statistical Notes for Health Planners*, Vol. 2 (Washington, D.C.: National Center for Health Statistics, July 1976), 4.

11

The Epidemiology of Health Services Utilization*

Determinants of Service Utilization

Preceding chapters examined the relevance to health services management of the principles and techniques of epidemiology—the science concerned with the occurrence, distribution, and determinants of health and disease in a population. This chapter discusses how the occurrence of disease is translated into utilization of health services, focusing on determinants, recent trends, and the epidemiological (population-based) analysis of utilization for health services management.

The utilization of health services is an interaction between consumers and providers of care. It is a complex behavior determined by a wide range of factors. There has been a great deal of research on this topic. A 1979 bibliography lists approximately 1,500 reports of studies related to the utilization of health services, most of them published between 1960 and 1976.[1] This discussion is based on the models by Donabedian[2] and by Andersen and Newman,[3] as well as on a critical review by McKinlay.[4]

A new report from CDC's National Center for Health Statistics presents trends for the past decade in the utilization of health services across the spectrum of care—from ambulatory care, to hospitalization, to nursing home and home health and hospice care. In this report, they list approximately 225 reports on the studies and trends of utilization for a wide variety of diseases, conditions, and resources. The report tracks levels and patterns of use and examines aspects of the health care delivery system that

---

*Much of the material in this chapter is abridged and utilized liberally from *Health Care in America: Trends in Utilization* by A. B. Bernstein et al. (Hyattsville, Md.: National Center for Health Statistics, 2003) to reinforce the major trends in health care utilization in the United States. Please see *http://www.cdc.gov/nchs/data/misc/healthcare.pdf*

influence health care utilization, such as developments in medical practice, new technologies, changes in payment and delivery systems, new health policy initiatives, and the aging of the U.S. population. Information is presented in easy-to-read charts accompanied by brief text that highlights key findings.[5]

The report integrates data from all of the components of the National Health Care Survey (NHCS), a family of surveys conducted by NHCS on health care establishments and providers. The NHCS documents and monitors health care provided in physicians' office practice, hospital emergency and outpatient departments, short-stay hospitals, nursing homes, and home health and hospice care agencies.

The report is organized around determinants of health care utilization (such as the aging of the U.S. population, supply of health care providers, and changes in technology); selected trends in the utilization of health care services (including ambulatory, inpatient, and long-term care services); and trends in utilization of procedures, drugs, and health care outcomes. Within these major sections of the report, selected diagnoses and conditions (such as diabetes, cancer, ischemic heart disease, and chronic obstructive pulmonary disease) are presented. Also highlighted are topics of interest to public health and health services researchers and policymakers such as injuries, medications ordered or provided during ambulatory care visits, preventive care services, and adverse effects following medical treatment.[6]

The purpose of the chartbook is to provide an overview of health care utilization in America, as well as information to help understand utilization patterns in light of factors that affect the delivery of these services.[7,8] A recent edition of the book by A. R. Kovner and D. Neuhauser presents updated concepts and thoughts on the nature of health services management. Although not focused on the epidemiologic perspectives of health services management, they do provide an in-depth review of the management, accountability, and organizational design of an organization and the relationship to health services management.[9]

Donabedian has noted the different types of determinants of health services utilization.[10] Donabedian's description of the medical care process and its environment reflects perceived and evaluated need. The perceived need relates to consumer factors such as sociodemographic, sociopsychological, and eipdemiological; whereas the evaluated need represents the provider factors. In turn, these factors influence the utilization of health care services. The set of interactions between health professionals and their clients takes place not within a vacuum but within an organizational environment that in turn is surrounded and penetrated by social and cultural features.[10] Health services utilization therefore is influenced by sociocultural, organizational, consumer-related, and provider-related factors. Although these categories are discussed as independent entities, keep in mind that they often are indissociable.

McAlearney recently updated the Donabedian perspective based on the determinants of health services utilization. As noted in Table 11-1, the

TABLE 11-1 Defining Populations in Population Health Management

Factor	Rationale for Segmentation in Population Health Management	Example Groups
Age	Permits development of age-appropriate health behavior and wellness strategies	Federal Medicare program uses age 65 as cutoff point to determine eligibility for elderly
Income	For low-income individuals, increases access to lower-cost clinics and care options; used as justification for sliding fee scales	Among criteria used for Medicaid eligibility; can define low-income groups for health centers and clinics
Geography	Creates natural boundaries for defining populations	Proximity to a hospital for pregnant women; Medicaid programs defined by state
Community	A subset of geographic segmentation, helps organize outreach, funding, and health information network development; provides foundation to develop community-based health indicators and health goals for local populations	Healthy Cities Project of the World Health Organization; Community Health Status Indicators Project with the Health Resource and Service Administration (HRSA) of the U.S. Department of Health and Human Services; Healthwise Healthy Communities Project in Idaho
Employer	Employers providing health insurance and disability coverage can also target employee groups for population health management interventions	Employee population
Insurance Coverage	Insurance carriers are responsible for medical care costs of enrolled populations, thus their incentives are aligned with population health management goals	Enrolled population; health plan members
Health	Targeting groups on the basis of disease or health status permits stratification into groups who will most benefit from specific population health management interventions	Groups defined by disease status or other health criterion

Source: A. S. McAlearney, "Population Health Management in Theory and Practice," in *Advances in Health Care Management*, vol. 3, ed. G. T. Savage, J. Blair, and M. Fottler (New York: JAI Press/Elsevier Science Ltd., 2002) p. 37.

basis for analyzing utilization patterns has been expanded to include specific factors, but the overall concepts vary minimally from the early Donabedian model.[11,12] In fact, the Donabedian model suggests a much more comprehensive approach consequentially while embracing the specifics as defined by McAlearney.

Sociocultural Factors

Sociocultural determinants of health care utilization include technology and values.[13] Technology is considered a sociocultural as opposed to an organizational factor to denote the relatively little control health services managers have over it. Technology influences the utilization of services. In some cases, it reduces utilization by decreasing the illness levels or the need for medical care.

This is what Lewis Thomas calls the "genuinely decisive technology of modem medicine,"[14] exemplified by modern methods of immunization against diphtheria, pertussis, and so on, and the contemporary use of antibiotics and chemotherapy for bacterial infections. For example, the prevalence of tuberculosis hospitals has declined as a result of the high technology of medicine that has affected illness levels, which in turn have influenced utilization of some specialized hospitals.

In other cases, technology actually increases the utilization of services. Thomas calls this "half-way technology," represented by such developments as transplantations of hearts, kidneys, and other organs and by the invention of artificial organs. Progress in radiology and nuclear medicine also can be considered half-way technology. This technology is designed to compensate for the incapacitating effects of certain diseases that the medical profession is unable to do very much about—in other words, to "make up for disease" or to postpone death.

Societal values also influence the utilization of health services. Although this is a rather difficult field of study because societal values, norms, and beliefs influence all other aspects and determinants of the medical care process, some specific examples can be helpful.

In the United States, the use of the hospital as a place to be born and to die is almost totally determined by social norms, with technological factors of second importance.[15] This is attested by the fact that 97 percent of all live births in the United States in 2000 occurred in hospitals,[16] while for various races the percentage of in-hospital births was less.[17] Obviously in other countries the percentage of in-hospital births is much lower. Another example is the financing of health care discussed in the next section of organizational determinants.

Several sociological studies have looked at the patterns of health services utilization by different subgroups of society.[18] Zola compares the presenting symptoms of Italian and Irish patients in the outpatient clinics of a Boston hospital.[19] He reports very different sets of complaints (more eye, ear, nose, and throat complaints from the Irish; more pain experienced by the Italians) and concludes that the particular symptoms individuals act upon—those for which they are going to use health services and seek medical care—are determined by their cultural, ethnic, or reference group.

Suchman, in a study of the effect of the social structure of various ethnic and cultural subgroups in New York on their utilization of health services,[20,21] defines that structure as being either parochial or cosmopolitan. He finds that highly cosmopolitan groups tend to seek medical care earlier and more often, whereas parochial groups rely more on other lay persons in their group (Friedson's lay referral system[22]). As McKinlay's later analysis points out, Suchman was crudely measuring the impact of "social networks" on health services utilization.[23] These social networks (family, kinship, and friendship) to which individuals belong probably determine, to a large extent, their health services utilization behavior.

Forces That Affect Health Care Utilization

Multiple forces determine how much health care people use, the types of health care they use, and the timing of that care. Table 11-2 identifies some, but certainly not all, major forces that affect trends in overall health care utilization over time. Some forces encourage more utilization; others deter it. For example, antibiotics and public health initiatives have dramatically reduced the need for people to receive health care for many infectious diseases, even though overuse can also increase antibiotic-resistant strains.[24] However, other factors, such as increases in the prevalence of chronic disease, can contribute to increases in overall utilization. Consumer preferences can alter the amount of treatment obtained outside hospital and nursing home settings. New therapeutic technologies provided in new types of settings, such as corrective eye surgeries, can increase demand. Aging is also associated with increased health care utilization.[25,26,27,28] Provider practice patterns can shift from emphasizing one type of treatment (e.g., psychotherapy) compared to another (e.g., drug treatment for mental illness). Some factors affect utilization per person (e.g., guidelines that recommend preventive anticholesterol or antidiabetes medications on an ongoing basis or that recommend more preventive services per person). Other factors can have more effect on the total number of people, or percentage of the population, who are able to receive the service. For example, less invasive cardiac procedures now are performed on very frail or old

TABLE 11-2   Forces That Affect Overall Health Care Utilization

Factors That Can Decrease Health Services Utilization	Factors That Can Increase Health Services Utilization
Decreased supply (e.g., hospital closures, large numbers of physicians retiring)	Increased supply (e.g., ambulatory surgery centers, assisted living residences)
Public health/sanitation advances (e.g., quality standards for food and water distribution)	Growing population
	Growing elderly population:
Better understanding of the risk factors of diseases and prevention initiatives (e.g., smoking prevention programs, cholesterol-lowering drugs)	■ more functional limitations associated with aging
	■ more illness associated with aging
	■ more deaths among the increased number of elderly, which is correlated with high utilization
Discovery/implementation of treatments that cure or eliminate diseases	New procedures and technologies (e.g., hip replacement, stent insertion, MRI)
Consensus documents or guidelines that recommend decreases in utilization	Consensus documents or guidelines that recommend increases in utilization
Shifts to other sites of care can cause declines in utilization in the original sites:	New disease entities (e.g., HIV/AIDS, bioterrorism)
■ as technology allows shifts (e.g., ambulatory surgery)	New drugs, expanded use of existing drugs
	Increased health insurance coverage
■ as alternative sites of care become available (e.g., assisted living)	Consumer/employee pressures for more comprehensive insurance coverage
Payer pressures to reduce costs	Changes in practice patterns (e.g., more aggressive treatment of the elderly)
Changes in practice patterns (e.g., encouraging self-care and healthy lifestyles; reduced length of hospital stay)	Changes in consumer preferences and demand (e.g., cosmetic surgery, hip and knee replacements, direct marketing of drugs)
Changes in consumer preferences (e.g., home birthing, more self-care, alternative medicine)	

Source: A. B. Bernstein et al., *Health Care in America: Trends in Utilization* (Hyattsville, Md.: National Center for Health Statistics, 2003).

people or people with many co-morbid conditions when in the past it was considered too risky to perform the previously more invasive procedures on these populations.[5]

It has been documented that people who cannot pay for health care services—either out-of-pocket, through private or social health insurance (such as Medicare), through public programs such as Medicaid, or through some other means—might not receive needed services in the United States, and there is a large body of literature on the topic.[29,30,31] Still, factors other than ability to pay also affect access to health care services. One paradigm of health care utilization identifies predisposing, enabling, and need determinants of care.[32,33] Predisposing factors include the propensity to seek care (such as whether an individual's culture accepts the sick role or encourages stoicism) and what types of care are preferred for specific symptoms. Enabling factors include depth and breadth of health insurance coverage, whether an individual can afford copayments or deductibles, whether services are located so that they can be conveniently reached, and other factors that allow someone to receive care. Need for care also affects utilization, but need is not always easily determined without expert input. Many people do not know when they need care and what the optimal time to seek care is, and many conditions are not easily diagnosed or treated. If all people could obtain unlimited health care, perceived need—by both patient and provider—might be the only determinant of health care utilization, but unfortunately barriers to needed care, such as availability or supply of services, ability to pay, or discrimination, have an impact on utilization overall.[5]

Aging of the Population

The number of persons age 65 and older increased from about 31 million to about 34 million between 1990 and 2000. The percentage of the population age 65 and older remained fairly constant during this period— about 12.4 percent (Figure 11-1). The number of the oldest old, age 85 and older, increased from about 3 million to over 4 million in 2000, or from 1.2 percent to 1.5 percent. In short, although the number of elderly increased during this decade, it did not increase at a very rapid rate.[34] Baby boomers are still under age 65, but as they age, both the number and percentage of elderly in the United States will accelerate rapidly. However, baby boomers are currently in their forties and fifties and are beginning to experience the onset of chronic conditions such as diabetes and heart disease.

Aging is associated with an increase in functional limitation and in the prevalence of chronic conditions. As people age, they tend to use more hospital services and prescription medicines. In 1999, people over the age of 65 years experienced nearly three times as many hospital days per thousand than the general population. This ratio goes up to nearly four times for people over the age of 75.[35]

However, the relationship between aging (or any correlate of utilization) and overall health care utilization is not a direct one. Increased longevity can be a result of the postponement of disease onset or a steady rate of functional loss.[36,37,38,39] The elderly do have a higher rate of many procedures and are prescribed more drugs, but the increase in the use of some drugs can reduce the prevalence of some other conditions and their associated utilization. For example, increased use of glucose-lowering and

Millions of Persons in Age Group

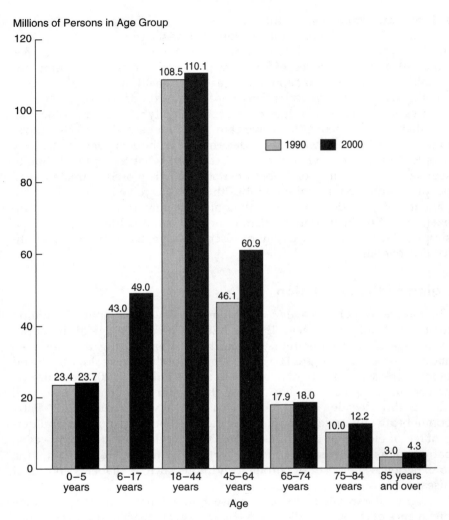

FIGURE 11-1 Change in Age Distribution of the U.S. Population: United States, 1990–2000. *Source:* A. B. Bernstein et al., *Health Care in America: Trends in Utilization* (Hyattsville, Md.: National Center for Health Statistics, 2003), 9.

antihypertensive drugs can reduce complications of diabetes and associated care for some elderly, but it can also be associated with increased utilization of physicians' services. There is also some evidence that the rate of acute care, in general, decreases with advanced age because of co-morbid conditions or unwillingness to perform invasive or traumatic therapies on the very old.[40] The independent effect of aging of the population on health services utilization, therefore, is not immediately apparent.[5]

Major Policy Initiatives Affecting Health Care Utilization

In the United States, there are at least three major payers for health care: governments (federal, state, and local); employers, through employer-based health insurance; and health care consumers themselves, through out-of-pocket payments. In general, services that are covered by insurance or payment programs are more likely to be utilized than services that must be paid for directly by consumers. Thus, the benefit and payment structure of Medicare and Medicaid programs, private insurers, and managed care plans tend to strongly influence utilization patterns.

Table 11-3 shows some of the major federal payment policy changes that have occurred since 1980. Major Medicare and Medicaid cost-containment efforts, such as the Prospective Payment System for hospitals and the Resource Based Relative Value Scale for physician payment, created incentives to shift sites of services provided.[41,42,43] Use of the hospice and ambulatory surgery benefits, as well as the supply of these providers, increased substantially after the Medicare program began to cover these services. Changes in payment policy also created incentives to provide services differently. For example, the increase in a capitated payment and the need to use gatekeepers has been associated with a changing mix of primary and specialty care.[44,45] Expansion of the Medicaid program and implementation of the State Children's Health Insurance Program share the goal of increasing utilization of services by poor children and their families.

Managed care in its many incarnations also affects the type and mix of health services available to its covered enrollees. Employers, in particular, work with managed care companies to determine benefit packages offered to employees. Because capitated managed care is paid on a per-person rather than a per-service basis, managed care organizations do not set payment rates for individual services; they have some freedom to substitute services across sites and to be somewhat flexible in the range of services they provide. There is some evidence that capitated managed care plans provided more physician services and fewer hospital services than fee-for-service plans during the first part of the 1990s; however, this differential seems to be leveling off as hospitalization and other provider payment rates decline for all payers.[5,46]

Acute Care Supply

Utilization of services is affected by availability of services. Health care providers can accommodate only a finite number of patients. Over the past decade, the overall supply of some types of health care services has remained relatively constant, although the services might be provided in different types of settings. The supply of many other types of providers increased substantially—in particular, facilities specializing in new technological procedures or tests and new types of long-term care residential facilities.[5]

TABLE 11-3   Selected Major Federal Policy Initiatives Affecting Health Care Utilization

1982	■ Medicare hospice benefits added on a temporary basis.
1983	■ Change from "reasonable cost" to prospective payment system based on diagnosis-related groups for hospital inpatient services begins under Medicare.
1985	■ Medicare coverage mandated for newly hired state and local government employees.
	■ Emergency Medical Treatment and Labor Act (EMTALA) passes as part of the Consolidated Omnibus Budget Reconciliation Act (COBRA) of 1985 to address the problem of "patient dumping" from emergency departments.
	■ The Consolidated Omnibus Budget Reconciliation Act (COBRA) of 1985 requires most employers who provide employees with group health plans to offer to continue that coverage under certain circumstances.
1986	■ Medicare hospice benefits become permanent.
1987	■ Federal Nursing Home Reform Act (part of the Consolidated Omnibus Budget Reconciliation Act) passes, which creates a set of national minimum standards of care and rights for people living in certified nursing facilities.
1988	■ Major overhaul of Medicare benefits is enacted, aimed at providing coverage for catastrophic illness and prescription drugs.
	■ Medicare adds coverage for routine mammography.
1989	■ Medicare catastrophic coverage and prescription drug coverage are repealed.
	■ Medicare coverage is added for pap smears.
1992	■ Medicare physician services payments are based on fee schedule (Resource Based Relative Value Scale, or RBRVS).
1993	■ Under Medicaid, states are required to provide additional assistance to low-income Medicare beneficiaries under the State Children's Health Insurance Program (SCHIP).
1996	■ Health Insurance Portability and Accountability Act (HIPAA) enacted to provide health insurance protection for people leaving employment.
1997	■ The Balanced Budget Act (BBA) of 1997 creates a new program (SCHIP) and funding source for states to provide health insurance to children.
	■ Medicare+Choice is enacted under the BBA. Major payment adjustments are proposed for nursing homes, home health care, and other covered services.
	■ The BBA also mandates changes in payment to nursing homes, home health agencies, and hospital outpatient departments.
	■ FDA relaxes its rules on mass media advertising for prescription drugs.
1999	■ Prospective payment for skilled nursing homes under Medicare (passed with the BBA of 1997) enacted.
2000	■ Medicare+Choice Final Rule takes effect.
	■ Prospective payment systems for outpatient services and home health agencies take effect.

Source: A. B. Bernstein et al., *Health Care in America: Trends in Utilization* (Hyattsville, Md.: National Center for Health Statistics, 2003), 11.

Hospital Supply The number of community hospitals in the United States decreased from 5,384 in 1990 to 4,915 in 2000. The number of beds per 1,000 population also declined from 4.2 to 3.0 between 1990 and 2000. This reduction in hospital capacity was accompanied by increased staffing. Full-time equivalent personnel increased from about 3,420,000 to about 3,911,400 between 1995 and 2000.[47] Many of the additional staff are not devoted to patient care but to management or administration. Hospitals are also providing a greater percentage of their care on an outpatient basis. Data from the American Hospital Association shows that outpatient department visits increased from 860 to 1,852 per 1,000 persons between 1990 and 2000, indicating that their capacity has been expanded over time.[48,49] The number of hospital emergency departments (EDs), however, has decreased by about 8 percent between 1994 and 1999, with a large percentage of ED closures in rural areas.[50,51]

Physician Supply Unlike hospitals, the number of physicians serving the U.S. population continues to increase. There are also more specialists of all types, except general surgeons and radiologists.[52] However, physicians are not evenly distributed throughout the nation; they are concentrated in urban areas, causing considerable shortages in some rural areas. The federal government estimates that more than 2,200 physicians would be needed in nonmetropolitan areas to eliminate primary care health professional shortage areas.[53]

New Types of Acute-Care Facilities Not only is the supply of physicians increasing, physicians and other health care providers are also increasingly providing services in new types and sites of care. Table 11-4 shows some of the relatively new types of facilities that the Joint Commission on Accreditation of Healthcare Organizations (JCAHO) accredits. The number of ambulatory surgery centers, for example, has grown rapidly since the 1980s.[54] The number of Medicare-certified ambulatory surgery centers alone increased from 1,197 in 1990 to 2,644 in 1998.[5]

Long-Term Care Supply—Nursing Homes

Long-term care (LTC) is defined as a continuum of medical and/or social services designed to help people who have disabilities or chronic care needs. Long-term care services include traditional medical services, social services, and housing. In contrast to acute care, LTC is designed to prevent deterioration of the recipient and to promote social adjustment to stages of decline. Unlike rehabilitation care, there is not necessarily an expectation that the recipient will "get better." Services can be short- or long-term and can be provided in a person's home, in the community, or in residential facilities (e.g., nursing homes or assisted living facilities).[55]

TABLE 11-4   Selected Acute Care Providers Accredited by the Joint Commission on Accreditation of Healthcare Organizations (JCAHO)

Ambulatory surgery centers	Mobile services
Birthing centers	MRI centers
Cardiac catheterization labs	Multispecialty group practices
Community health centers	Occupational health centers
Dialysis centers	Office-based surgery offices
Endoscopy centers	Ophthalmology/eye practices
Group medical practices	Oral and maxillofacial centers
Hospitals (general, psychiatric, rehabilitation, children's)	Physician offices
Imaging centers	Prison health centers
Indian health clinics	Radiation/oncology clinics
Infusion therapy centers	Sleep centers
Laser centers	Student health services
Lithotripsy services	Urgent/emergency care centers
Military clinics	Women's health centers

Source: A. B. Bernstein et al, *Health Care in America: Trends in Utilization* (Hyattsville, Md.: National Center for Health Statistics, 2003), 13.

Because LTC is a concept, not a facility or place, it is difficult to quantify either the number of LTC providers or the number of people receiving such care. Home health care agencies (see "Postacute, Rehabilitation, and End-of-Life Care Supply") provide some LTC, although they provide more post-acute care. Nursing homes provide the bulk of formal LTC. Data from the National Nursing Home Survey (NNHS) shows that there has been a slight increase in the number of nursing homes providing nursing care between 1985 and 1999, from 16,900 to 17,900.[†]

Enactment of The Nursing Home Reform Act of 1987—part of the 1987 Omnibus Budget Reconciliation Act (OBRA87)—also created incentives for Medicaid-certified nursing homes to be certified by Medicare. NNHS data shows that, between 1985 and 1995, the percentage of nursing homes certified only by Medicaid declined by 55 percent (from 45 percent to 20 percent in 1995), although the percentage dually certified by Medicare and Medicaid increased by 94 percent (from 36 percent to 70 percent in 1995, data not shown). By 1999, 82 percent of nursing homes were dually certified by Medicare and Medicaid (data not shown).

[†]The 1985 NNHS excludes an estimated 2,200 residential care homes.

Medicare certification requirements include mandated services, often requiring nursing facilities to hire or contract with additional staff. The percentage of nursing homes providing nursing services, medical services, physical therapy, speech and hearing therapy, occupational therapy, and nutritional services also increased drastically between 1985 and 1995 (Figure 11-2). These trends continued into 1999. The number of full-time

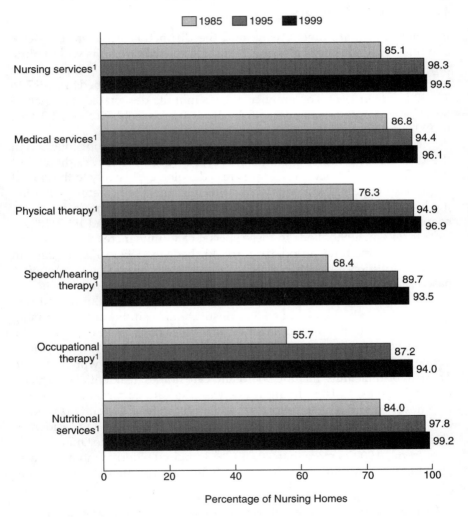

¹Time trend is significant (P < 0.05)

FIGURE 11-2   Rehabilitative and Other Services Offered by Nursing Homes: United States, 1985, 1995, 1999. *Source:* Centers for Disease Control and Prevention, National Center for Health Statistics, National Nursing Home Survey (NNHS).

equivalent patient care staff per 100 beds increased by 15 percent between 1985 and 1999, although the number of full-time equivalent registered nurses per 100 beds increased by 49 percent between 1985 and 1999 (data not shown).[‡]

Special Care Units and Other Long-Term Care Residences

Nursing homes are diversifying, and the distinction between long-term and other types of care is blurring. Although special care units within nursing homes are relatively new, their number is increasing. Nursing home beds devoted to special care units increased from 255,600 beds in 1997 to 343,300 beds in 1999. The number of beds in units designated for rehabilitative or subacute care increased from 105,200 beds in 1997 to 125,700 beds in 1999 (data not shown).

Data on special care units for Alzheimer's disease was not collected in the 1995 National Nursing Home Survey; however, the survey did collect information on distinct special care areas devoted exclusively to the care of cognitively impaired residents. Using this measure, the percentage of nursing homes with special care units for patients with Alzheimer's disease or cognitive impairments increased 35 percent between 1995 and 1999 (18% in 1995 to 24% in 1999). Beds in these special care units increased 44 percent during the same time period, from 108,400 beds in 1995 to 156,300 beds in 1999. In addition, nursing homes are increasingly providing community-based services (e.g., adult day care, home health care) to nonresidents.

With technological advances that allow more chronically ill and disabled people to be treated outside of institutional settings such as nursing homes, and with the development of new types of assisted living and life care facilities (and communities), it is becoming increasingly difficult to define and describe long-term care and the types of people who receive it. These hybrid facilities include board and care homes, residential care facilities and homes, assisted living residences, life care communities, congregate housing, and other categories that vary by state and locality (see Table 11-5 for examples). Estimates of the number of assisted living residences alone (as defined by the state in which they are located) in the United States vary from 10,000 to more than 40,000.[56,57] Impaired elderly who previously might have been confined to a nursing home because alternative care sites

---

[‡]Patient care staff includes administrative, medical, and therapeutic staff (dentists, dental hygienists, physical therapists, speech pathologists and/or audiologists, dieticians or nutritionists, podiatrists, and social workers) and nursing staff (registered nurses, licensed practical nurses, nurse's aides, and orderlies).

TABLE 11-5 Some Names of Long-Term Care Residences

Selected Long-Term Care Facilities Regulated by the State of California	*Other Names for Long-Term Care Residences*
Alzheimer's facilities or units	Adult foster care
Assisted living facilities	Adult homes
Congregate living	Adult living facilities
Continuing care retirement communities	Board and care homes
	Community-based retirement facilities
Home health care services	Domiciliary care
Life care communities	Enhanced care
Nursing homes	Group homes
Retirement housing	Homes for the aged
Residential care	Personal care adult living facilities
Senior apartments	Personal care homes
Selected Long-Term Care Facilities/Care Regulated by the State of New Jersey	Sheltered housing elder care homes
	Supportive care
Adult day care	
Assisted living programs	
Assisted living residences	
Comprehensive personal care homes	
Nursing homes	
Residential health care facilities	

Source: A. B. Bernstein et al., *Health Care in America: Trends in Utilization* (Hyattsville, Md.: National Center for Health Statistics, 2003), 17.

did not exist increasingly enter these new types of places. These facilities are not consistently defined, and no standard or validated national estimates currently exist for them.

Postacute, Rehabilitation, and End-of-Life Care Supply

The supply of subacute and postacute services has increased rather dramatically over the past decade, in part because of improvements in technology that allow care to be provided outside of a hospital setting, and in part because payment policy encourages reductions in inpatient hospital care. Often conditions cannot be successfully cured all at once, and postacute recovery or rehabilitation care is needed to prevent further deterioration in health status, to restore functioning, or to maximize quality of life for those with fatal illnesses.

Medicare pays for postacute or subacute care in a hospital or nursing unit that provides skilled nursing care. Medicare and Medicaid also cover home health care services (in the patients' homes); end-stage renal disease services provided at freestanding dialysis centers; and rehabilitation services in nursing homes, rehabilitation hospitals, rehabilitation units of acute-care hospitals, and Comprehensive Outpatient Rehabilitation Facilities (CORFs). The number of these facilities, some of which are shown in Table 11-6, shows a particularly rapid proliferation and an equally dramatic disenrollment from certification during the decade. Fifty-nine CORFs became Medicare-certified between 1997 and 1998 alone, and the number dropped substantially between 1998 and 1999.[5,58]

The trend of shorter hospital stays (following Medicare's change to a prospective hospital payment system in 1983), combined with technological and pharmaceutical advances and relaxation of Medicare eligibility requirements for home health care in the late 1980s, was associated with a shift of services from hospitals to the community and dramatic growth in the home health industry.[59] Figure 11-3 shows that the total number of home health agencies varied with the supply of Medicare-certified agencies between 1992 and 2000. In 2000, Medicare-certified home health agencies comprised nearly three-fourths of all home health agencies, and Medicare was the single largest payer for home health services. Since 1997, after the Balanced Budget Act of 1997 reduced home health payment rates, the number of Medicare-certified home health agencies declined by 26 percent.[60] Through the 1990s, however, the home health industry was the fastest growing sector in the health care industry. The hospice concept of palliative care was introduced to the United States around 1974. The hospice industry grew as Medicare began covering these services in 1982, and in particular, after a Congressional mandate increased reimbursement rates in the late 1980s. The number of Medicare-certified hospices grew substantially between 1990 and 1999, from 825 to 2,326 (Table 11-6).[5]

Geographic Accessibility   Definitions of the concept of accessibility vary widely. Opinions differ concerning which factors should be included within this concept and whether access is a characteristic of the resources

TABLE 11-6   Number of Medicare-Certified Providers: United States, 1985–2000

Type of Medicare-Certified Provider	1985	1990	1997	1998	2000
End-stage renal disease facilities	1,393	1,937	3,367	3,531	3,787
Comprehensive outpatient rehabilitation facilities	72	186	531	590	522
Hospices	164	825	2,344	2,317	2,326

Source: Centers for Medicare & Medicaid Services, *HCFA Statistics,* 1998, 1999, and 2000.

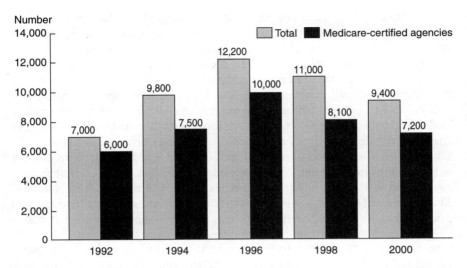

FIGURE 11-3   Home Health Agencies and Medicare-Certified Home Health Agencies: United States, 1992–2000. *Sources:* B. Haupt, E. Hing, and G. Strahan. The National Home and Hospice Survey (NHHS): 1992 summary. National Center for Health Statistics. *Vital Health Stat* 13 (117). 1994; Jones, A., Strahan, G. The National Home and Hospice Care Survey (NHHCS): 1994 summary. National Center for Health Statistics. *Vital Health Stat* 13(126). 1997; Haupt, B., Jones, A. The National Home and Hospice Care survey (NHHCS): 1996 summary. National Center for Health Statistics. *Vital Health Stat* 13(141). 1999; The National Home and Hospice Care Survey (NHHCS), 1998, 2000. National Center for Health Statistics; basic statistics about home care available in an online report at *http://www.nahc.org/Consumer/hcstats.html.*

or of the clients.[61] Accessibility is considered here—following Dona-bedian's definition[62]—as referring to the characteristics of the resource that facilitate or obstruct use by potential clients. Two of these are related: geographic accessibility and temporal accessibility.

Geographic accessibility refers to spatial factors that facilitate or obstruct utilization. It is the relationship between the location of supply and the location of clients[63] (or of need). It can be measured by distance (mileage), travel time, or travel cost. These measures of accessibility have been studied extensively elsewhere.[64,65,66,67]

The relationship between geographic accessibility and utilization of services, however, is less clear-cut than generally thought. The relationship between geographic accessibility and volume of services consumed seems to depend on the type of care and type of resource considered. Increased access (decreased distance, travel time, or travel cost) probably means increased use associated with milder complaints.

In other words, the use of preventive services is more highly associated with geographic accessibility than is the use of curative services; as is the use of generalist care as compared to specialists; and of physician services as compared to hospital services. The more severe the illness or complaint, and the more sophisticated or specialized the resource or service, the less important or strong is the relationship between geographic accessibility and volume of services utilized. There seems to be a stronger but still rather limited relationship between geographic accessibility and the choice of the site visited.[68] In a study of a prepaid group plan in an urban setting, in which equivalent services (internal medicine and pediatrics) were offered at three alternative clinics, Weiss, Greenlich, and Jones reported that 69 percent of the visits were made to the clinic nearest to the patients' homes.[69] That 31 percent of the visits were not made at the closest clinic illustrates the point that other factors, such as prestige, also influence the choice of site.

However, as should be clear from the discussion of place in Chapter 7, investigation of place (and, therefore, of accessibility) should not be limited to place of residence. In the example just cited, place of work might explain some of the 31 percent of visits not made to the closest clinic. In fact, in performing an accessibility analysis, health services managers should always consider whether place of residence is the most appropriate indicator of the location of clients. In some instances, other indicators might be more useful.

The concept of temporal accessibility is closely related to geographic accessibility. Temporal accessibility refers to the limitations in the time the resources are available (as opposed to the space limitations in the case of geographic accessibility). As Donabedian puts it, "The hours during which the physician holds office sessions, or the ambulatory care facility remains open, influence the ability of clients, especially working people, to obtain care."[70] Penchansky and Thomas[71] refer to temporal accessibility as "accommodation," which they define as "the relationship between the manner in which the supply resources are organized to accept clients and the clients' ability to accommodate to these factors and the clients' perception of their appropriateness."

Social Accessibility Social accessibility refers to the other nonspatial and nontemporal characteristics of resources that may facilitate or obstruct use of services. Social accessibility can be divided into two dimensions: acceptability and affordability. Acceptability refers to psychological, social, and cultural factors, affordability to economic factors.

Penchansky and Thomas define acceptability as "the relationship of clients' attitudes about personal and practice characteristics of providers to the actual characteristics of existing providers, as well as to provider attitudes about acceptable characteristics of clients."[72] Few studies have been done on acceptability of care. It seems, however, that consumers are unwilling to use available and geographically accessible services because of provider attributes such as sex (reluctance of some men to see a woman physician), age, race, ethnicity, and religious affiliation.

Some of these same attributes can influence the willingness of providers to treat (or not want to treat) some patients. The refusal of certain providers to serve welfare patients is an example. Hospitals or other such facilities can have formal or informal admission policies that exclude patients. Donabedian even mentions exclusions on the basis of some diagnoses such as alcoholism, drug addiction, mental illness, tuberculosis, or contagious diseases as further examples of acceptability barriers to utilization.

On the other hand, the impact of affordability on utilization has been well documented. Affordability is "the relationship of prices of services and providers' insurance or deposit requirements to the clients' income, ability to pay, and existing health insurance."[73] Some authors consider affordability a characteristic pertaining to the individual. It is the opinion here, however, that affordability is a modality of the organization of health services, intimately linked to societal norms.

The relationship of affordability to health services utilization is best seen when comparing insured and noninsured patients where voluntary health insurance is available (in the United States) or, even better, when comparing utilization before and after the introduction of a universal (national) health insurance plan (in Canada).

In the United States, studies show that people with voluntary health insurance tend to consume more physician services than those without it.[74] They also are admitted to hospitals more often and have higher rates of hospitalized surgery. In Canada, an analysis of the effects of the introduction of a universal health insurance plan in Quebec shows that when economic barriers are removed, lower income groups considerably increase their utilization of physician services.[75] At what cost for this increase in utilization is not well documented or clear as to who bears the cost. There are still significant analyses to be completed.

Consumer-Related Factors

As noted, health services utilization is an interaction between consumers and sources or providers of care in a social and organizational environment. Many characteristics and attributes of consumers (clients or patients) are related to utilization. The illness level or need for health care obviously is one. Others include such indicators of need as mobility status, perceived symptoms of illness, chronic activity limitation status, disability days, and diagnosis.

Perception of illness or of its probability of occurrence is almost always a necessary (although not sufficient) factor in the use of health services. More specifically, it is a factor in the decision to seek care. As the next section (on providers factors) shows, once care is sought, consumer factors become much less important in the subsequent utilization of services.

Other consumer-related factors can be divided into two categories: sociodemographic and sociopsychologic. In the terminology of Andersen and Newman,[76] all of these are predisposing factors. Those authors also include in the individual determinants of utilization what they call enabling factors. These include family-related variables such as income, health insurance, type of and access to regular source of care, as well as community-related factors such as availability of care, price of health services, region of the country, and urban-rural character.

The opinion here is that these enabling factors pertain to the social and organizational environment of the medical care process and were discussed as such.

Sociodemographic Factors   The same demographic and social variables described in Chapter 5 as they relate to mortality and morbidity also are related to utilization of services. These variables include age, sex, race, ethnicity, marital status, and socioeconomic status (education, occupation, income). It often is difficult to know whether these sociodemographic variables really influence utilization; that is, whether they bring about differences in inclination toward use of health services or merely reflect differences in illness levels (mortality and morbidity patterns). Both of these aspects of the relationship between sociodemographic characteristics and use of services are important.

A descriptive epidemiologic investigation for administrative, planning, or health policy purposes should describe the utilization of services specifically for each of the sociodemographic attributes (as was described in the mortality and morbidity patterns in Chapter 5). Analytic epidemiology is concerned with sociodemographic factors as determinants of health services use. For a given illness level, would certain age, sex, race, marital status, or socioeconomic groups tend to use more health services, assuming equal geographic and economic accessibility? Unfortunately, little research has been done on this topic.

The relationship between age and volume of physician visits is best described by a weak U-shaped curve.[77] Infants and older individuals consume more services than other age groups, a major factor for health services managers to consider when expanding or developing new services. This, too, seems simply to reflect the mortality and morbidity patterns described in Chapter 5. Hospital admission rates are lower for children and highest in the reproductive years, then decline until age 65 when they peak again. Middle-aged adults have higher surgery rates. The length of hospital stay increases steadily with age, as does the consumption of prescribed and nonprescribed drugs.

Women use more health services than men, beginning with the childbearing years (ages 15 to 44) and continuing through old age.[78] Much of the difference involves obstetrical care. However, females also have more surgery, more dental care, more preventive physical examinations and use more drugs and medications. Men outnumber women in mental hospitals. Because the need for dental care and preventive services is higher for females, their higher utilization seems to indicate that they do tend to seek more health services (or at least some types of services) than do men, regardless of morbidity patterns.

Income differences aside, whites consume more health services of all kinds than blacks, although the latter do have overall higher mortality and morbidity rates. This and the fact that blacks have longer average lengths of stay in hospitals indicates a racial/ethnic difference in the level of severity of symptoms and illnesses at which care is sought.

The literature does not report any specific effect of marital status on utilization; indeed, usage seems to reflect the expected age and sex composition and morbidity status of the various marital status categories.[79]

It is not easy to examine the relationship of socioeconomic status to utilization because it is confounded by at least two important variables—health status and social accessibility (more precisely, affordability). Furthermore, the literature reports many contradictory results. Most studies say that the high socioeconomic groups traditionally have used more physician services.[80]

In any case, all agree that the gap between the poor and the nonpoor has been narrowing since the introduction of Medicare and Medicaid. Data published in *Health U.S. 2003* show higher hospital admission rates and more physician visits per year among the poor than the nonpoor. A 1981 study relates this higher utilization to the fact that the poor tend to have more serious, especially chronic, illnesses compared to the nonpoor.[81] An analysis of the 1976 to 1978 National Health Interview Surveys shows that the poor have more physician visits than those with higher income but that after adjustment for age and health status these differences are reversed.[82]

The variation in the results of all these studies might stem from two factors. First, many studies fail to distinguish between different types of services. Different groups utilize similar sources of care for entirely different reasons or, given the same need, turn to different services.[83] For example, the 1981 Canada Health Survey[84] and a 1978 study in France[85] show that although those with higher levels of income consult health professionals somewhat more frequently than those with lower incomes, these consultations often take place when no associated health problem is reported (for example, for preventive services).

In the United States, a 1980 study of children's utilization of medical care in a community with "generous Medicaid benefits and a university-sponsored pediatric project" shows that children in higher income families are taken to private practitioners more frequently but that youngsters below the poverty line go to health centers and clinics more often.[86]

The second factor in the wide variation in results is that, as McKinlay points out,[87] most researchers fail to consider that socioeconomic status can be associated only indirectly with utilization of health services. The relationship between that status and utilization can be ameliorated not only by the variables' affordability and health condition but also by participation in certain social institutions or social networks that dictate or suggest "acceptable" patterns of use. The studies mentioned earlier about the cultural factors in utilization patterns indirectly support such a hypothesis of "reference group" influence.

Sociopsychological Factors   Another set of consumer-related factors can be termed "sociopsychologic." Researchers have long been aware that persons perceive illness symptoms differently. It is logical to propose that different persons therefore behave differently in seeking care according to their perceptions. Some individuals act on a set of symptoms, whereas others choose to totally disregard them or fail to act on them.[88] In addition to illness perception, attitudes or beliefs about medical care, physicians, and disease influence utilization.

Although it is easy to see conceptually how sociopsychologic factors could have an impact on use of health services, past studies of these variables show little accuracy in predicting utilization. It should be pointed out, however, that these findings are far from conclusive.[89]

Researchers have failed to distinguish between different types of services. Psychosocial factors related to the use of care might be expected to have a different impact on the use of different services.

Researchers generally have looked at the relation between sociopsychologic factors and total utilization of services. It would be much more appropriate to look at the initial visit per illness episode because the patient has much less control over the subsequent utilization of services.[90] In other words, perceptions, attitudes, and beliefs can have a high impact on the first decision to seek care, but the relationship between sociopsychologic factors and utilization can be obscured when looking at total use.

Finally, psychosocial factors are only some of the numerous factors related to utilization of services. Most studies failed to control for the impact of these other variables. The relationship between sociopsychologic variables and utilization thus can often be masked by the impact of other variables.[91]

Provider-Related Factors

A last category of determinants of health services utilization consists of factors related to health care providers, mainly physicians. These factors can be divided into two groups: economic and provider characteristics.

Economic Factors   There is a growing belief among health economists that the traditional interaction between supply and demand does not hold true in the medical marketplace. On the contrary, the alternative "demand-shift" or inducement hypothesis states that medical practitioners have the ability to generate demand for their services or (in economic terms) that they can shift the position of the consumers' demand curve.[92]

One of the first studies to suggest such a hypothesis was in 1972 by Fuchs and Kramer, who report that supply factors, technology, and number of physicians appear to be of decisive importance in determining the utilization of and expenditures for doctors' services.[93] Several studies have since reported similar findings,[94,95] although numerous criticisms also have been made:[96]

- Consumers of care are not really aware of their health services needs or, put another way, the professional and consumer definitions of need often differ. Furthermore, in many cases such as emergencies and mental illness, persons other than the consumer make decisions regarding the care to be received.

- Consumers often are not able to evaluate which providers may offer "better" care or which substitutes may be warranted.

- The occurrence of disease at a given point is a random, involuntary phenomenon—often of an urgent nature. Because of this and of the fact that the benefits received from utilization of services are unknown before treatment actually occurs, consumers are unable to make "rational" decisions to utilize services.

- Consumers do not know which services to request. They simply demand to be treated and leave it up to the physicians to decide which services are appropriate. Consequently, the physicians are in the paradoxical position of being producers of services who must decide for the client which ones must be consumed.[97]

- Most treatments require full patient compliance over the episode of care.

As mentioned in the previous section, some of the contradictory results in the analysis of demand and utilization of medical care can come from the failure to distinguish between the first and subsequent visits. The utilization process could be viewed, for simplification purposes, as consisting of a patient-initiated stage (the initial visit) and a physician-generated stage (the subsequent visits). Some authors suggest restricting the use of the term *demand* to the patient-initiated stage, and *utilization* referring to the physician-generated stage.[98] Such a distinction certainly would facilitate the investigation of the respective influence of provider-related factors and others on the use of health services.

Provider Characteristics   Provider characteristics also have been related to utilization of services. Physicians' behavior in generating utilization of services is related to their degree of specialization, to the medical school from which they graduated, to the hospital of residency, and to the number of years that have elapsed since completion of residency training.

For example, it has been shown that physicians trained in medical schools and hospitals with a scientific-medical orientation generally use fewer clinical and technical resources; however, under conditions of uncertainty (when diagnosis is unknown), they tend to use more services.[99]

The setting in which physicians actually work also has an influence on their professional activity.[100] Furthermore, norms and rules develop and influence physicians' behavior. Finally, other factors such as number and types of auxiliary health personnel and other workers, equipment, and use of technological innovations are related to physicians' behavior.

Trends in Health Services Utilization

It is imperative to understand the trends in health services utilization if appropriate use is to be made of the ensuing epidemiologic methods. This section describes trends in utilization at the turn of the century, first health resources in terms of personnel and facilities, then health care expenditures and ambulatory and inpatient care.

Overall Use of Health Services

Health care utilization rates are important indicators of what general types of care specific populations seek, and they also indicate how services are shifting. Despite major changes in the health care delivery system, the aging population, managed care incentives, and visits to physicians' offices rates per 1,000 population were relatively stable over the decade, neither increasing nor decreasing significantly between 1990–91 and 2000 (Table 11-7). The emergency department (ED) visit rate has not increased significantly since 1992; however, the decrease in the number of hospital EDs in the United States has resulted in a concentration of ED visits in the remaining EDs. At the same time, the rate for illness-related visits to EDs rose from 21.0 to 24.0 visits per 100 persons.[5,101]

By contrast, the overall rates of visits per 1,000 persons to hospital outpatient departments (OPDs) increased by 29 percent from 1992 through 2000. In part, this reflects hospitals' greater emphasis on expanding their outpatient services. Visits to OPDs, however, still comprise a relatively small percentage of the overall number of visits made to physicians.[102]

Hospital utilization in the United States, as measured by the number of hospital discharges, peaked in the early 1980s, declined until the late 1980s, then stabilized between 1990 and 2000.[103] The 2000 rate of 114 hospital discharges per 1,000 population has not changed significantly from the 122 per

TABLE 11-7 Use of Health Care Services: United States, 1990–2000

Year	Office-Based Physician Visits	Hospital Outpatient Department Visits*	Hospital Emergency Department Visits	Short-Stay Hospital Discharges
		Rate per 1,000 population		
1990–91	2,777	–	–	122
1992–93	2,925	236	356	119
1994–95	2,643	256	364	117
1996–97	2,865	271	349	114
1998–99	2,931	296	375	117
2000	3,004	304	394	114

– Data not available.

*Time trend is significant ($p < 0.05$).

Source: Centers for Disease Control and Prevention, National Center for Health Statistics, National Ambulatory Medical Care Survey (NAMCS), National Hospital Ambulatory Medical Care Survey (NHAMCS), and National Hospital Discharge Survey (NHDS).

1,000 population rate of 1990 and 1991. Declining hospital use and length of stay is attributed to cost-containment measures instituted by Medicare and Medicaid programs, other payers, and employers, as well as to scientific and technologic advances that allow a shift in services from hospitals to ambulatory outpatient settings, the community, home, and nursing homes.[104] Because certain types of care currently can be provided only in inpatient settings, hospitalization rates cannot decrease indefinitely.

Overall utilization rates do not tell exactly what services are provided to specific persons and cannot serve as proxies for either access to specific services or quality of care. A physician's office visit could include tests, procedures, and even surgery, or it could consist entirely of a discussion with a physician. A hospital or nursing home stay could be for diagnostic, palliative, or recuperative care, or conversely for medical or surgical interventions. These trends can, however, spotlight areas that should be investigated in greater depth.[5]

Primary Care and Specialty Physician Visits

On average, 72 percent of Americans visit an office-based setting for ambulatory care 6.5 times during a year.[105] In 2000, about one-half of the approximately 756.7 million visits to office-based physicians were to one of the three types of primary care practices: general and family practice (24 percent), internal medicine (15 percent), and pediatrics (13 percent).[106] According to a recent report by the Institute of Medicine, primary care is defined as "the provision of integrated, accessible, health care services by clinicians who are accountable to address a large majority of personal health care needs, develop a sustained partnership with patients, and practice in the context of the family and the community."[107] The same report states that, within the parameters of today's health care system, physicians trained in family medicine, general internal medicine, and general pediatrics are most likely to provide primary care. Specialists, however, provide primary care to some patients.

Overall, the visit rate to primary care physicians—defined here as general and family practitioners, general internists, and pediatricians—was statistically similar between 1992–93 (1,488 per 1,000 population) and 2000 (1,560 per 1,000 population). Within specific primary care specialties, visit rates to general and family practice physicians or to pediatricians did not change, but the visit rate per 1,000 population to internists increased from 400 in 1992–93 to 458 in 2000 (Figure 11-4).

Figure 11-4 also shows similar visit rates to nonprimary care physicians (that is, physicians other than general and family practice doctors, internists, and pediatricians) in 1992–93 and 2000. A previous study noted that efforts to increase primary care rates fostered greater growth in the number of primary care physicians versus nonprimary care physicians during the 1990s.[108] It is of interest that the visit rate to nonprimary care

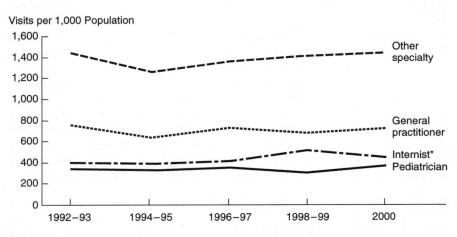

*Time trend is significant ($p < 0.05$).

FIGURE 11-4   Office Visits to Primary Care and Specialty Physicians: United States, 1992–2000. *Source:* Centers for Disease Control and Prevention, National Center for Health Statistics, National Ambulatory Medical Care Survey (NAMCS).

specialties increased from 1994–95 through 2000. This is somewhat unexpected because the spread of managed care during the 1990s was hypothesized to discourage use of specialists.[5,109]

Physician Office and Hospital Outpatient Department Visits

People of all ages visit physicians' offices and hospital outpatient departments (OPDs) to receive preventive and screening services, diagnosis, treatment, medical counseling, and other ambulatory care. In general, visits to hospital OPDs are found to be more commonly associated with imaging studies (e.g., mammography, scans), minor surgery, and specialty referrals than those made to physicians' offices.[110]

Examining only overall utilization rates for the entire U.S. population, however, masks important differences in use by population subgroups, such as particular age or racial groups. Between 1992 and 2000, overall utilization rates in physicians' offices for children or young adults ages 18 to 44 years did not change (Figure 11-5). However, the rate of visits to physicians' offices among the population 65 years of age and older increased by about 12 percent between 1992–93 and 2000 (from 5,470 to 6,125 visits per 1,000 persons). Persons 45 to 64 years of age also had significantly more visits per population over the 1990s. Increases in utilization rates for the population 45 years of age and older can be associated, in part, with greater emphasis on use of cholesterol- and glucose-lowering drugs that require

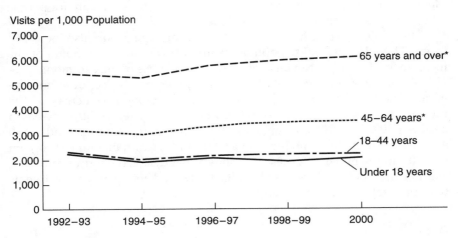

*Time trend is significant ($p < 0.05$).

FIGURE 11-5   Physician Office Visits by Age: United States, 1992–2000. *Source:* Centers for Disease Control and Prevention, National Center for Health Statistics, National Ambulatory Medical Care Survey (NAMCS).

Visits per 1,000 Population

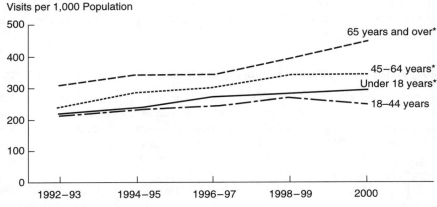

*Time trend is significant ($p < 0.05$).

FIGURE 11-6   Hospital Outpatient Department Visits, by Age: United States, 1992–2000. *Source:* Centers for Disease Control and Prevention, National Center for Health Statistics, National Hospital Ambulatory Medical Care Survey (NHAMCS).

monitoring by a physician or on diagnostic testing such as mammography that consensus guidelines recommend commence after age 50. Note that almost all Americans 65 years of age and older become eligible for Medicare coverage, which can improve access to physician care for people who were previously uninsured or underinsured.[111]

The OPD visit rate for the 45- to 65-year-old age group also increased from 241 to 343 per 1,000 population in 2000 (Figure 11-6). Some of the increase for this group can be related to increased use of the commonly provided outpatient services described, such as imaging services or minor surgeries. The rate for persons 65 years of age and older also increased. The rate of OPD visits per 1,000 for children (under age 18) also increased between 1992 and 2000, from 220 to 291. This increase corresponds with expansions in Medicaid and the State Children's Health Insurance Program (SCHIP) in the mid-1990s. Research shows that disabled children and poor children are more likely to visit hospital OPDs and emergency departments than privately insured children.[112,113]

Race

In 1999, white persons represented 82 percent of the U.S. civilian noninstitutionalized population but made 86.5 percent of all office-based physician visits.[114] As shown in Figure 11-7, the visit rate for white persons for 2000 was about 48 percent higher than for black persons (3,161 versus 2,139 vis-

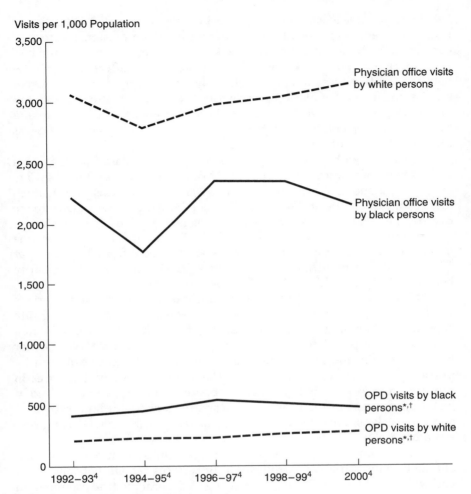

Visits per 1,000 Population

FIGURE 11-7   Physician Office and Hospital Outpatient Department Visits, by Race: United States, 1992–2000. *Source:* Centers for Disease Control and Prevention, National Center for Health Statistics, National Ambulatory Medical Care Survey (NAMCS), and National Hospital Ambulatory Medical Care Survey (NHAMCS).

its). Some possible reasons behind these race disparities in the utilization of health care services include historical patterns of the provision of care, perceptions of both providers and care-seekers, and financial and cultural barriers to care.[115] For black and white persons, the differential in rates between the two races remained relatively stable over the decade. Other studies document that black Americans are more likely to use hospital outpatient departments (OPDs) and clinics as their usual source of care and that a greater percentage of white persons use private physicians' offices as their usual source of care.[116,117]

Consistent with greater dependence on hospital-based settings as a usual source of medical care, National Hospital Ambulatory Medical Care Survey data shows that, from 1992 to 2000, black persons had a much higher utilization rate of hospital OPDs than did white persons. During the decade, the OPD visit rate for black persons increased, from 418 visits per 1,000 population in 1992–93 to 483 in 2000. During this same period, the outpatient visit rate for white persons also increased, from 210 visits per 1,000 population in 1992–93 to 280 visits in 2000. However, the disparity between black and white OPD utilization did not change.[5]

An Institute of Medicine Report documents that racial minorities receive different, often lower quality medical care than do white Americans. Although some racial, ethnic, and other disparities in care across different population groups have narrowed over time, other major health care utilization disparities remain that are not easily explained by prevalence, incidence, or risk factors. The sources of these differences in care are complex and not immediately apparent, and they can be rooted in historical patterns of the provision of care, perceptions of both providers and care-seekers, financial and cultural barriers to care, as well as numerous other factors.[118]

One example of (past or present) disparities in use shows that, although many variables in utilization of services remain between black and white populations, some are lessening. A general medical examination is the most frequent reason cited for visits to office-based physicians.[119] The differential between rates of general physical examinations (as defined by the patients' reason for visit) in physicians' offices for black and white populations has been decreasing over time (Figure 11-8).[5,120]

Hospital Emergency Department Visits—Age and Race

Hospital emergency departments (EDs) serve a wide range of medical needs, from treatment of seriously ill patients and life-threatening, injury-related conditions to less serious health conditions, minor injuries, and other nonemergency care. The past decade saw a notable increase in the volume of ED visits, a 20 percent increase between 1992 and 2000, although the number of these types of facilities was actually decreasing. Seeking care

Visits per 1,000 Population

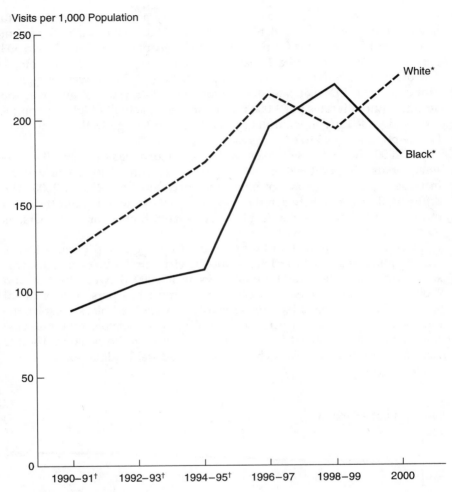

*Time trend is significant ($p < 0.05$).

†Difference between black and white population is significant ($p < 0.05$).

FIGURE 11-8 Office Visits with General Medical Exam as Primary Reported Reason for Visit, by Race: United States, 1990–2000. *Source:* Centers for Disease Control and Prevention, National Center for Health Statistics, National Ambulatory Medical Care Survey (NAMCS).

at an ED is associated with several factors, such as possession of health insurance, access to health care providers, and seriousness of condition.[121]

Patterns of use of hospital EDs differ by patient age. Younger people are more likely to visit an emergency room for injuries, although older people are more likely to visit EDs for medical conditions that respond to nonsurgical treatment, in large part because elderly people are more likely to have chronic conditions.[122] Between 1992 and 2000, there was a 19 percent increase in ED visit rates for persons 45 to 64 years of age (from 254 to 303 per 1,000 population) and a 21 percent increase for persons 65 years of age and older (from 409 to 496 per 1,000 population).[123] There was no significant change in ED visit rates for persons under 45 years of age over the decade, although rates per 1,000 population were actually higher throughout the decade for young adults and children under age 18 than they were for the population 45 to 64 years old.

In 2000, the rate of ED visits for black persons was 617 per 1,000 persons versus 370 per 1,000 for white persons (Figure 11-9). There was no increase in overall ED use for either race between 1992–93 and 2000. The differential visit rate between the two races also remained about the same throughout the decade, that is, about 68 percent higher for black persons than for white persons overall.

Trends in ED utilization by race varied by age group (Figure 11-10). Among persons ages 45 to 64 years, the ED visit rate for black persons was almost twice the rate found for white persons in 2000. Between 1992–93 and 2000, ED visit rates increased for both black and white persons 45 years of age and older. Among elderly (65 years of age and older) black persons, the rate increased by about 51 percent (from 478 to 721 visits per 1,000 persons) compared to a 19 percent increase among elderly white persons. The ED visit rate for white and black children remained stable (data not shown).

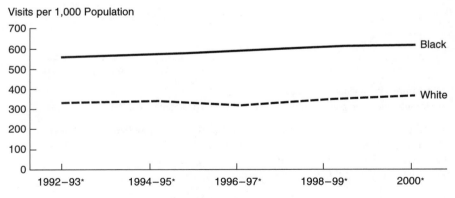

Visits per 1,000 Population

*Difference between black and white population is significant ($p < 0.05$).

FIGURE 11-9 Hospital Emergency Department Visits, by Race: United States, 1992–2000. *Source:* Centers for Disease Control and Prevention, National Center for Health Statistics, National Hospital Ambulatory Medical Care Survey (NHAMCS).

Visits per 1,000 Population

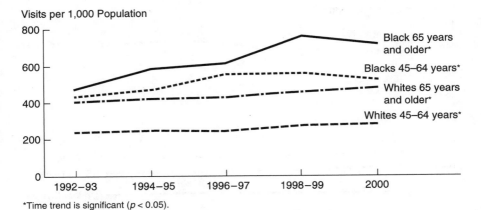

*Time trend is significant (*p* < 0.05).

FIGURE 11-10 Hospital Emergency Department Visits, by Race and Age: United States, 1992–2000. *Source:* Centers for Disease Control and Prevention, National Center for Health Statistics, National Hospital Ambulatory Medical Care Survey (NHAMCS).

Factors contributing to this difference may include the fact that black seniors are more likely to have only Medicare coverage and thus not have drug coverage; this limits their ability to purchase drugs, which, in turn, contributes to poorer outcomes. In addition, black seniors are likely to encounter greater difficulty finding office-based physicians who are willing to accept new patients.[5,124,125]

Hospital Discharges—Age and Race

Although spending for hospital care as a share of all personal health care spending in the United States is falling—from 41 percent in 1993 to 37 percent in 1999—hospital care still accounts for a larger percentage of health care expenditures than any other health care service.[126] In 1996, about 7 percent of Americans spent one or more nights in a hospital, a slight decrease from 1987, when 9 percent of the population had any expense for inpatient hospital services.[127,128]

The rate of hospital discharges per 1,000 population declined between 1992–93 and 2000 for persons 18 to 64 years of age (Figure 11-11). For persons 45–64 years of age, the discharge rate fell about 12 percent, even with increasing rates of cardiac procedures performed on this age group, from a rate of 129 to 114 per 1,000 population over the past decade. The hospital discharge rate for children did not change significantly during this period.

Although it appears that there is a slight upward trend in utilization rates for the population ages 65 years and older, this trend is not significant.

Discharges per 1,000 Population

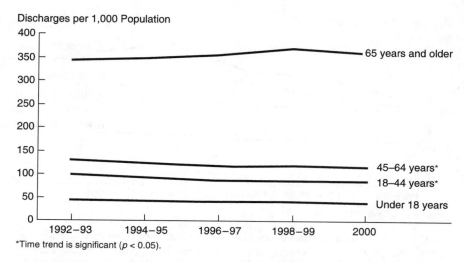

*Time trend is significant (*p* < 0.05).

FIGURE 11-11   Hospital Discharges, by Age: United States, 1992–2000. *Source:* Centers for Disease Control and Prevention, National Center for Health Statistics, National Hospital Discharge Survey (NHDS).

Elderly patients use more health care services, including hospital care, than do younger populations in large part because of greater need. Other research shows that they are being treated for more chronic conditions than in the past, and they are receiving an increasing number of medications and complex surgical interventions (e.g., cardiac surgeries such as percutaneous transluminal coronary angioplasty and stent insertion), which may explain why their hospitalization rates did not decrease.[129] Between 1992 and 1998, the percentage of elderly Medicare beneficiaries, who comprise over 90 percent of all elderly, who had at least one inpatient stay remained fairly constant, hovering around 18 percent of the population in both years.[130]

Black Americans had higher hospitalization rates than white Americans during the 1990s, and the difference remained constant across the decade. Although hospitalization rates for both groups appeared to have declined over time, these trends are not statistically significant. The hospital discharge rate per 1,000 population for black persons was 111 in 1992–93 and 98 in 2000. The hospital discharge rate per 1,000 population for white persons was 93 in 1992–93 and 84 in 2000 (Figure 11-12). Medicare program data show that black, Hispanic, and Native American beneficiaries 65 years of age and older have higher hospitalization rates than white beneficiaries, although Asian American beneficiaries have lower hospitalization rates.[5,131]

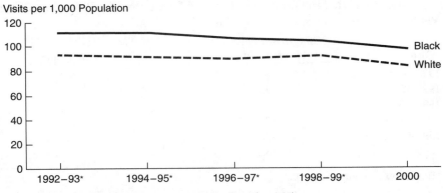

Visits per 1,000 Population

*Difference between black and white population is significant ($p < 0.05$).

FIGURE 11-12   Hospital Discharges, by Race: United States, 1992–2000. *Source:* Centers for Disease Control and Prevention, National Center for Health Statistics, National Hospital Discharge Survey (NHDS).

Duration of Hospitalizations, Physician Office Visits, and Hospital Outpatient Department Visits

Time spent with a physician has been found to influence health care costs and patient satisfaction.[132,133] Between 1990–91 and 2000, the mean duration for office-based physician visits increased slightly, from 16.7 minutes to about 18 minutes (Table 11-8).[*] This result is somewhat surprising given perceptions of shorter visits associated with managed care and employer and insurer focus on reducing costs and increasing productivity.[134]

Mean time spent with physicians at outpatient departments (OPDs) remained constant at an average of slightly longer than 18 minutes from 1997–2000 (data not shown). Although the overall average duration of physician and hospital outpatient visits did not decrease, this may mask differences in duration of visit for specific populations and for specific conditions. For example, between 1985 and 1995, office-based psychiatry visits became shorter, and the proportion of visits that lasted 10 minutes or less increased.[135] Other research has concluded that, on average, physicians

---

[*]Duration of visit to a physician's office or to a physician in a hospital outpatient department refers to the amount of time spent in face-to-face contact between the physician and the patient. This time is estimated and recorded by the physician and does not include time spent waiting to see the physician, time spent receiving care from someone other than the physician without the presence of the physician, or time spent by the physician in reviewing patient records and/or test results. In cases where the patient received care from a member of the physician's staff but did not actually see the physician during the visit, the duration was recorded as "zero" minutes.

TABLE 11-8   Mean Duration of Medical Encounters for Physician Office
Visits And Hospital Stays: United States, 1990–2000

Year	Office-Based Physician Visits (minutes)*	Short-Stay Hospital Length of Stay (days)*
1990–91	16.7	6.4
1992–93	17.7	6.1
1994–95	17.4	5.6
1996–97	17.2	5.2
1998–99	18.0	5.0
2000	18.1	4.9

*Time trend is significant ($p < 0.05$).

Source: Centers for Disease Control and Prevention, National Center for Health Statistics, National Ambulatory Medical Care Survey (NAMCS), and National Hospital Discharge Survey (NHDS).

who rely on capitated plans for a large percentage of their income spent slightly less time with their patients compared to physicians who do not.[136]

In recent years, the backlash against real or perceived hospital length-of-stay restrictions imposed by managed care policies and insurance companies has resulted in legislation mandating insurance coverage for longer stays for maternity and neonatal patients.[137] Transfers of selected procedures from inpatient to outpatient settings also may have contributed to a higher average length of stay for the more complex procedures still treated in the hospital setting. Nevertheless, the length of stay in nonfederal, short-stay hospitals peaked in the early 1980s and has been decreasing ever since.[138] The average length of stay declined from 6.4 days for the combined years 1990–91 to slightly less than 5 days in 2000.[5]

Use of Home Health Care Services

Home health care is the provision of services to individuals and their families in their homes for the purpose of promoting, maintaining, or restoring health. Persons using home health care services provided by a home health care agency include the chronically ill and disabled of all ages, those recuperating from a hospitalization or acute illness, and the terminally ill.

Between 1992 and 1996, the rate of elderly persons using home health services rose from 29.6 per 1,000 persons to 52.5 per 1,000 persons, respectively. After 1996, the rate declined to 27.7 per 1,000 persons in 2000 (Figure 11-13). Because 7 out of 10 home health patients were elderly, rates of home health use for all age groups followed a similar pattern. The overall rate of home health utilization for every 1,000 persons increased from 4.8 in 1992 to 9.1 in 1996 before dropping to 4.9 in 2000 (Figure 11-14).[5]

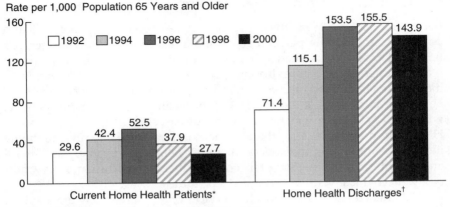

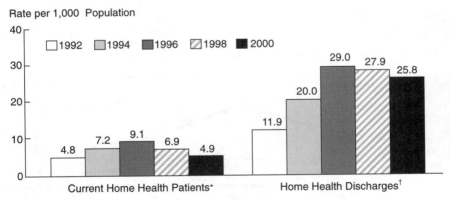

FIGURE 11-13 Use of Home Health Care by the Population 65 Years of Age and Over: United States, 1992–2000. *Source:* Centers for Disease Control and Prevention, National Center for Health Statistics, and National Home and Hospice Care Survey (NHHCS).

FIGURE 11-14 Use of Home Health Care, by the Population of All Ages: United States, 1992–2000. *Source:* Centers for Disease Control and Prevention, National Center for Health Statistics, and National Home and Hospice Care Survey (NHHCS).

Home Health Patient Characteristics

Between 1992 and 1998, the types of services received by home health patients changed. The percentage of home health patients who received homemaker services peaked at 26 percent in 1996, when Medicare payment was most generous, before dropping back to 22 percent in 1998. Similarly, more patients received high-tech home care services in 1996 than in 1998.[139] High-tech home care is the application of technology at home to patients with acute, subacute, or chronic organ diseases, dysfunction, or failure. High-tech diagnostic and therapeutic services available in the home include IV antibiotics, transfusion therapy, chemotherapy, dialysis, enteral and parenteral nutrition, long-term oxygen therapy, hydration, x ray/radiology, mechanical ventilation, and sleep studies.[140]

Patients receiving home health services on any given day are a subset of all users during the year. Data from this sample of current patients, however, present a cross-sectional picture of typical users. In 2000, 4.9 of every 1,000 persons in the United States were enrolled in a home health program. Among these users, women used home health services (6.2 per 1,000 females) twice as often as men (3.5 per 1,000 males), particularly at 85 years of age and over (data not shown). Across time (Figure 11-15), rates of home health use for all age groups peaked in 1996, then declined through 2000.

Rates of home health use among white persons also peaked in 1996, increasing from 3.9 per 1,000 white persons in 1992 to 7.1 in 1996, before dropping to 4.5 per 1,000 population in 2000. Previous studies found that

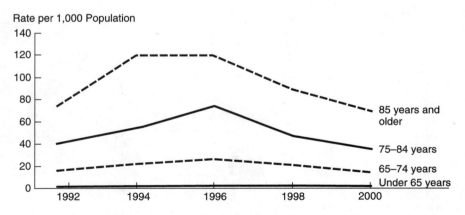

Rate per 1,000 Population

FIGURE 11-15 Current Home Health Patients, by Age: United States, 1992–2000. *Source:* Centers for Disease Control and Prevention, National Center for Health Statistics, and National Home and Hospice Care Survey (NHHCS).

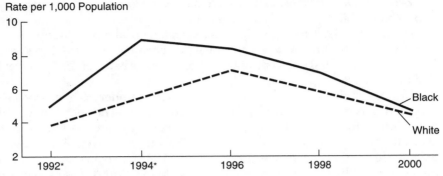

Rate per 1,000 Population

*Difference between black and white population is significant ($p < 0.05$).

FIGURE 11-16   Current Home Health Patients, by Race: United States, 1992–2000. *Source:* Centers for Disease Control and Prevention, National Center for Health Statistics, and National Home and Hospice Care Survey (NHHCS).

during the early 1990s, black persons were more likely than white persons to use postacute care services provided by home health agencies than nursing homes.[141,142] During 1992–94, rates of current home health use among black persons exceeded that for white persons (Figure 11-16). After 1994, racial differences in rates of home health use narrowed and were practically eliminated by 2000 (4.5 per 1,000 white persons compared with 4.7 per 1,000 black persons). The rate of home health use among black persons peaked earlier in 1994, increasing from 5 per 1,000 black persons in 1992 to 8.9 per 1,000 in 1994 before declining to 4.7 per 1,000 black persons in 2000.[5]

Health Care Expenditures

Health insurance coverage is an important and critical determinant of access to health care and thus important in utilization.[143,144,145] Uninsured children and nonelderly adults are substantially less likely to have a usual source of health care or a recent health care visit than their insured counterparts. Uninsured persons are more likely to forgo needed health care due to cost concerns.[146] The major source of coverage for persons under 65 years of age is private employer-sponsored group health insurance. Private health insurance may also be purchased on an individual basis, but it costs more and generally provides less coverage than group insurance. Public programs such as Medicaid and the State Children's Health Insurance Program provide coverage for many low-income children and adults.

Between 1984 and 1994 private coverage declined among the nonelderly population while Medicaid coverage and the percentage of uninsured increased. Since 1994 the age-adjusted percentage of the nonelderly population with no health insurance coverage has been between 16–17 percent, Medicaid between 9–11 percent, and private coverage between 70–73 percent (Figure 11-17).

In 2001 more than 16 percent of Americans under 65 years of age reported having no health insurance coverage. The percentage of nonelderly adults without health insurance coverage decreases with age. In 2001 adults 18–24 years of age were most likely to lack coverage and those 55 to 64 years of age were least likely (Figure 11-18). Persons with incomes below or near the poverty level were at least three to four times as likely to have no health insurance coverage as those with incomes twice the poverty

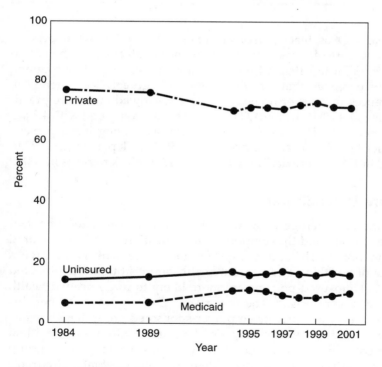

FIGURE 11-17   Health Insurance Coverage among Persons under 65 Years of Age: United States, 1984–2001. *Source:* Centers for Disease Control and Prevention, National Center for Health Statistics, and National Health Interview Survey.

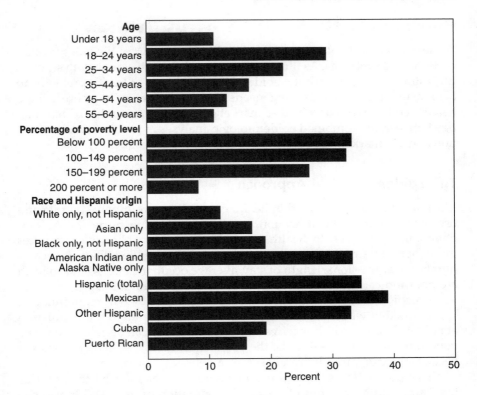

FIGURE 11-18   No Health Insurance Coverage among Persons under 65 Years of Age, by Selected Characteristics: United States, 2001. *Source:* Centers for Disease Control and Prevention, National Center for Health Statistics, and National Health Interview Survey.

level or higher. Hispanic persons and non-Hispanic black persons were more likely to lack health insurance than non-Hispanic white persons. Persons of Mexican origin were more likely to be uninsured than non-Hispanic black persons or other Hispanics. Access to health insurance coverage through employment is lowest for Hispanic persons.[7,147]

It becomes obvious that these trends demonstrate major problems in the utilization of health services. If health care managers are to be able to have an impact on these trends, they must begin an epidemiologic analysis of their data. This approach relates the epidemiology of a population group to its utilization of health services.

Management has long ignored this most important association.

Epidemiologic Analysis of Utilization

As described in Chapter 3, analysis of utilization is part of the identification of needs and problems. As illustrated in Table 3-3, analysis of health services utilization combines with the epidemiologic analysis of health problems to help managers in determining needs. For management purposes, these health needs can be conceived as market gaps and opportunities. This analogy between the combined epidemiologic analyses of problems and utilization and the marketing process is developed in a subsequent chapter.

The Epidemiological Approach

Most organizations involved in health care delivery routinely compile and use data on consumer utilization, mostly for reporting purposes. An epidemiologic approach to health services management, however, requires more than this simple accounting of the services provided. Figures such as number of admissions, length of stay, average occupancy rates, and so forth are poor indicators of the actual rate of health services utilization.[148]

An epidemiologic analysis of such utilization is, by nature, population based. In other words, utilization data need to be related to the population at risk of needing health services so that rates of use can be calculated. The denominator for rates—that is, the population at risk—often is unknown because the care provider rarely serves a defined population.[149]

This population at risk of needing services was referred to earlier as the "surrounding community" or the "population of interest." It also has been called the "constituency"[150] or the "health services area." Several methods for the determination of health services areas are described in detail elsewhere.[151,152,153]

Organizational Services   The aim of an epidemiologic analysis of health services utilization is to determine which of the health issues previously identified in the area are not currently met and need to be addressed by the organization.

The organization's existing services should be analyzed first. This is done by looking at specific services and programs and includes a sociodemographic description of the users. It also provides information on case mix—what types of morbidity (diagnosis) results in a patient who seeks care. Analysis of patient origin (a detailed breakdown of where patients are coming from) is included. Such an analysis of patient origin provides data on what has been called "organizational commitment," that is, the proportional distribution of all clients coming from given areas.[154]

Constituent Service Use   The second step is the analysis of the services used by the constituents (population of interest). This includes all the elements just described (sociodemographic characteristics, case mix, and patient origin). It produces information on who uses health services, for what problems (diagnosis), and where. This indicates the organization's market share for different services.

The proportion of a given area's admissions that go to one hospital as opposed to others has been called the "organizational relevance."[155] The terms *commitment* and *relevance* in this context are attributed to Robert Sigmand. Table 11-9 illustrates the relevance and commitment of an organization (Hospital A) whose constituency is composed of five census tracts. The commitment means that, for example, 30 percent of the inpatients of Hospital A come from census tract 02, and 25 percent come from census tract 04. These two areas are the major sources of inpatients for Hospital A. The relevance is an indicator of market penetration: In a given area, what proportion of admissions does Hospital A receive? In this example, it is census tract 05 that is the most relevant to Hospital A; although admissions from this area make up only 10 percent of its admissions, this still represents 90 percent of the total from the area. Overall, Hospital A receives 33 percent of the admissions from its constituency.

In performing this second step in the epidemiologic analysis of health services utilization, data from all the providers used by people in the areas of interest (constituency) must be compiled. In many situations these are almost impossible to gather unless a special survey can be done—except when the whole constituency is covered under a comprehensive health insurance plan such as in Canada or in prepaid settings.

When community-wide utilization data is not available, Medicare (Part B) data can be of value in describing utilization as well as listing variations in morbidity (diagnostic case mix).[156] Medicare data is available for virtually the total population over age 65 so that utilization of health services for that subset can be described and analyzed fully. Some data such as patient

TABLE 11-9   Hospital A's Commitment and Relevance

| Census Tract | Total Admissions | Hospital A | | | Other Hospitals |
		Admissions	Commitment: % of A's Admissions	Relevance: % of Admissions to A	Relevance: % Admissions to Others
01	10,000	4,000	20%	40%	60%
02	10,000	6,000	30%	60%	40%
03	13,332	2,000	10%	15%	85%
04	25,000	5,000	25%	20%	80%
05	2,222	2,000	10%	90%	10%
Others	–	1,000	5%	–	–
Total	60,554	20,000	100%	33%	–

origin (relevance) can be extrapolated to the whole population. Similarly, mortality and morbidity data from vital statistics are reasonable alternatives for estimating overall patient origin.[157,158]

The Epidemiologic Process

Figure 11-19 illustrates the process of epidemiologic (population-based) analysis of utilization. The purpose is to identify gaps in use of health services. This is done by comparing the institution's current utilization and constituents' overall use of health services with the previously identified needs and problems. As Figure 11-19 indicates, current utilization of services is a subset of overall constituency use, which in turn is a subset of the total (ideal, potential) that could result.

The sociodemographic characteristics of the users of the target organization can be compared to those of all the individuals from the constituency who used services (at this institution or elsewhere) and to the characteristics of all the constituents (users and nonusers). This indicates which constituents the organization serves, which ones use health services, and which are not served by the institution and/or other facilities.

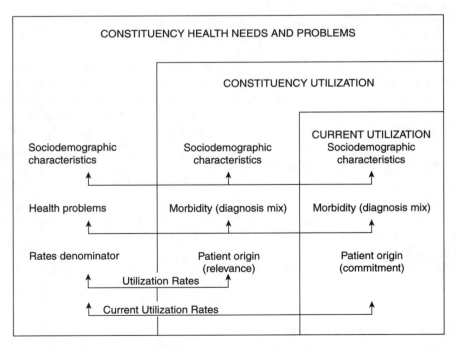

FIGURE 11-19   Epidemiologic Analysis of Health Services Utilization.

The health problems that resulted in utilization of the institution's services can be compared with those for which constituents sought care and with those identified previously—that is, all the health problems that potentially and ideally could result in consumption of services.

Current constituency rates also can be calculated. These rates are as specific as possible (e.g., age, race, sex) and calculated for specific services, programs, and diagnosis (i.e., morbidity and mortality). These rates can be adjusted (standardized) for comparison purposes. They then can be used to compare utilization from different areas of the constituency as well as from other areas, for example, the county, the state, or the nation.

The Epidemiologic Analysis: An Example   Through this epidemiologic analysis of utilization, health services managers can identify underserved constituents as well as underserved problems. Table 11-10 presents a simplified epidemiologic analysis of utilization for a hypothetical Hospital A. Hospital A's constituency is composed of five census tracts. Its commitment and relevance were described in Table 11-9. This example is limited to the distribution of three sociodemographic attributes (age, race, and sex) of the constituency population, of the constituents users of services, and of the clients of Hospital A. It also presents a general analysis of health problems.

TABLE 11-10   Age, Sex, and Race Distribution and Representation Indexes[*]

		Constituency	Constituency Users		Current Users		
						Representation Index	
Age	Sex	%	%	Representation Index	%	Constituency	Users
Under 20	Male	16.1	7.0	43.5	5.4	33.5	77.1
	Female	15.7	6.5	41.4	5.1	32.5	78.5
20–44	Male	19.0	4.3	22.6	4.9	25.8	114.0
	Female	18.3	15.1	82.5	9.2	50.3	60.9
45–64	Male	9.6	12.7	132.3	15.6	162.5	122.8
	Female	10.1	17.0	168.3	19.4	192.1	114.1
Over 65	Male	4.0	17.3	432.5	18.2	455.0	105.2
	Female	7.2	20.1	279.2	22.2	308.3	110.4
Race	White	72.3	80.2	110.9	88.4	116.2	110.2
	Black	24.2	17.1	70.7	10.3	42.6	60.2
	Other	3.5	2.7	77.1	1.3	37.1	48.1

[*]A representation index is the ratio of the percentage of population in a particular sociodemographic population to the similar percentage in any other population, multiplied by 100. When a group is overrepresented in a population, the index exceeds 100, and vice versa.

To simplify comparisons, a representation index (RI), adapted from Gerbner and Signorielli,[159] is used. This is defined as the ratio of the percentage of a population in a given sociodemographic group to the corresponding percentage in another population, multiplied by 100. When a group is overrepresented in a population, the index will be greater than 100, and vice versa. Thus, representation in the constituency user groups and in the current user groups can be measured, as well as constituency users among current users.

In Table 11-10, there are more than four times more males over 65 among the constituent users of services than among the overall constituency (representation index = 432.5) and even more among the hospital's patients (RI = 445.0). On the other hand, females under 20 are underrepresented (RI = 32.5). These relationships between age-sex and use of services are consistent with both morbidity patterns (Chapter 5) and determinants of utilization.

This is not true, however, for the race distribution of the users of services in this constituency. Whites are overrepresented both among constituency users and current users; blacks and others are underrepresented. Because this cannot be explained by morbidity patterns, it can be concluded that blacks and others definitely are underserved as compared to whites.

The last column in Table 11-10 compares the patients of Hospital A with the constituency users. This is similar to a measure of that facility's market share. That hospital thus serves proportionally fewer of the under-20-year-old users and considerably fewer females ages 20 to 44. This indicates that a potential for expansion lies in obstetrical and pediatric services. Because Hospital A serves even fewer blacks and others than the other hospitals, they too offer a potentially larger market.

Similarly, the health problems of the constituency can be compared with the morbidity that resulted in use of services by constituents and by Hospital A's patients. However, this can be done in only a relatively "soft" manner because utilization statistics relate to encounters, not to incidence of disease (for which many encounters are necessary).[160]

The comparison of constituency and current utilization can be done in a more straightforward manner. The diagnosis distribution of constituency users and current users can be compared using representation indexes. For example, if 10 percent of the use of hospital services by constituents is attributed to deliveries whereas only 7 percent of Hospital A's patients were hospitalized for deliveries, the representation index is 70, meaning that there are 30 percent fewer deliveries in Hospital A. Using fairly broad diagnostic groupings, Hospital A's market shares for different diagnoses (and services) also can be analyzed.

A final component of the epidemiologic analysis of health services utilization involves Hospital A's commitment and relevance, using patient origin data. Table 11-9 indicates, for example, that the hospital is not doing well at serving patients from census tracts 03 and 05. It should investigate possible social and geographic accessibility barriers in these tracts.

Obviously, this type of epidemiologic analysis in health services management is not limited to urban analysis; it can be accomplished just as easily in a rural setting.

Summary

This chapter examines the determinants of health services utilization. The translation of the occurrence of disease into use of health services is shown to be mediated by many sociocultural, organizational, consumer-related, and provider-related factors. Current trends in health services utilization are discussed, followed by description of an epidemiologic model for the analysis of health services utilization.

Health services managers should adopt an epidemiologic population-based perspective of utilization, relating it to their constituency and to their health problems. Analysis of utilization is part of the identification of the needs of the population.

References

1. L. C. Freeburg et al., *Health Status, Medical Care Utilization, and Outcome: An Annotated Bibliography of Empirical Studies*, 4 vols. (Washington, D.C.: National Center for Health Services Research, Publication No. PHS80-3263, November 1979).
2. A. Donabedian, *Aspects of Medical Care Administration: Specifying Requirements for Health Care* (Cambridge, Mass.: Harvard University Press, 1973), 61.
3. R. Andersen and J. F. Newman, "Societal and Individual Determinants of Medical Care Utilization in the United States," *Milbank Memorial Fund Quarterly* 51 (1973):95–124.
4. J. B. McKinlay, "Some Approaches and Problems in the Study of the Use of Services—An Overview," *Journal of Health and Social Behavior* 13 (1972):115–152.
5. A. B. Bernstein et al., *Health Care in America: Trends in Utilization* (Hyattsville, Md.: National Center for Health Statistics, 2003). Much of the material in this chapter is abridged and utilized liberally from *Health Care in America: Trends in Utilization*. Please see *http://www.cdc.gov/inchs/data/misc/healthcare.pdf*
6. Bernstein, *Health Care in America*.
7. New Chartbook Examines Health Care Utilization in America: Documents Major Trends and Shifts in Health Care, *http://www.cdc.gov/nchs/pressroom/04facts/healthcare.htm*.

8. Health Care in America: Trends in Utilization, *http://www.cdc.gov/nchs/data/misc/healthcare.pdf.*

9. A. R. Kovner and D. Neuhauser, eds., *Health Services Management: Reading and Commentary*, 7th ed. (Chicago: Health Administration Press, and Washington, D.C.: AUPHA Press, 2003).

10. Donabedian, *Aspects*, 60–61.

11. Kovner and Neuhauser, *Health Services Management.*

12. A. S. McAlearney, *Population Health Management: Strategies to Improve Outcomes* (Chicago: Health Administration Press, and Washington, D.C.: AUPHA Press, 2003).

13. Andersen and Newman, "Societal Determinants," 99.

14. L. Thomas, *The Lives of a Cell* (New York: Bantam Books, Inc., 1975), 39.

15. Andersen and Newman, "Societal Determinants," 104.

16. J. A. Martin et al., "Births: Final Data for 2002," *National Vital Statistics Report* 52, no. 10 (2003).

17. National Center for Health Statistics and S. Taffel, "Midwife and Out-of-Hospital Deliveries, United States," *Vital and Health Statistics* 21, no. 40 (Washington, D.C.: U.S. Government Printing Office, 1984).

18. McKinlay, "Some Approaches," 128–132.

19. I. K. Zola, "Culture and Symptoms: An Analysis of Patients Presenting Complaints," *American Sociological Review* 31 (October 1966):615–630.

20. E. A. Suchman, "Sociomedical Variations among Ethnic Groups," *American Journal of Sociology* 70 (November 1964):319–331.

21. E. A. Suchman, "Health Orientation and Medical Care," *American Journal of Public Health* 56 (January 1966):97–105.

22. E. Friedson, *Patients' Views of Medical Practice* (New York: Russell Sage Foundation, 1961).

23. McKinlay, "Some Approaches," 131.

24. "Ten Great Public Health Achievements—United States, 1900–99," *Morbidity and Morality Weekly Report* 48, no. 12 (1999):241–243.

25. J. F. Fries, "Aging, Cumulative Disability, and the Compression of Morbidity," *Comprehensive Therapy* 27, no. 4 (2001):322–329.

26. T. T. Perls, "Centenarians Prove the Compression of Morbidity Hypothesis, but What About the Rest of Us Who Are Genetically Less Fortunate?" *Medical Hypotheses* 49, no. 5 (1997):405–407.

27. C. D. Mathers, "Gains in Health Expectancy from the Elimination of Diseases among Older People," *Disability Rehabilitation* 21, nos. 5–6 (1999):211–221.

28. W. J. Nusselder, K. van der Velden, J. L. van Sonsbeck et al., "The Elimination of Selected Chronic Diseases in a Population: The Compression and Expansion of Morbidity," *Amican Journal of Public Health* 86 (1996):187–94.

29. M. C. McCormick, R. M. Winick, A. Elixhauser et al., "Annual Report on Access to and Utilization of Health Care for Children and Youth in the United States—2000," *Ambulatory Pediatrics* 1, no. 1 (2001):3–15.

30. R. W. Broyles, L. Narine, E. N. Brandt Jr., "The Temporarily and Chronically Uninsured: Does Their Use of Primary Care Differ?" *Journal of Health Care for the Poor and Underserved* 13, no. 1 (2002):95–111.

31. R. C. Bradbury, J. H. Golec, and P. M. Steen, "Comparing Uninsured and Privately Insured Hospital Patients: Admission Severity, Health Outcomes and Resource Use," *Health Service Management Research* 14, no. 3 (2001):203–210.

32. R. Andersen and L. A. Aday, "Access to Medical Care in the U.S.: Realized and Potential," *Medical Care* 16, no. 7 (1978):533–546.

33. R. Andersen, "Revisiting the Behavioral Model and Access to Medical Care: Does It Matter?" *Journal of Health and Social Behavior* 36(March 1995):1–10.

34. Administration on Aging, "A Profile of Older Americans: 2002." *http://www. aoa.gov/default.htm, http://www.aoa.gov/prof/statistics/profiles2002.asp.*

35. AHA Trendwatch (by The Lewin Group), *American Hospital Association* 3, no. 3 (2001).

36. Fries, "Aging, Cumulative," 322–329.

37. Perls, "Centenarians Prove," 405–407.

38. Mathers, "Gains in," 211–221.

39. Nusselder et al., "The Elimination," 187–194.

40. J. Lubitz, L. G. Greenberg, Y. Gorina et al., "Three Decades of Health Care Use by the Elderly, 1965–1998," *Health Affairs* 19, no. 3 (2000):178–184.

41. A. A. Okunade and A. A. Miles, "Medicare Physician Reform and the Utilization of Cardiovascular Procedures," *Journal of Health and Social Behavior* 11, no. 1 (1999):37–52.

42. B. H. Gilman, "Hopsital Response to DRG Refinements: The Impact of Multiple Reimbursement Incentives on Inpatient Length of Stay," *Health Economics* 9, no. 4 (2000):277–294.

43. N. McCall, A. Petersons, S. Moore, and J. Korb, "Utilization of Home Health Services Before and After the Balanced Budget Act of 1997: What Were the Initial Effects?" *Health Serv Res* 38, no. 1 (2003):85–106.

44. C. Chaix-Couturier et al., "Effects of Financial Incentives on Medical Practice: Results from a Systematic Review of the Literature and Methodological Issues," *International Journal of Quality Health Care* 12, no. 2 (2000):133–142.

45. A. B. Beinstein et al., "Trend Data on Medical Encounters: Tracking a Moving Target," *Health Affairs* 20, no. 2 (2001):5873.

46. R. Weinick and J. Cohen, "Leveling the Playing Field: Managed Care Enrollment and Hospital Use, 1987–1996," *Health Affairs* 19, no. 3 (2000):178–84.

47. The Lewin Group, *The Trendwatch Chartbook 2001* (Chicago: American Hospital Association, 2001), *http://www.hospitalconnect.com/ahapolicyforum/ trendwatch/chartbook2001.html.*

48. The Lewin Group, *Trendwatch Chartbook 2001.*

49. *Hospital Statistics, 2002 Edition* (Chicago: American Hospital Association, 2002).

50. L. R. Brewster, L. S. Ruddell, and C. A. Lesser, "Emergency Room Divisions: A Symptom of Hospitals under Stress," *Center for Studying Health Systems Change Issue* Brief No. 38 (2001).

51. The Lewin Group, "AHA TrendWatch: Emergency Departments—An Essential Access Point to Care," *American Hospital Association* 3, no. 1 (2001).

52. National Center for Health Statistics, *Health, United States, 2001 with Urban and Rural Health Chartbook* (Hyattsville, Md.: National Center for Health Statistics, 2001).

53. Office of Rural Health Policy, *Facts about Rural Physicians* (Rockville, Md.:, 1997).

54. American College of Physicians and Surgeons, *Socio-economic Factbook for Surgery 1991–92* (Chicago: Health Administrative Press, 1991).

55. N. McCall, ed., "Who Will Pay for Long Term Care? Insights from the Partnership Program," *Chapter 1: Long Term Care: Definition, Demand, Cost, and Financing* (Chicago: Health Administration Press, 2001).

56. R. T. Hodlewsky, (1998). *Facts and trends: 1998 The assisted living sourcebook.* Washington, DC: National Center for Assisted Living, American Health Care Association.

57. The National Investment Conference for the Senior Living and Long Term Care Industries (NIC), *National Housing Survey of Adults Age 60+: Opinions, Attitudes, Perceptions and Behaviors,* 1997; executive summary at *http://www.ncal.org/about/vital.htm,* accessed on 8/28/03.

58. Health Care Financing Administration, *1999 HCFA Statistics* (Baltimore, Md.: Corporate author: Institute of Medicine, 1999).

59. G. S. Wunderlich, F. A. Sloan, and C. A. Davis, eds., "Nursing Staff in Hospitals and Nursing Homes: Is It Adequate?" *Institute of Medicine* (Washington, D.C.: National Academy Press, 1996).

60. National Association of Home Care, "Basic Statistics about Home Care," 2000, *http://www.nahc.org/Consumer/hcstats.html,* accessed on 8/28/03.

61. National Association of Home Care, "Basic Statistics about Home Care."

62. Donabedian, *Aspects,* 419.

63. R. Penchansky, and J. W. Thomas. 1981. "The Concept of Access: Definition and Relationship to Consumer Satisfaction." *Medical Care* 19 no. 2 (981): 127-40.

64. G. E. Alan Dever, *Community Health Analysis* (Rockville, Md.: Aspen Systems Corporation, 1980), 251–261.

65. G. W. Shannon and G. E. Alan Dever, *Health Care Delivery: Spatial Perspectives* (New York: McGraw-Hill Book Company, 1974), 141.

66. Donabedian, *Aspects,* 425–463.

67. E. M. Bosanac et al., "Geographic Access to Hospital Care: A 30-Minute Travel Time Standard," *Medical Care* 14, no. 7 (July 1976):616–624.

68. L. A. Aday and R. Eichhom, *The Utilization of Health Services: Indices and Correlates. A Research Bibliography* (Washington, D.C.: U.S. Public Health Service, Health Services and Mental Health Administration, DHEW Publication No. (HSM) 73-3003, 1973), 27.

69. J. E. Weiss, M. R. Greenlich, and J. F. Jones, "Determinants of Medical Care Utilization: The Impact of Spatial Factors," *Inquiry* 8 (December 1971):50–57.

70. Donabedian, *Aspects,* 425.

71. Penchansky and Thomas, "Concept of Access," 128.

72. Penchansky and Thomas, "Concept of Access," 129.

73. Penchansky and Thomas, "Concept of Access."

74. Aday and Eichhom, *Utilization of Health Services,* 24.

75. P. E. Enterline, A. D. McDonald, and J. C. McDonald, *Some Effects of Quebec Health Insurance* (Washington, D.C.: U.S. Public Health Service, National Center for Health Services Research, DHEW Publication No. PHS 79-3238, January 1979).
76. Andersen and Newman, "Societal and Individual Determinants."
77. D. K. Chessy et al., National Ambulatory Medical Care Survey: 2001 Summary, *Advance Data from Vital and Health Statistics* no. 337 (2003): 5.
78. Chessy et al. "National Ambulatory Medical Care Survey."
79. Chessy et al. "National Ambulatory Medical Care Survey."
80. National Center for Health Statistics, *Health, United States, 2003* (Hyattsville, Md.: National Center for Health Statistics, 2003), 8–10.
81. National Center for Health Statistics, *Health, United States, 2003*, 14.
82. J. C. Kleinman, M. Gold, and D. Makuc, "Use of Ambulatory Medical Care by the Poor: Another Look at Equity," *Medical Care* 19, no. 10 (October 1981): 1011–1022.
83. McKinlay, "Some Approaches," 120.
84. Health and Welfare Canada and Statistics Canada, *The Health of Canadians— Report of the Canada Health Survey* (Ottawa: Minister of Supply and Services, 1981), 167.
85. P. Flamme and J. C. Portonnier, "Le systeme de sante face aux risques graves," *Revue Francaise des Affaires Sociales* (October–December 1978):352–361.
86. L. B. Wolfe, "Children's Utilization of Medical Care," *Medical Care* 18, no. 12 (December 1980):1196–1207.
87. McKinlay, "Some Approaches," 120.
88. McKinlay, "Some Approaches," 126.
89. J. B. McKinlay and D. B. Dutton, "Social-Psychological Factors Affecting Health Service Utilization," in *Health Care Consumers, Professions and Organizations*, ed. J. B. McKinlay, Milbank Reader Series no. 2 (New York: Milbank Memorial Fund, 1978), 118–170.
90. R. M. Battistella, "Factors Associated with Delay in the Initiation of Physicians' Care among Late Adulthood Persons," *American Journal of Public Health* 61 (July 1968):1348–1361.
91. R. M. Battistella, "Limitations in the Use of the Concept of Psychological Readiness to Initiate Health Care," *Medical Care* 6 (July–August 1968):308–319.
92. J. Richardson, "The Inducement Hypothesis: That Doctors Generate Demand for Their Own Services," in *Health, Economics, and Health Economics*, ed. J. Van Der Gaag and M. Perlman (Amsterdam: North Holland Publishing Company, 1981), 189–214.
93. V. P. Fuchs and M. J. Kramer, *Determinants of Expenditures for Physicians' Services in the United States 1948–1968*. DHEW Publication No. (HSM) 73-3013 (Washington, D.C.: U.S. Government Printing Office, December 1972).
94. R. G. Evans, "Supplier-Induced Demand: Some Empirical Evidence and Implications," in *The Economics of Health and Medical Care*, ed. M. Perlman (New York: John Wiley & Sons, Inc., 1974), 162–173.
95. Richardson, "Inducement Hypothesis," 189–214.
96. J. P. Newhouse, "The Demand for Medical Care Services: A Retrospect and Prospect," in *Health, Economics*, 85–102.

97. A. P. Contandriopoulos, *Un modele de comportement des medecins en tant que producteurs de services*, doctoral diss., Universite de Montreal, 1976, 295.

98. G. L. Stoddart and M. L. Bares, "Analysis of Demand and Utilization through Episodes of Medical Service," in *Health Economics*, 149–170.

99. R. Pineault, "The Effect of Medical Training Factors on Physicians' Utilization Behavior," *Medical Care* 15, no. 1 (January 1977):51–67.

100. R. Pineault, "The Effect of Medical Training Factors on Physicians' Utilization Behavior," *Medical Care* 14, no. 2 (February 1976):121–137.

101. C. W. Burt and L. F. McCaig, "Trends in Hospital Emergency Department Utilization: United States, 1992–99," *Vital Health Stat* 13, no. 150 (2001):1–34.

102. N. Ly and L. F. McCaig, "National Hospital Ambulatory Medical Care Survey: 2000 Outpatient Department Summary," *Advance Data from Vital and Health Statistics*, no. 327 (Hyattsville, Md.: National Center for Health Statistics, 2002).

103. M. J. Hall and M. F. Owings, "2000 National Hospital Discharge Survey," *Advance Data from Vital and Health Statistics*, no. 329 (Hyattsville, Md.: National Center for Health Statistics, 2002).

104. G. S. Wunderlich et al., "Nursing Staff."

105. N. A. Krauss, S. Machlin, and B. L. Kauss, "Use of Health Care Services, 1996," *Medical Expenditures Panel Survey Research Finding #7*, online report located at *http://www.meps.ahrq.gov/paper/r7_99–0018/RF7.html*.

106. D. K. Cherry and D. A. Woodwell, "National Ambulatory Medical Care Survey: 2000 Summary," *Advance Data from Vital and Health Statistics*, no. 327 (Hyattsville, Md.: National Center for Health Statistics, 2002).

107. Institute of Medicine, "Primary Care: America's Health in a New Era," (Washington, D.C.: National Academy Press, 1996).

108. E. S. Salsberg and G. J. Forte, "Trends in Physician Workforce, 1980–2000," *Health Affair* 21, no. 5 (2002):165–73.

109. Kaiser/Health Research Education Trust, "Employee Health Benefits, 1999 Annual Summary," online at *http://www.kff.org*.

110. C. B. Forrest and E. M. Whelan, "Primary Care Safety-Net Delivery Sites in the United States: A Comparison of Community Health Centers, Hospital Outpatient Departments and Physicians' Offices," *JAMA* 284, no. 16 (2000):2077–2083.

111. Medicare Payment Advisory Commission, "Report to the Congress: Selected Medicare Issues" (Washington, D.C.: MedPAC, June 1999).

112. Forest and Whelan, "Primary Care," 2077–2083.

113. G. T. Ray, T. Lieu, R. M. Weinick et al., "Comparing the Medical Expenses of Children with Medicaid and Commercial Insurance in an HMO," *American Journal of Management Care* 6, no. 7 (2000):753–760.

114. D. K. Cherry, C. W. Burt, and D. A. Woodwell, "National Ambulatory Medical Care Survey: 1999 Summary," *Advance Data from Vital and Health Statistics*, no. 322 (Hyattsville, Md.: National Center for Health Statistics, 2001).

115. Institute of Medicine, B. D. Smedley, A. Y. Smith, and A. R. Nelson, eds., *Unequal Treatment: Confronting Racial and Ethnic Disparities in Health Care (2002)* (Washington, D.C.: National Academy Press, 2002).

116. L. Shi, "Experience of Primary Care by Racial and Ethnic Groups in the United States," *Medical Care* 37, no. 10 (1999):1068–1077.

117. V. M. Freid, D. M. Makuc, and R. N. Rooks, "Ambulatory Health Care Visits by Children: Principal Diagnosis and Place of Visit," *Vital Health Stat* 13, no. 137 (1998):1–23.

118. B. D. Smedley et al., "Unequal Treatment."

119. D. K. Cherry et al., "National Ambulatory Medical Care Survey: 1999."

120. D. Schneider, L. Appleton, and T. McLemore, "A Reason for Visit Classification for Ambulatory Care," *Vital Health Stat* 2, no. 78, (National Center for Health Statistics, 1979).

121. N. Ly and McCaig, "National Hospital."

122. N. Ly and McCaig, "National Hospital."

123. L. F. McCaig and N. Ly, "National Ambulatory Medical Care Survey: 2000 Emergency Department Summary," *Advance Data from Vital and Health Statistics*, no. 327 (Hyattsville, Md.: National Center for Health Statistics, 2002).

124. N. Ly and McCaig, "National Hospital."

125. E. S. Salsberg and Forte, "Trends," 165–173.

126. S. Heffler, K. Levit, S. Smith et al., "Health Spending Growth Up in 1999; Faster Growth Expected in the Future," *Health Aff* 20, no. 2 (2001):193–203, 2001.

127. H. Hahn and D. Lefkowitz, "Annual Expenses and Sources of Payment for Health Care Services," *National Medical Expenditure Survey Research Finding* 14, AHCPR Pub. No. 93-0007 (Rockville, Md.: Agency for Health Care Policy and Research, 1992).

128. N. Krauss, S. Machlin, and B. Kass, "Medical Expenditure Panel Survey Research Finding #7: Use of Health Care Services," AHCPR Pub. No. 99-0018 (Rockville, Md.: Agency for Health Care Policy and Research, 1999).

129. J. Lubitz et al., "Three Decades," 19–32.

130. H. Liu and R. Sharma, "Health and Health Care of the Medicare Population: Data from the 1998 Medicare Current Beneficiary Survey," prepared under the U.S. Department of Health and Human Services, Center for Medicare and Medicaid Services, to Westat (Rockville, Md.: USDHHS, March 2002).

131. P. W. Eggers and L. G. Greenberg, "Racial and Ethnic Differences in Hospitalization Rates among Aged Medicare Beneficiaries, 1998," *Health Care Finance Rev* 21, no. 4 (2000):91–105.

132. K. H. Dansky and J. Miles, "Patient Satisfaction with Ambulatory Healthcare Services: Waiting Time and Filling Time," *Hosp Health Serv Adm* 42, no. 2 (1997):165–7.

133. C. T. Lin, G. A. Albertson, L. M. Schilling et al., "Is Patients' Perception of Time Spent with the Physician a Determinant of Ambulatory Patient Satisfaction?" *Arch Intern Med* 161, no. 11 (2001):1437–1442.

134. D. Mechanic, "The Managed Care Backlash: Perceptions and Rhetoric in Health Care Policy and the Potential for Health Care Reform," *Milbank Q* 79, no. 1 (1999):35–54, III-IV.

135. M. Olfson, S. C. Marcus, and H. A. Pincus, "Trends in Office-Based Psychiatric Practice," *Am J Psychiatry* 156, no. 3 (1999):451–457.

136. R. Balkrishnan, M. A. Hall, D. Mehrabi et al., "Capitation Payment, Length of Visit, and Preventive Services: Evidence from a National Sample of Outpatient Physicians," *Am J Manag Care* 8, no. 4 (2002):332–340.
137. Newborn and Mothers' Patient Protection Act of 1996; see *http://hippo.find-law.com/newborn.html.*
138. M. J. Hall and Owings, "2000 National Hospital."
139. A. B. Bernstein, "Trend Data," 5873.
140. Department of Geriatric Health, *Medical Management of the Home Care Patient: Guideline for Physicians,* 2d ed. (Chicago: American Medical Association, 1998).
141. K. Liu, D. Wissoker and C. Rimes, "Determinants and Cost of Post-Acute Care Use by Medicare SNFs and HHAs," *Inquiry* 35, no. 1 (1990):49–61.
142. A. Steiner and C. R. Neu, "Monitoring the Changes in Use of Medicare Posthospital Services," report prepared for the Health Care Financing Administration (Santa Monica, Calif.: RAND), 1993.
143. The State of Health Care in America 2002, *Business and Health* (Montvale, N.J.: Medical Economics, 2002).
144. National Center for Health Statistics, *Health, United States, 2003* (Hyattsville, Md.: National Center for Health Statistics, 2003).
145. Metro Public Health Department of Nashville/Davidson County, Access to Care, *Community Health Behavior Survey 2001, http://healthweb.nashville.gov/Web%20Docs/pdf%20copies/AccesstoCare.pdf.*
146. J. Z. Ayanian, J. S. Weissman, E. C. Schneider et al., "Unmet Health Needs of Uninsured Adults in the United States," *JAMA* 285, no. 4 (2000):2061–2069.
147. National Center for Health Statistics 2003, *Health,* 28.
148. J. E. Wennberg, "A Small Area, Epidemiological Approach to Health Care Data" (paper presented at the sixth national meeting of the Public Health Conference on Records and Statistics, St. Louis, June 14–16, 1976).
149. P. E. Sartwell and J. M. Last, "Epidemiology," in *Maxcy-Rosenau Public Health and Preventive Medicine,* 11th ed., J. M. Last, ed. (New York: Appleton-Century-Crofts, Inc., 1980), 29.
150. R. E. MacStravic, *Determining Health Needs* (Ann Arbor, Mich.: Health Administration Press, 1978), 186–187.
151. R. E. MacStravic, *Determining Health Needs.*
152. G. E. Alan Dever, *Community Health Analysis* (Rockville, Md.: Aspen Systems Corporation, 1980), Chapter 8.
153. G. W. Shannon and G. E. Alan Dever, *Health Care Delivery Spatial Perspectives* (New York: McGraw-Hill Book Company, 1974), 14.
154. Dever, *Community Health Analysis,* Chapter 8.
155. Dever, *Community Health Analysis.*
156. Wennberg, "A Small Area, Epidemiological Approach."
157. MacStravic, *Determining,* 186–187.
158. P. K. New, "Use of Birth Data in Delineation of Medical Service Areas," *Rural Sociology* 20 (September–December 1955):272–281.
159. G. Gerbner and N. Signorielli, "The World According to Television," *American Demographics* (October 1982):15–17.
160. Sartwell and Last, "Epidemiology," 29.

12

Geographic Information Systems

Introduction

A Geographic Information System (GIS) is a computer system capable of capturing, storing, analyzing, and displaying geographically referenced information; that is, data identified according to location. A GIS also includes the procedures, operating personnel, and spatial data that go into the system.[1]

GISs are driving dramatic changes throughout society. They make it possible for people to see whatever they wish—county boundaries, school and doctor locations, population densities, open space, and many other topics of interest. All that is needed is the proper data, and a map can be created using the GIS software.[2]

The power of a GIS comes from the ability to relate different information in a spatial context and to reach a conclusion about this relationship. Most of the information known about the world contains a location reference, placing that information at some point on the globe. For example when information on sexually transmitted diseases (STDs) is collected, it is important to know where the infections are distributed geographically. Comparing this information with other information, such as the per capita income, age distribution, health, education, clinics, and policies pertaining to the location, can demonstrate the relationship between areas of higher risk for STDs and inadequate health education and/or socioeconomic levels.

The STD example is one of many that can be presented that exhibits an application of the spatial analysis to health management problems. Table 12-1 illustrates recent GIS applications in the areas of disease prevalence, immunization, pregnancy rates and prenatal care, injury monitoring and surveillance, public health control programs, environmental problems

TABLE 12-1 Examples of Epidemiologic Applications Using a GIS

Disease Prevalence	Health Application	Figure	Location	Spatial Content	GIS Software	Brief Description of Application
	Lead Poisoning	12-1	Duval County, Florida	Census block	ArcView GIS 3.0a	To target blood lead screening for childhood lead poisoning based on CDC screening guidelines, the map combines information about lead poisoning cases with data on the year of house construction, a census variable highly correlated with the use of lead-based paint.
	Lead Poisoning	—	Santa Clara County, California	Census tract	Atlas GIS for Windows 3.0	Lead Hot Zones in Santa Clara County; criteria for establishing these zones were determined by census tracts that ranked above the fiftieth percentile in pre-1950s housing, children under six years of age, and poverty.
	Lead Poisoning	—	Kellogg, Idaho	City/town	ArcView GIS 3.0a	Characterize community environmental exposures to lead, displayed trends in mean blood levels for children over a ten-year period following a major release of lead at a smelter; historical measurements provide a basis for considering a medical monitoring program for the affected communities.

TABLE 12-1 (continued)

	Health Application	Figure	Location	Spatial Content	GIS Software	Brief Description of Application
Disease Prevalence (continued)	Immun- ization	12-2	Hillsborough County, Florida	Census block	ArcView GIS 3.0a	Surveys of immunization levels in two-year-old children can be combined with birth certificate and census data to help target immunization pockets of need.
	Immun- ization	—	Salt Lake County, Utah	ZIP code	ArcView GIS 3.0a	Direct hepatitis A immunization program efforts to ZIP codes with children at highest risk.
Birth Outcomes	Pregnancy/ Prenatal Care	12-3	Georgia	ZIP code	Atlas GIS for Windows 3.0 ArcView GIS 3.0a	Cocaine use by pregnant women in Georgia, dried blood-spot specimens collected from newborns were used to identify Benzoylecgonine (a cocaine metabolite) in ZIP codes with more than 50 births.
	Pregnancy/ Prenatal	—	Lancaster County, South Carolina	Census block	ArcView GIS 3.0a	Use of geostatistical techniques and a logistic regression model to predict high-risk areas for teen live births; combining GIS and census data, they successfully predicted high-risk areas compared with the patterns for actual live birth data.

TABLE 12-1 (continued)

	Health Application	Figure	Location	Spatial Content	GIS Software	Brief Description of Application
Birth Outcomes	Pregnancy/ Prenatal Care	—	North Dakota	ZIP code	Atlas GIS 3.03	To characterize the adequacy of prenatal care defined by the Kessner Index; to eliminate statistically unstable rates as a result of small numbers, home address ZIP codes for patients with live births were aggregated to the county level and five years of data were analyzed.
Morbidity Surveillance	Injury	12-4	Ventura County, Santa Barbara	Map grid	ArcView GIS 3.0a with Spatial Analyst	Used kernel filtering (gridded density surface) techniques to map motor vehicle injuries requiring emergency transport; staff used the map to help target education and prevention efforts.
	Injury	—	Kansas City, Missouri	ZIP code	MapInfo Professional 4.0	To identify ZIP codes with the highest age-adjusted homicide rates within a city.
	Injury	—	Boston, Massachusetts	ZIP code	MapInfo Professional 4.0	To show maps of hospital discharge data can provide insights into the pattern of injuries among adults in a community.

TABLE 12-1 (continued)

	Health Application	Figure	Location	Spatial Content	GIS Software	Brief Description of Application
Public Health Control Programs	Animal Rabies Control	—	Central Palm County, Florida	Street address	Atlas GIS for Windows 3.0	Used to plot animal rabies cases by animal type, date of case, and over time to help target interventions.
	Animal Rabies Control	12-5	Mahoning County, Ohio	Latitude-longitude	Atlas GIS 2.1 with hand-held Global Positioning Satellite units	Determine points for surveillance and oral vaccine baiting for raccoons infected with rabies.
Environmental Problems	Toxic Emissions	12-6	Hanford Nuclear Reservation, Washington	Toxic plume	ARC/INFO 7.0 for Unix	To evaluate risk from exposure to Iodine-131 released into the air from a U.S. government plutonium production facility from 1945 to 1951. Individuals who were exposed through consumption of contaminated milk as young children might now be at risk for developing thyroid cancer and other conditions; their map was used to help define who is eligible for medical evaluation and referral services.
	Water Pollution	—	Clymer, New York	Water district	AutoCad Map 2.0	To caution families about the risk of methemoglobinemia (resulting in low blood oxygen) from using water with elevated levels of nitrate-nitrogen to prepare baby formula.

TABLE 12-1 (continued)

	Health Application	Figure	Location	Spatial Content	GIS Software	Brief Description of Application
Environmental Problems	Water Pollution	—	Linn County, Iowa	Bedrock depth	ArcView GIS 3.0a	To document that many private wells with high nitrate levels in Linn County are located in areas where bedrock is relatively shallow.
	Water Pollution	—	Harford County, Maryland	Tax parcel	ArcView GIS 3.0	To monitor potential groundwater pollution plumes around a landfill and to help target areas of concern.
	Water Pollution	12-7	Hutchinson, Kansas	Groundwater zones	ArcInfo 7.1.1, ArcView GIS 3.30a, and ESRI Data Automation Kit 3.5.1	To project public water withdrawal from the community aquifer by five-year zones of groundwater capture and in 300-day intervals.
Distance Learning	Distance-based Learning	12-8	Eastern North Carolina	Telemedicine areas	MapInfo Professional 4.5	To plan where telemedicine sites might be located in relation to medically underserved areas; although their map is targeted toward improving education for personal health care providers, analogous maps could be drawn for national and state distance-based training programs for many different types of public health practitioners.

TABLE 12-1 (continued)

Health Application	Figure	Location	Spatial Content	GIS Software	Brief Description of Application
Community Needs Assessment and Access	Community Profiles / Access	—	Austin, Texas	Street address	MapInfo Professional 4.5	To demonstrate the use of population pyramids to profile how clinic clientele in an area can vary spatially; understanding such differences in social and health characteristics of client populations is important from the perspective of improving efficiency in the delivery of public health services.
	Community Profiles / Access	—	Columbia, South Carolina	Street address	ArcView GIS 3.0	To improve access to health and public services that are vital to employable welfare recipients.
	Community Profiles / Access	—	Akron, Ohio	Street address	MapInfo Professional 4.0	To show how local health departments can identify the "market areas" for their clinics by plotting the home addresses of active patients at each clinic location. This type of analysis can be used to make decisions about optimal locations for clinics, clinic consolidations, and staffing arrangements, and to evaluate access to health care.

TABLE 12-1 (continued)

Health Application	Figure	Location	Spatial Content	GIS Software	Brief Description of Application
Community Needs Assessment and Access	12-9	Ingham County, Michigan	Map grid	Atlas GIS 3.1, SPSS 6.1, and Quattro Pro 6.01	To develop a GIS "surface" map of the estimated distribution of the percentage of adults without health insurance in local community areas of the county using synthetic estimates.
Community Profiles / Access	12-10	DeKalb County, Georgia	Census tract	ArcView GIS 3.0a	To illustrate how information about consumer behavior (developed to help businesses target commercial products) can also have implications for targeting community health prevention efforts. For example, an area with a cluster group characterized by high cigarette consumption and sales might be a prime candidate for a smoking cessation program.
Community Profiles / Access	—	Northern New Castle County, Delaware	Census tract	Atlas GIS 3.0	To identify community priority areas; relevant census tract-level variables provided the basis for ranking small areas and ultimately assigning them to priority groups.

TABLE 12-1 (continued)

Health Application	Figure	Location	Spatial Content	GIS Software	Brief Description of Application
Integrated Data/GIS Systems					
Data System	—	King County, Washington	ZIP code	MapInfo Professional 4.5 and VISTA/PH 8.0	To help users analyze the types of information typically needed for a community health profile using software; analysis can range from simple (crude- or age-specific rates) to more complex (age-adjusted rates, 95% confidence intervals, and a statistical test for trends over time). The results can be imported into GIS packages.
Data System	—	Clackamas County, Oregon	High school district	ArcView GIS 3.0a	To describe development of a Community Health Mapping Engine (CHiME). Their ultimate goal is a Web-based system that could be used by community members and epidemiologists.
Data System	12-11	Maryland	County	ArcView GIS 2.1 and Maryland automated GIS system	To describe a system in which LHDs potentially could access a state health department Web site, import tabular information, use GIS to map the data, and then export the results either to print a hard copy of the map or to include an electronic copy in a computerized slide show.

Source: Adapted from T.B. Richards, C.M. Croner, and L.F. Novick, "Atlas of State and Local Geographic Information Systems (GIS) Maps to Improve Community Health," *Journal of Public Health Management and Practice* 5, no. 2 (1999):2–8.

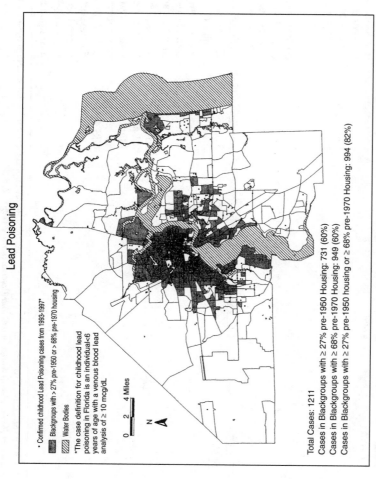

Lead Poisoning

· Confirmed childhood Lead Poisoning cases from 1993-1997"

▓ Blackgroups with > 27% pre-1950 or > 68% pre-1970 housing

▨ Water Bodies

"The case definition for childhood lead poisoning in Florida is an individual<6 years of age with a venous blood lead analysis of ≥ 10 mcg/dL

N

0 2 4 Miles

Total Cases: 1211

Cases in Blackgroups with ≥ 27% pre-1950 Housing: 731 (60%)
Cases in Blackgroups with ≥ 68% pre-1970 Housing: 949 (60%)
Cases in Blackgroups with ≥ 27% pre-1950 housing or ≥ 68% pre-1970 Housing: 994 (82%)

FIGURE 12-1 Development of Childhood Blood Lead Screening Guidelines, Duval County, Florida, 1998. *Source:* C. Duclos, T. Johnson, and T. Thompson, *Journal of Public Health Management Practice* 5, no. 2:9–10.

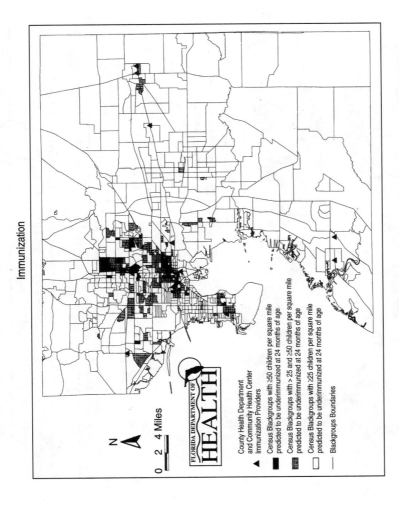

Immunization

FIGURE 12-2 Identifying Predicted Immunization "Pockets of Need," Hillsborough County, Florida, 1996–1997. *Source:* J. Devine, W.K. Gallo, and H.T. Janavski, *Journal of Public Health Management Practice* 5, no. 2:15–16.

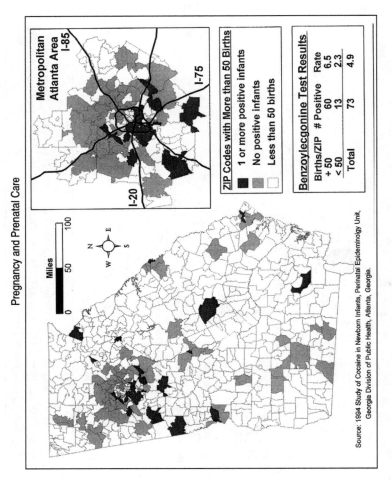

Pregnancy and Prenatal Care

Source: 1994 Study of Cocaine in Newborn Infants, Perinatal Epidemiology Unit, Georgia Division of Public Health, Atlanta, Georgia.

FIGURE 12-3 Prevalence of Benzoylecgonine (a Cocaine Metabolite) in Newborn Infants by ZIP Code, Georgia, February 22 through April 23, 1994. *Source:* M. D. Brantley, *Journal of Public Health Management Practice* 5, no. 2 (1999):19–20.

Injury

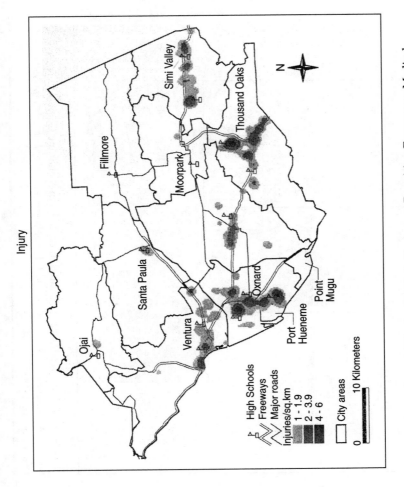

FIGURE 12-4 Automobile Accidents to Teenagers Requiring Emergency Medical Transport, Ventura County, California, 1996. *Source:* P. Van Zuyle, *Journal of Public Health Management Practice* 5, no. 2 (1999):25–26.

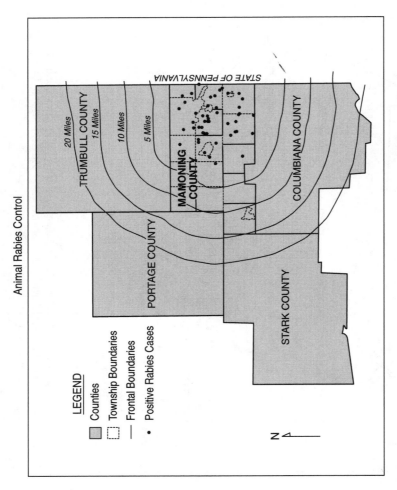

FIGURE 12-5 Positive Raccoon-Strain Rabies Cases in Mahoning County, Ohio, 1997. *Source:* M. Stefanak, K. A. Vaughn, and J. F. Shaheen, *Journal of Public Health Management Practice* 5, no. 2 (1999):33–34.

Toxic Emissions

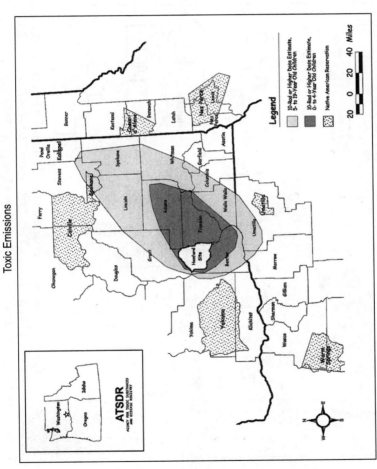

FIGURE 12-6 Locations around the Hanford Nuclear Facility Where Average Milk Consumption by Children in 1945 Would Have Resulted in an Estimated Median Iodine-131 Dose to the Thyroid of 10 Rad or Higher, Washington. *Source: W. D. Henriques and R. F. Spengler, Journal of Public Health Management Practice 5, no. 2 (1999):35–36.*

Water Pollution

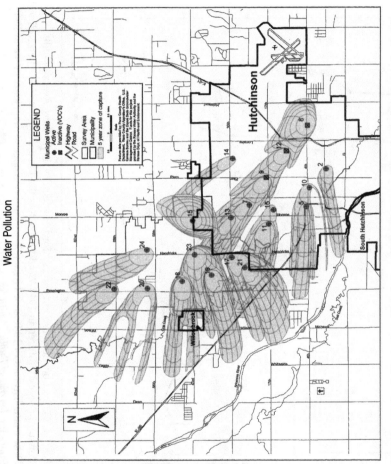

FIGURE 12-7   A Computer Simulation of Groundwater Withdrawal Patterns for Public Water Supply Wells, Hutchinson, Kansas, 1998–2003. *Source:* D. L. Partridge and M. D. Mathews, *Journal of Public Health Management Practice* 5, no. 2 (1999):43–44.

Distance-Based Training

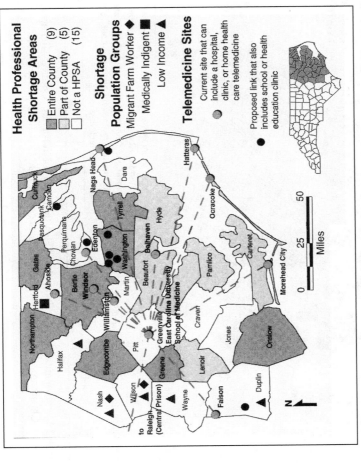

FIGURE 12-8 Location of East Carolina University School of Medicine Telemedicine Sites in Relation to Primary Care Health Professional Shortage Areas for North Carolina's Health Service Area VI, 1997. *Source:* J. L. Wilson and A. Branigan, *Journal of Public Health Management Practice* 5, no. 2 (1999):45–46.

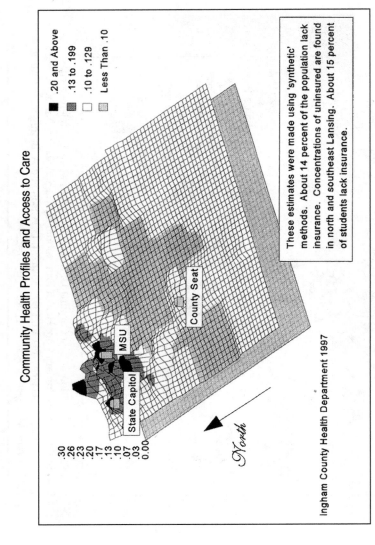

FIGURE 12-9 Percentage of Adults without Health Insurance in Ingham County, Michigan, 1994. *Source:* M. Cheatham, *Journal of Public Health Management Practice* 5, no. 2 (1999):53–54.

Community Health Profiles and Access to Care

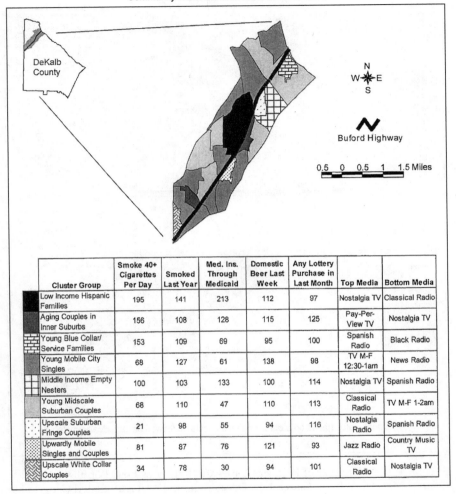

Cluster Group	Smoke 40+ Cigarettes Per Day	Smoked Last Year	Med. Ins. Through Medicaid	Domestic Beer Last Week	Any Lottery Purchase in Last Month	Top Media	Bottom Media
Low Income Hispanic Families	195	141	213	112	97	Nostalgia TV	Classical Radio
Aging Couples in Inner Suburbs	156	108	128	115	125	Pay-Per-View TV	Nostalgia TV
Young Blue Collar/ Service Families	153	109	69	95	100	Spanish Radio	Black Radio
Young Mobile City Singles	68	127	61	138	98	TV M-F 12:30-1am	News Radio
Middle Income Empty Nesters	100	103	133	100	114	Nostalgia TV	Spanish Radio
Young Midscale Suburban Couples	68	110	47	110	113	Classical Radio	TV M-F 1-2am
Upscale Suburban Fringe Couples	21	98	55	94	116	Nostalgia Radio	Spanish Radio
Upwardly Mobile Singles and Couples	81	87	76	121	93	Jazz Radio	Country Music TV
Upscale White Collar Couples	34	78	30	94	101	Classical Radio	Nostalgia TV

FIGURE 12-10   Using Marketing Information to Focus Smoking Cessation Programs in Specific Census Block Groups along the Buford Highway Corridor, DeKalb County, Georgia, 1996. *Source:* M. Y. Rogers, *Journal of Public Health Management Practice* 5, no. 2 (1999):55–57.

Data Analysis Systems

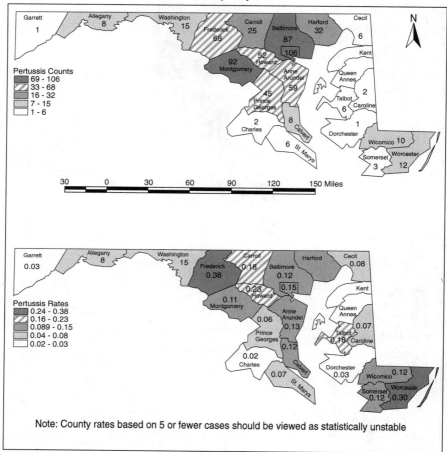

FIGURE 12-11   Number of Pertussis Cases and Rates per 1,000 Population by County, Maryland, 1997. *Source:* J. K. Devasundaram, "An Automated Geographic Information System for Local Health Departments," *Journal of Public Health Management Practice* 5, no. 2 (1999):70–72.

including water pollutants, distance-based learning, community health profiles, transportation and access issues, and the development of data systems. The examples illustrated in the table are quite representative of the current application of geographical information systems to basic health services management problems and public health issues.[3]

A GIS, therefore, can reveal important new information for the health services managers and public health analysts that leads to better decision making.

The depiction of information through maps makes patterns and relationships visible that are not seen in spreadsheets. This makes the data more interesting and more accessible to individuals who do not have the time or expertise to wade through data table after data table. Additionally, through the use of color and patterning it can show the relationship of the data in comparison to a normal value. For example, counties with infant mortality rates higher than the state average are one color, while counties with rates lower than the state average are another color. Seeing the patterns of color allows health managers to recognize areas in need of more services and/or prevention programs.

For health services managers who want to start the process of implementing or installing a GIS system, it is suggested that they initiate certain internal elements and then external areas to consider where assistance is needed (Table 12-2).

GIS—The Basics

GIS organizes and stores large amounts of multipurpose information. GIS adds the geographic dimension to perform analyses and display data using information technology by providing the interface between information and a map. This makes it easy to present information to key decision makers quickly, efficiently, and effectively in the health care environment.[4]

There are several GIS software choices available. Many of them can be used generally, while some of them are specifically made for certain professionals such as hydrologic scientists or petroleum industry specialists. General-use GIS software is listed in Table 12-1 along with various applications in the health field.

Rogers points out, "For purposes of local decision makers responsible for authorizing funds to support GIS activities, the bottom line is how GIS adds value to local public health performance." The heart of GIS is that information can be referenced geographically and analyzed spatially at a subcounty level. The system allows public health problems to be mapped by individual streets, local neighborhoods, or any other subcounty area of interest to the community. With GIS, maps can be created easily, linked with data, revised, and combined with other maps to give new relational

TABLE 12-2 Health Services Management Creating Standards with GIS

Internal Activities (by Managers)	External Activities (with Assistance)
1. Build a library of local geographic files related to the health services area.	1. Assess the availability of basic reference files for secondary and other mapping components.
2. Identify basic files, primarily births, deaths, cases of reportable disease, discharge diagnoses, and basic demographic files.	2. Make an effort to increase geography of existing databases, which are available to your organization (e.g., births, deaths, hospital discharges).
3. Develop projects, such as market area analyses and community profiles.	3. Implement efforts to ensure confidentiality and comply with HIPAA regulations.
4. Develop community GIS partnerships to evaluate the systemwide parameters (e.g., traffic accidents and breast screening programs).	4. Provide training for identified staff to implement quality GIS services into the mainstream of evaluation.
5. Develop community GIS partnerships to evaluate data for hospitals and/or managed care plans.	5. Be sure data being used is identified as to source, quality, timelines, and reliability. Currently, national statistics are very few and, in many cases, lacking.
6. Develop partnerships to evaluate clinic service areas and client community-service-area market, which are key to effective hospital planning and evaluation of proposed services.	6. Assure appropriate interpretation of the maps. Distortion with maps can be as frequent as distortion with statistics.

Source: Adapted from M. Y. Rogers, "Getting Started with Geographic Information Systems (GIS): A Local Perspective," *Journal of Public Health Management and Practice* 5, no. 4 (1999):22–23.

views of information about a community. In addition, GIS enables users to employ a wide range of spatial statistical analysis methods to provide exploration and potentially new insights into data relationships.[5]

Data Capture

Putting the information into the system involves identifying the objects on the map, the absolute location on the earth's surface, and their spatial relationships. Software tools that automatically extract features from satellite images or aerial photographs are gradually replacing what has traditionally been a time-consuming capture process (Figure 12-12). Objects are identified in a series of attribute tables—the "information" part of a GIS. Spatial relationships, such as whether features intersect or whether they are adjacent, are the key to all GIS-based analyses.

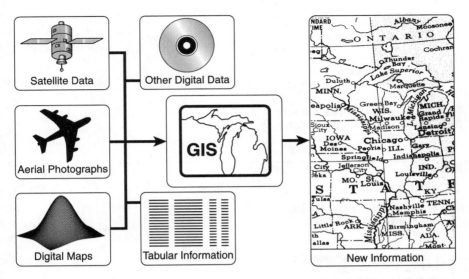

FIGURE 12-12 GIS Data Capture Methods. *Source:* USGS, Science for a Changing World. Eastern Region Geography, *http://erg.usgs.gov/isb/pubs/gis_poster/*.

Specifically, GIS requires a geographic file and an attribute database. A geographic file consists of the information needed to create and name points, lines, and areas (Figure 12-13). Points (e.g., health center locations, sites of motor vehicle facilities) are exact locations. Lines (such as roads, street segments between intersections with cross streets) connect two or more points. Areas require actual space (such as the boundaries of counties, service areas, toxic plumes, or census tracts). The information in the geographic database (points, lines, and areas) is "georeferenced" with longitude and latitude coordinates that enable the points, lines, and areas to be correctly positioned on any GIS map.[6]

Data Integration

A GIS makes it possible to link, or integrate, information that is difficult to associate through any other means. Thus, a GIS can use combinations of attribute databases for mapping variables to build and analyze new patterns and relationships.

Attribute databases consist of the additional information that needs to be displayed on the map (such as a name, measurement, or characteristic). The attribute database needs to be linked with the geographic database before the attribute database information can be displayed on the map. The process of linking the information in the attribute database to the geographic database is referred to as geocoding.[7]

Points

cases of disease, septic tanks, motor vehicle crashes, hospitals, health clinics, swimming pools, restaurants

The points represent the Health Centers operated by the DeKalb County Board of Health.

⊙ Health Centers

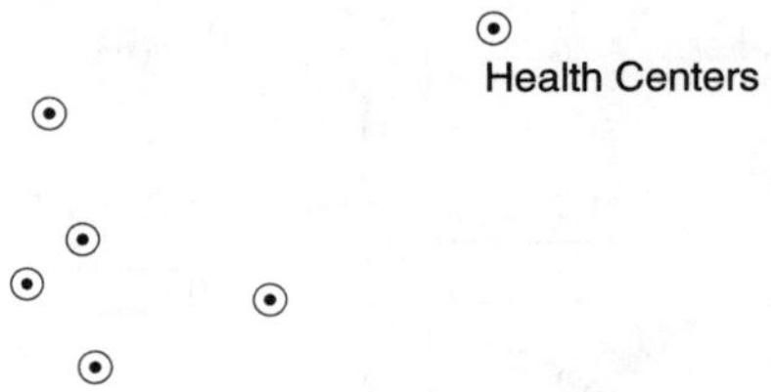

Lines

streets, interstates, sewer lines, power lines, railroads, rivers, sidewalks

Lines are used to represent the highways and interstates in DeKalb County, Georgia.

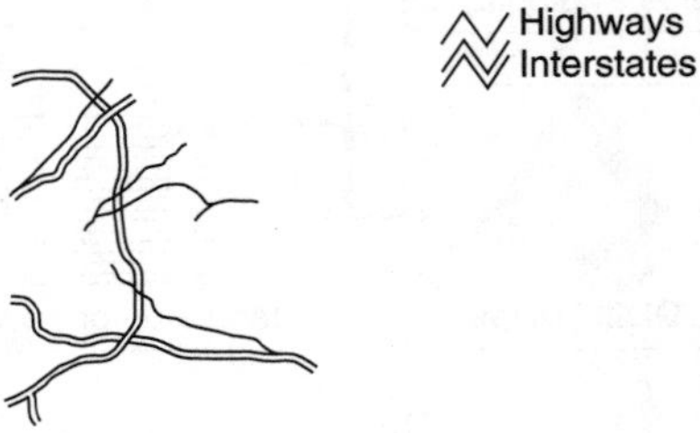

∿ Highways
∿ Interstates

Areas

states, counties, census tracts, ZIP codes, service areas, cities, towns, political districts, school districts, tax parcels, parks

Polygons show the service areas covered by the Health Centers operated by the DeKalb County Board of Health.

Service Areas
▨ Central
▦ East
☐ North
☐ South
▨ West
☐ County Bondary

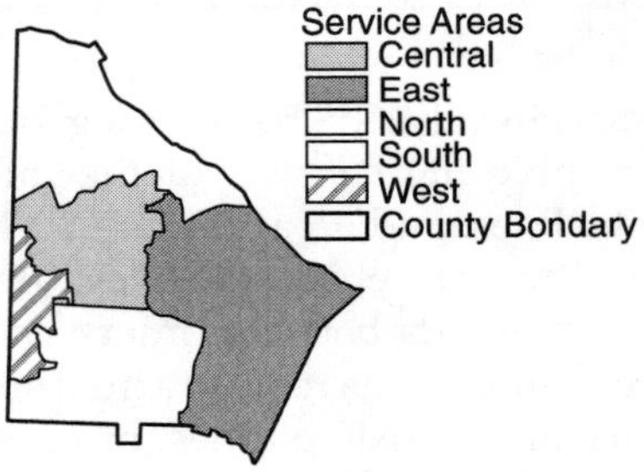

Layers

points, lines, and polygons

Map of DeKalb County Health Centers and their service areas are created by layering points, lines, and areas together.

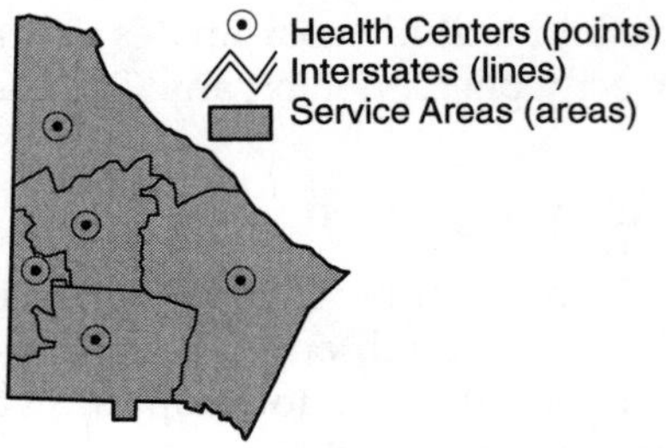

⊙ Health Centers (points)
∿ Interstates (lines)
▮ Service Areas (areas)

FIGURE 12-13   Points, Lines, and Areas Become Multiple Layers in a GIS. *Source:* Office of Assessment, Surveillance, and Epidemiology, Population Based Services, DeKalb County Board of Health.

Geocoding

Geocoding may be a very time-consuming process, especially in (1) areas with rapid growth and development and (2) rural locations. However, there are private vendors who provide this service for a very minimal cost.

In high-growth areas issuing permits for new subdivisions with more streets can present a problem. Rapid growth and new construction can soon lead to inaccuracies in the GIS street reference file. When cases need to be geocoded individually or by review through noncomputerized sources of information, the geocoding process can be time-consuming.

Similarly, geocoding cases in rural areas can be problematic. Rural locations often lack city-style addresses and are hard to pinpoint on a map. For example, a trailer park address can be acceptable for U.S. Postal Service mail delivery but cannot be included in the GIS street-based file.[8]

The Application of GIS in Health Services Management

By the year 2010, GIS applications in public health practice will no longer consist of the ad hoc approaches that were seen in the 1990s. By the year 2010, GIS technology will be customized for public health applications. This GIS health software will offer applications that "know" which data systems are needed and where they are located. After loading the appropriate data and performing relevant analyses, the system will offer alternative courses of action ranging from informing other people in the public health system, to issuing health advisories.

Several examples are illustrated of the way public health practitioners are likely to routinely use technology in the year 2010, organized according to the ten consensus "essential public health services" identified in 1994 by U.S. Public Health Service agencies and major national public health organizations.[9] The Centers for Disease Control and Prevention (CDC) is currently pilot-testing performance standards for state and local public health systems based on this framework.[10]

GIS and Health Services Management

The analysis and understanding of health care problems from an epidemiologic perspective includes the concept of place or geography. Knowing where people, problems, and resources are is paramount to delivery of efficient and effective health care services in a community that is represented by a fairly well defined service area.

In 1854 an English physician, John Snow, provided the classic example of how a map can be used to identify an etiologic agent. From an epidemiologic research perspective, he identified the water source responsible for an outbreak of cholera in London by mapping the locations of those afflicted with the disease and the pumps that provided the water. Subsequent removal of the handle from the pump proved to be the clue to the etiology and transmission of the agent.

The trend to use GIS to benefit the health care industry has been slow to develop but currently is experiencing a significant upward spiral. Both public and private sectors are developing innovative ways to harness the data, integrate the information, and spatially visualize the results. The types of agencies and organizations adopting GIS span the health care spectrum—from public health departments and public health policy and research organizations, to hospitals, medical centers, and health insurance organizations.[11]

Epidemiology focusing on place (geography) plays a major role in understanding the dynamics of health, the causes, consequences, and the spread of disease. The classic public health triad composed of man, agent/vehicle, and environment emphasizes the importance of geographic location (environment or space) in health and disease. Interactions within this triad can also change with time.[12] However, with the more modern holistic models of lifestyle, environment, biology, and health care delivery system, the GIS has wider appeal and significantly more applications.

The GIS continues to be used in public health and health services management for epidemiologic and health services utilization studies by analysts and managers. By tracking the sources of diseases and the movements of contagions, understanding variation in utilization patterns, and identifying patterns of use, agencies can respond more effectively to outbreaks of disease, assess resource availability, and monitor health services utilization by identifying at-risk populations, targeting intervention, and evaluating patterns of distribution.[13]

Researchers, public health professionals, policymakers, health services managers, and others use GIS to better understand spatial relationships that affect health outcomes, public health risks, disease transmission, access to health care, and other public health concerns. The system is being used with greater frequency to address neighborhood, local, state, national, and international public health issues.[14]

From a community health perspective, GIS could potentially serve as a powerful evidence-based tool for early problem detection and solution. When properly used, GIS can inform and educate (professionals and the public); empower decision making at all levels; help plan and tweak clinically and cost-effective actions by predicting outcomes before making any financial commitments and ascribing priorities in a climate of finite resources; change practices; and continually monitor and analyze changes, as well as sentinel events.[15]

Whether an epidemiologist tries to track and contain the expansion of an epidemic, a health services manager tries to make better decisions concerning the use of scarce resources, or a physician tries to better manage time or patients in a population-based medical setting—GIS offers a comprehensive line of concepts, methods, and applications to assist in solving health services problems.

The success of a public health agency and the development of prevention programs can certainly depend on the timely acquisition, management, analysis, and dissemination of information.

To respond to the importance of the GIS as a requisite tool for improvement in the problem health areas, the CDC is currently pilot-testing performance standards for routinely using GIS technology in state and local public health systems based on the ten consensus "essential public health services."

Examples of applications of GIS in the health services management areas are noted here. These activities are indicative of the widespread application of GIS:

- Community health assessment and surveillance
- Environmental risk assessment
- Program planning and evaluation
- Community health education
- Identification of disparities in health care[16]
- Infectious disease analysis
- Tracking of immunization status (children)
- Event response
- Resource utilization and allocation
- Health care planning
- Workforce analysis
- Health policy development
- Definition of health service areas[17]

Table 12-3 gives a more detailed report of actual programs that have been implemented using the GIS approach. Thus, such applications as health status assessment, surveillance, preventive programs, linking health services to resources, and researching new and innovative solutions are all typical uses of GIS to aid in the management of health services.

A GIS incorporated surveillance system would

- Make it possible to evaluate many indicators of a bioterrorism event simultaneously, compare variations, and identify common trends
- Facilitate the rapid recognition of a disease outbreak
- Assist in determining exposure sites
- Improve data transmission and analysis speed

TABLE 12-3   GIS Applications for Health Services Management

Applications	Project Description
Monitor health status to identify community problems	As part of a community health report card, a local public health department serving a county with 300,000 population and ten high schools wants to map adolescent pregnancy rates for each high school's attendance area. In a secure environment in which the confidentiality of individuals and individual households is protected, the department codes the street address of each pregnant adolescent and prepares a smoothed (spatially filtered) map of adolescent pregnancy rates using a set of overlapping circles of fixed size. Next, using GIS software, school attendance boundaries are superimposed over the smoothed map. In addition to maps displaying the entire jurisdiction, higher magnification views are developed for each school attendance area, accompanied by a chart with summary statistics on use of prenatal care services, by trimester of pregnancy, to engage parents, faculty, and students in dialogue about how to best develop and target specific interventions for each district.[20]
Diagnose and investigate health problems and hazards in the community	An epidemiologist in a large urban hospital uses data from medical records for asthma cases to map the current week and prior time periods. Inspecting the maps for unusual case clusters or patterns, she finds a new pattern of increased asthma hospitalizations. She expediently "visits" the hospital with the highest rate and reviews the cases. Eight of ten affected individuals work at the same factory. Subsequently, using GIS technology linked to a "worker right to know" database about workplace chemical exposures, the epidemiologist reviews the potential exposures at the factory and identifies the agents associated with asthma-related hospital admissions. The epidemiologist then requests that an industrial hygienist visit the plant the same day.[21]
Inform, educate, and empower people about health issues	One of a community's identified priorities is to develop an anti-smoking campaign. An anti-smoking coalition uses GIS technology and commercial lifestyle segmentation profiles (or a public health analog developed by CDC by 2010) to identify subgroups that are most likely to include active smokers, the Census blocks where active smokers are most likely to reside, and the most effective communication media and times of day to deliver anti-smoking messages to these subgroups.[22]

TABLE 12-3 (continued)

Applications	Project Description
Mobilize community partnerships and action to identify and solve health problems	A community identifies childhood immunization levels as a priority. The local public health department wants to engage the faith community as part of an initiative to increase immunization rates. The department maps the locations of churches in areas with the highest numbers of young children. The ministers of these churches are invited to a meeting, where they decide to join as a work group to develop appropriate health promotion materials and intervention strategies. During a subsequent meeting, the work group uses GIS technology to map locations of school clinics and childcare centers within an inner-city area. Additional maps are used to assign church volunteers to school clinics and childcare facilities so travel distance is minimized. Maps are also developed to evaluate geographic patterns of children with missed immunization appointments, to help target educational interventions.[23]
Develop policies and plans that support individual and community health efforts	The local public health department prepares a map to show the location of each health clinic in the community (including those run by hospitals and managed care plans, as well as those run by public health agencies). Another map is prepared that shows the residences of Medicaid-eligible individuals who use each clinic location. Using GIS technology, community decision makers overlay these maps and use the resultant patterns to help develop plans for better utilization of existing health care resources.[24]
Enforce laws and regulations that protect health and ensure safety	To better provide neighborhood services, a local public health agency organizes its services by geographic areas, with a different subdivision of the agency responsible for each service area. Under this new system, environmental complaints need to be assigned to the correct service area. In some cases, an address on one side of the street belongs to one service area while an address on the other side of the street belongs to a different area. Using a Web-enabled public access GIS database, the agency GIS manager extracts geographic boundary files for street addresses and for the boundaries of the service areas. Using a GIS program, the manager creates a geographic polygon for each area and uses "point-in-polygon" assignment procedures to allocate street addresses to the correct service areas. When the agency receives an environmental complaint, the street address is initially processed through a computer program that standardizes the address in conformance with U.S. Postal Service standards (correcting spelling errors, verifying the existence of the address on the computerized system, and so on). The complaint is then automatically assigned to the appropriate service area based on the standardized street address.[25]

TABLE 12-3 (continued)

Applications	Project Description
Link people to needed personal health services and assure the provision of health care when otherwise unavailable	A non-English-speaking, foreign-born person entering the United States is identified as having tuberculosis (TB). This individual also has a severe heart problem that requires medication. A TB outreach worker uses a GIS health care access map to identify the nearest cardiologist who speaks the same language as the patient. Again using GIS technology, the TB outreach worker also produces a public transportation map printed both in English and in the patient's language that shows the patient how to travel to the physician's office.[26]
Assure a competent public health and personnel health care workforce	CDC plans a distance-based training program (via satellite) on TB prevention in foreign-born people who have recently entered the United States. CDC uses a GIS map to identify public health departments in areas with large numbers of such individuals; these departments are invited to participate. During the teleconference, the geographic origins of phone calls are automatically displayed on a GIS map to help identify callers and to monitor the number and locations of the callers on "hold."[27]
Evaluate effectiveness, accessibility, and quality of personal and population-based health services	A local public health department prepares GIS maps showing its service delivery points as well as other community health resources. These maps include details about: units of service provided at each location; expenditures; and demographic information such as poverty level for each program participant. By linking clinical data with these maps, the department is able to evaluate whether resources are being deployed optimally to address priority health needs and to effect of services on selected preventable health outcomes.[28]
Research for new insights and innovative solutions to health problems	A graduate student in geography conducts an urban morphology study, mapping the history of population growth and forecasting the evolving shape of the city and public transportation needs. Several high-resolution digital earth images, taken over a period of one year, are available for an area under development. The student electronically imports these images and uses automated change detection to determine the changes over a one-year period, for example, the addition to housing developments, roads, landfills, and other features. This information is included in a community health report card and used to help establish community priorities and plans.[29]

TABLE 12-3 (continued)

Applications	Project Description
Disease surveillance using GIS	CDC works with state and local health departments and information system contractors to develop a real-time or almost real-time surveillance system incorporating GIS. Many city and state public health agencies begin to invest substantial sums to develop and implement such surveillance systems.[30]
Vital statistics, tabulation, interpretation, and publication of the essential facts of births, deaths, and reportable diseases	GIS can maintain relevant health care and demographic statistics by geographic area. These areas commonly range from census tracts to ZIP codes to counties upward to states and nations. GIS allows visualization of the data via maps for comparison between the geographic units, which assists in the interpretation as well as publication bf health related facts.[31]
Control of communicable diseases including tuberculosis	GIS can document the locations of populations at risk based on their behavior and environment. People with similar demographic characteristics also have similar lifestyles. GIS technology allows for the creation of LSP indexes, categorizing population into behavioral and demographic groups. Communicable disease patterns can be influenced by population behavior. Some diseases are environmentally related (for example methemoglobinemia in newborns from drinking water exposure). GIS can document geographic areas at high risk (for example ground water with elevated levels of nitrate). GIS can locate newborns in the affected area, then use that information to develop a program to warn families of the potential risk and prevent environmentally related disease.[31]
Environmental sanitation including supervision of milk and milk processing, food processing, and public eating places and maintenance of sanitary conditions of employment. Protect against environmental hazards and prevent injuries.	GIS can map the location of facilities and geographically associate those facilities to the natural and built environments. GIS can characterize the location and LSP of the work force likely to be employed at restaurants. GIS can map locations of restaurants and food processing units to help establishing the frequency for inspecting these facilities. GIS can evaluate the impact of failing septic systems on municipal water supplies. GIS can document the potential environmental hazard to people from naturally occurring radon emission.[31]
Public health laboratory services	Geocoding surveillance data can provide new insights for surveillance programs.[31]

TABLE 12-3 (continued)

Applications	Project Description
Hygiene of maternity, infancy, and childhood including supervision of the health of school children. Assure the quality and accessibility of health services.	GIS can answer such questions as where are newborns located, what locations have high risk for teenage pregnancy? What are neighborhoods with highest infant mortality rate? Do low-income teenage mothers have access to health care facilities for prenatal care?[31]
Health education of the general public so far as this is not covered by the functions of the departments of education.	GIS can promote healthy behavior by documenting where the populations are located that have the greatest need of improved information, then using GIS enabled internet sites as an out reach vehicle for health education.
Respond to disasters and assist communities in recovery.	As hurricanes, floods, or earthquakes demolish human-built environments, GIS can assist in recovery operations and reconstruction by documenting what the predisaster urban environment was and anticipating the likelihood of an environmental calamity occurring at the region.

■ Provide detailed information to assist with outbreak investigations.

■ Facilitate integration with other surveillance systems at all levels of government

■ Assist in providing efficient delivery of limited medical countermeasures, such as vaccines or antibiotics

■ Evaluate success in the areas of containment and mitigation

■ Provide historical and trend data to be used in baseline comparisons and long-term monitoring

Any surveillance system incorporating GIS could face many operational challenges such as the following:

■ Data collection and management being incomplete and untimely

■ Need for customization of each geographic region

■ Maintenance of efficient training and technical support

■ High costs of start-up and equipment

■ GIS software, while having many advantages, could be notoriously difficult to use[18]

■ Establishment of area coalitions and partnerships with the many contributors of patient care and services

■ Security and confidentiality, record matching and merging, detection, data presentation and automated notification[19]

Environmental Health Protection

Gonorrhea

A geographic information analysis of gonorrhea cases was conducted at the neighborhood level. It was an analysis of environmental risk in search of evidence for geographic clustering of reported gonorrhea cases. The objective was to look for evidence of the existence of a disease "core," an important concept in the design of preventive interventions.

Using the geocoded home address of reported gonorrhea cases for 1994, 1995, and 1996 in New Orleans, census tract maps detailing the sociodemographic and structural risk factors for gonorrhea and maps of clustered gonorrhea cases were overlaid. The primary structural risk factor evaluated was the availability of alcohol. Alcohol availability was measured both as on-sale (bars and restaurants) and off-sale (liquor stores and convenience stores) outlet density. By aggregating the geocoded gonorrhea cases into concordant census tracts ($n = 120$) and block groups ($n = 474$), gonorrhea rates were obtained at both these levels of analysis for the same areas. Small area analysis using gonorrhea rates as the dependent variable in multiple regression analyses revealed a similar pattern of association among the covariates, but the total amount of variance explained varied significantly from the census tract ($f = .85$) to the block group ($f = .62$) levels. The results also indicated percentages of gonorrhea cases among African Americans; in populations less than 18 years of age; in unmarried households; in rental households; and by off-sale alcohol outlet density. These were the strongest predicators of gonorrhea rates, once other covariates were controlled. These results suggest gonorrhea cases are geographically clustered and that clustering is best represented at the Census tract level. The results also indicate the clustering of gonorrhea cases can be predicted by a small number of socio-demographic and structural predictors.[31]

Lead Poisoning

The spatial distribution of pediatric lead poisoning cases in relation to environmental indicators of lead, housing, and the demographic attributes of block groups was conducted in Binghamton, New York. Primary data on childhood blood lead levels was based on screening records from July 1991 to June 1995. Approximately 17 percent of all children tested within this period had elevated blood lead levels. A number of GIS and statistical operations were used to determine (1) whether the distribution of lead poisoning cases reflects a consistent spatial pattern; and (2) the extent to which the pattern is linked to possible sources or pathways of exposure such as lead-emitting facilities, major transportation corridors, trace lead in soil, and municipal water supply and housing. The results revealed clearly defined clusters of lead poisoning cases along transportation lines within the urbanized and industrialized zones. Specifically, block groups in the central city that were characterized by old, subdivided, and rented properties and poverty had proportionately higher incidences than others. Nearly six out of every ten cases fell within these clusters. These results demonstrate how comprehensive health and environmental data can serve as input in delineating high-risk areas for lead monitoring and remediation programs.[32]

Bioterrorism

Given the terrorist attacks on the United States, the vulnerability revealed by the mailed anthrax spores, and evidence that the Al-Qaida terrorist network is trying to acquire biological weapons,[33] the prospects of a biological weapons attack seem greater today. A robust public health infrastructure for surveillance and response is critical to safeguard populations in the event of a bioterrorist attack. Following a bioterrorism event, it is crucial to record information pertaining to patient care, hospitalization, and laboratory results, quarantining patients, tracking contacts, vaccinations, administration of antibiotics, and allocation of equipment and personnel. Timely dispersal, sharing, and utilization of this information are vital to keep additional casualties from occurring in the wake of a bioterrorism event.[34]

In the event of a bioterrorist attack, visual analysis of case patterns, developed through GIS, can provide the means to react quickly and limit the number and sovereignty of those affected by the attack (Figures 12-14 to 12-16).[35]

GIS capabilities coupled with Web-based data resources create powerful techniques for accurate characterization of small population areas in ways that will be of enormous value to public health officials involved in planning and response activities.[36]

To explore these and other environmental problems, the GIS can provide a unique opportunity to exchange and share data across programs, sectors, and partners. Information on epidemiology, control, interventions, and health care resources are brought together to facilitate the development of a dynamic atlas of public health, which can be a platform for decision making.

An example of an online atlas type of program is GATHER. GATHER (Geographic Analysis Tool for Health and Environmental Research) is an

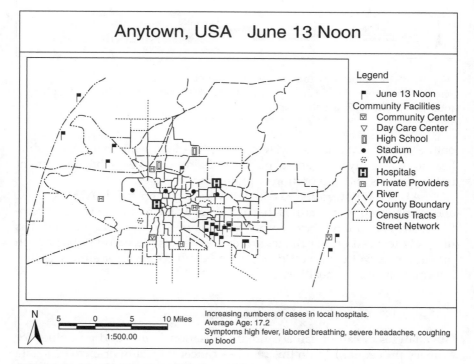

FIGURE 12-14   Bioterrorism Attack—at Noon.
Source: "Bioterrorism GIS Can Help Fight a New Threat," http://www.geoplace.com/gw/2002/0207/0207bio.asp

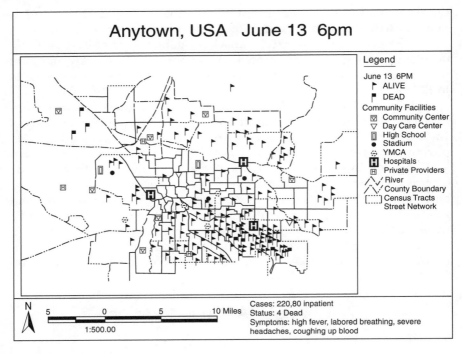

Anytown, USA   June 13   6pm

Legend

June 13 6PM
- ▶ ALIVE
- ▶ DEAD

Community Facilities
- ☑ Community Center
- ▽ Day Care Center
- 🏢 High School
- • Stadium
- YMCA
- 🅷 Hospitals
- ⊞ Private Providers
- /\\∿/ River
- /\\∿/ County Boundary
- [⋯] Census Tracts
- Street Network

N
5   0   5   10 Miles
1:500.00

Cases: 220,80 inpatient
Status: 4 Dead
Symptoms: high fever, labored breathing, severe
headaches, coughing up blood

FIGURE 12-15   Bioterrorism Attack—at 6:00 p.m.
Source: "Bioterrorism GIS Can Help Fight a New Threat," http://www.geoplace.
com/gw/2002/0207/0207bio.asp.

online spatial data access system that provides members of the public
health community and general public access to spatial data that is pertinent
to the analysis and exploration of public health issues.[37]

GATHER is powered by a GIS data warehouse hosted by ATSDR/CDC
and is enhanced with features that are of key value to members of the public health community. Not simply a "map my house" tool, GATHER is
uniquely focused on the challenges that are encountered by public health
professionals as they investigate public health concerns or simply gather
information about a health issue.[38]

GIS and Cancer Research

GIS analyses of cancer can accentuate causation factors and give clues for
primary prevention. To do this requires cancer mortality or incidence data
that covers all cancer patients and only cancer patient and, that is correct
and detailed enough. Few countrywide cancer registration systems exist.
Moreover, data collection methods and the items recorded, particularly

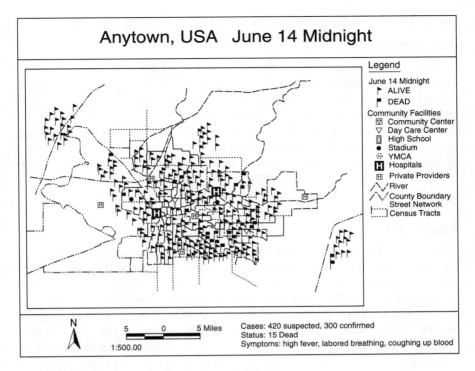

FIGURE 12-16   Bioterrorism Attack—at Midnight.
Source: "Bioterrorism GIS Can Help Fight a New Threat," http://www.geoplace.
com/gw/2002/0207/0207bio.asp.

data on patient residence, vary between registries. Diagnosis itself is problematic and diagnostic standards can vary between locations. Incidence
data are better than mortality data for most research purposes because survival rates vary substantially between populations, but incidence data is
available only for limited areas in the world.[39] Although residence address
is the ideal for GIS analysis, confidentiality constraints usually prevent
data reporting at that level. Moreover, place of residence at the time of
diagnosis is problematic in terms of causation unless the individual has
lived there for decades. Because latency periods vary substantially by cancer type and individual, a complete exposure history including all
addresses of all houses at which the individual has lived for ten to fifty
years prior to diagnosis is required. This information is seldom available.
Also because people do not stay home day and night, spatially and also
temporally accurate case histories based on the entirety of the activity
space in life are required to avoid erroneous conclusions and etiologic
hypotheses. Clearly, complete data sets of this nature are rare.[40]

GIS and the Business Side of Health Care

Managed Care

A managed care chief information officer (CIO) knows of a large national managed care company that has replaced its printed provider network directories with an online version, which allows anyone with a PC to locate an eligible provider and get printed driving instructions. The CIO also knows that the company previously outsourced all of its telephone directory service to a major long-distance telephone company. She believes that a managed care organization that is struggling to provide up-to-date provider and network information to its customers could make a strong case for using in-house GIS technology.[41]

Health System

A health system budget officer knows of a large geographically dispersed health system that, with the help of GIS, allocates "budgets" to each of its fifty-plus medical centers on the basis of time or distance to the center from customers' homes. The budget officer believes that any large hospital system that must plan, budget, and track resources over a wide geographic market and allocate patient resources to the medical facility closest to a patient's residence could use GIS technology to reduce staffing requirements and improve accuracy of the entire geographic budget allocation process.[42]

Pharmaceutical Sales

A sales executive knows of a pharmaceutical firm that, in response to new managed care and risk contracting incentives, is adjusting its sales strategy by incorporating geocoded age- and sex-adjusted disease data using GIS. The sales executive also knows that the company is arming all its field sales forces with GIS to allow sales personnel to act on information as they deem appropriate and to provide better intelligence to the providers they visit. The executive believes that any medical, pharmaceutical, and medical equipment firm that constantly tinkers with sales territories and large field sales forces could save millions of dollars annually by incorporating GIS technology.[43]

Public Health

A public health director knows of a county health department that created a data warehouse, allowing vital and health service data to be enabled geographically on-the-fly, thus making valuable information immediately available for dissemination within the agency and to the public via the Internet. The public health director envisions new agency functions that resemble nongovernmental health organization situations, such as improving customer service, enhancing interdepartmental data sharing, and dealing with daily geographic issues that relate to health services and agency program management. The director believes that GIS technology will allow any public health agency to leverage its scarce information system resources without sacrificing the quality of programs that presently collect and analyze the information.[44]

Confidentiality and Health Data in the United States

Whereas location data for GIS is easy to obtain in the United States, health data is not. Public policies and legal guidelines regarding confidentiality and privacy of health care information are neither clear nor complete but rather a patchwork of uncoordinated state and federal policies. Federal legislation has established restrictions on releasing federally held information on individuals, but individual state approaches to privacy vary greatly and frequently preclude the release of information at anything other than the most general level (e.g., county level instead of address level). Using such data in a GIS produces what is called spatial uncertainty. Using area centroids instead of exact locations can produce misleading results.[45]

For example, GIS and cancer research in Texas is plagued with data problems. Whereas mortality data is available for every cause of death from 1980 to 1996 at county level from EPIGRAM, mortality data at finer levels of spatial resolution is almost impossible to obtain due to confidentiality. Until recently, incidence data from the State Cancer Registry was both incomplete and not current. Of the eleven Public Health Regions in the state, incidence data was available for only three (Region 1, 1976–1985; Region 10, 1976–1984; Region 5, 1985) and partially for Region 8 (1976–1980). Efforts under way to improve the situation now require hospital cancer registries to report every diagnosed case or face a hefty fine. Time and maybe a legislation change can improve the situation. Until then, the ideal of "spatially and temporally accurate case histories" remains only a dream in Texas. These examples suggest that even where some data is available, suitability for GIS analysis is not always guaranteed.[46]

Through multivariate spatial statistical modeling of disease processes, GIS enables the evaluation of potentially true disease outbreaks and a more effective allocation of sparse remedial resources toward containment and prevention. GIS also assists users in better understanding the potential harmful effects of environmental pollutants, for example, toxic waste sites, and even in understanding the occurrence of pedestrian and other injuries and crimes. Today, environmental monitors measure air and water quality, solar irradiation, radon gas levels, and other exposures potentially deleterious to human health. These measurements can be brought into GIS and spatially referenced and integrated analytically with other health predictor variables and outcome data. In fact, any adverse (or positive) health-related phenomenon that can be defined spatially (atmospheric, aquatic or terrestrial) can lead to GIS analysis.[47]

The rationale for using GIS in public health management and practice is that it can be used as a descriptive and analytic technology allowing for viewing and better understanding geographic patterns, spatial associations, and related phenomena. GIS can also be adapted to use mathematic modeling to predict spatial trends and future occurrences. Because most health-related phenomena are inherently geographic, public health planners and managers need to consider the many uses of GIS and how those uses can in turn affect the paradigm of public health management and practice.[48]

Data Problems in GIS and Health

The analysis and interpretation of health data are influenced by many factors, the most important being those relating to boundaries, data quality, the size of study populations, and analytical methods. These factors are interrelated and cannot be considered in isolation. Boundaries, as well as census boundaries, are arbitrary from a health perspective. Boundaries also relate to data. Data from different sources can relate to different areas and populations so that they cannot satisfactorily be combined or compared. Data quality is in many cases more important than statistical precision. Small-area comparisons based on data that is not collected in a systematic and standardized fashion are potentially biased and cannot reliably be interpreted.

GIS in the Future

Federal, state, tribal, and local governments; private companies; academia; and nonprofit organizations are producing many computer databases that can be directly entered into a GIS. Different kinds of data in map form can be entered into a GIS. A GIS can also convert existing digital information, which might not yet be in map form, into forms it can recognize and use.

GIS and Public Health in Developing Countries

Whereas the developed countries are taking initiatives to establish a well-organized GIS-based health care system, the developing countries still face increasingly diverse and complex problems mainly due to rapidly growing populations and severe resource constraints. Rational allocation of scarce resources is difficult and is dependent on the size of the population. Expensive hospital-based health care systems are protected by strong vested interests, reorientation is mainly rhetorical, and primary health care is making only slow progress. The formulation of proper GIS faces some constraints, which include problems in the flow of information from the field, including delays, nonreporting, nonresponse, and a generally unsatisfactory quality of generated data from primary sources.[48]

References

1. United States Geological Survey (USGS); Publications; Geographic Information Systems. Available at *http://erg.usgs.gov/isb/pubs/gis_poster/*. Accessed on March 28, 2004.
2. Burlington County, N.J., Health Department, Geographic Information Systems Program. Available at *http://www.co.burlington.nj.us/departments/health/services/gis/*. Accessed on March 21, 2004.
3. T. B. Richards, C. M. Croner, and L. F. Novick, "Atlas of State and Local Geographic Information Systems (GIS) Maps to Improve Community Health," *Journal of Public Health Management and Practice* 5, no. 2 (1999):2–8.
4. World Health Organization, Communicable Disease Surveillance and Response (CSR), Public Health Mapping, Available at *http://www.who.int/csr/mapping/GPHM2pageflyerEng.pdf*. Accessed on March 26, 2004.
5. M. Y. Rogers, "Getting Started with Geographic Information Systems (GIS): A Local Health Perspective," *Journal of Public Health Management and Practice* 5, no. 4 (1999):22–33.
6. Rogers, "Geting Started."
7. Rogers, "Geting Started."
8. Rogers, "Geting Started."
9. E. L. Baker et al., "Health Reform and the Health of the Public," *JAMA* 272, no. 16 (1994):1276–1282.
10. T. B. Richards, C. M. Croner, G. Rushton, C. K. Brown, and L. Fowler. "Geographic Information Systems and Public Health: Mapping the Future," *Public Health Reports 1999*; 114:366–367.
11. Environmental Systems Research Institute (ESRI), News; Arc User, GIS for Health Care Today and Tomorrow. Available at *http://www.esri.com/news/arcuser/0499/umbrella.html*. Accessed on March 24, 2004.
12. Maged N. Kamel Boulos, "Toward Evidence-Based, GIS-Driven National Spatial Health Information infrastructure and surveillance services in the

United Kingdom," *International Journal of Health Geographics*. Available at *http://www.pubmedcentral.nih.gov/articlerender.fcgi?artid=343292*. Accessed on March 28, 2004.

13. ESRI, News.
14. Centers for Disease Control and Prevention, National Center for Health Statistics, GIS and Public Health. Available at *http://www.cdc.gov/nchs/gis.htm*. Accessed on April 7, 2004.
15. Maged N. Kamel Boulos, "Toward Evidence-Based, GIS-Driven National Spatial Health Information Infrastructure."
16. U.S. Department of Health and Human Services, Office of the Assistant Secretary for Planning and Evaluation (ASPE), GIS. Available at *http://aspe.hhs.gov/progsys/gis/fiscella.ppt*. Accessed on March 24, 2004.
17. Environmental Systems Research Institute (ESRI), Geographic Information System, Using GIS for Public Health. Available at *http://www.gis.com/specialty/healthandhumanservices/healthcare.html*. Accessed on March 25, 2004.
18. Maged N. Kamel Boulos, "Toward Evidence-Based, GIS-Driven National Spatial Health Information Infrastructure."
19. Burlington County, N.J., Health Department; Geographic Information Systems Program.
20. National Center Institute, "Linking GIS Technology with Essential Public Health Services" *Public Health Reports* 114 (1999):366–367. Available at: *http://www.healthgis-li.com/library/phr/linking.htm*. Accessed on March 21, 2004.
21. National Cancer Institute, "Linking GIS Technology," 366–367.
22. National Cancer Institute, "Linking GIS Technology," 366–367.
23. National Cancer Institute, "Linking GIS Technology," 366–367.
24. National Cancer Institute, "Linking GIS Technology," 366–367.
25. National Cancer Institute, "Linking GIS Technology," 366–367.
26. National Cancer Institute, "Linking GIS Technology," 366–367.
27. National Cancer Institute, "Linking GIS Technology," 366–367.
28. National Cancer Institute, "Linking GIS Technology," 366–367.
29. National Cancer Institute, "Linking GIS Technology," 366–367.
30. Centers for Disease Control and Prevention, "Updated Guidelines for Evaluating Public Health Surveillance Systems," *MMWR* 50 (July 27, 2001). Available at *http://www.cdc.gov/mmwr/PDF/RR/RR5013.pdf*. Accessed on February 12, 2004.
31. Agency for Toxic Substances and Disease Registry, GIS in Public Health, Disease Surveillance. Available at *http://www.atsdr.cdc.gov/GIS/conference98/homepage/abstracts.html*. Accessed on March 28, 2004.
32. Agency for Toxic Substances and Disease Registry, GIS in Public Health.
33. M. Popovich, R. Fiedler, S. Fiedler, and J. Massee, "Bioterrorism GIS Can Help Fight a New Threat," *Geoworld*. Available at *http://www.geoplace.com/gw/2002/0207/0207bio.asp*. Accessed in February 2004.
34. F. Mullan and L. Epstein, "Community-Oriented Primary Care: New Relevance in a Changing World." *American Journal of Public Health*, 92 (November 2002):1748–1755.
35. Popovich, "Bioterrorism: GIS Can Help Fight a New Threat."

36. A. C. Gatrell, *Geographies of Health* (Malden, Mass.: Blackwell Publishers, 2002), Chapters 1, 2, 3, 4, and 5.
37. Centers for Disease Control and Prevention, Geographic Analysis Tool for Health and Environmental Research, GATHER. Available at *http://gis.cdc.gov/*. Accessed on March 27, 2004.
38. CDC, Geographic Analysis Tool.
39. Department of Geography, Queen's University, Canada, and International Geographic Union (IGU), Commission on Health, Environment and Development, Agenda for Research on the Health and the Environment. Available at *http://geog.queensu.ca/h_and_e/healthandenvir/Finland%20Workshop %20Papers/OPPONG.DOC*. Accessed on March 28, 2004.
40. Department of Geography, Queen's University, and IGU, Agenda for Research.
41. W. F. Davenhall, "The Business Side of Healthcare: GIS," Virginia Geographic Information Network. Available at *http://www.vgin.vipnet. org/documents/articles/localgovt/The_business_side.htm*. Accessed on March 24, 2004.
42. Davenhall, "Business Side."
43. Davenhall, "Business Side."
44. Davenhall, "Business Side."
45. Department of Geography, Queen's University, and IGU, Agenda for Research.
46. Department of Geography, Queen's University, and IGU, Agenda for Research.
47. Maged N. Kamel Boulos, "Toward Evidence-Based, GIS-Driven National Spatial Health Information Infrastructure."
48. ESRI, GIS for Health Care.
49. D. A. Henderson, "The Looming Threat of Bioterrorism," *Science* 283 (1999):1279–1282;Wofford and Thrall TK.

13

Marketing, Epidemiology, and Management: Perinatal Application

The management of health services should be population-based; epidemiology offers principles and methods to guide such decision making. This chapter examines how marketing also can contribute to epidemiologically oriented health services management—utilizing a quality of life model that focuses on the improvement of perinatal health status.

This chapter is limited to a broad discussion of marketing and its application to health services delivery using perinatal health as an example. The object is to show that the same basic principles lie behind both the marketing and epidemiologic approaches to the management of health services, and that the combination of the two can lead to optimal population-based management of health services.

There is in fact a close affinity between epidemiology and marketing because they complement each other in relation to health services management. Both aim to strengthen the fit between the health services offered and the needs of the population. Both thus provide a set of principles and tools that can be used to manage the delivery of health services in a more equitable, appropriate, effective, and efficient way.

What Is Marketing?

Marketing can be conceived of as a set of methods that aims to reconcile the resources and production capacity of an organization with the needs and preferences of the consumers. Marketing theory is based on a systemic view of organizations in which their functioning is viewed in terms of exchanges.

An exchange relationship requires two things:[1] (1) a constituency—that is, some person, group, or organization with whom an exchange is to be accomplished; and (2) a value—that is, "something" that is exchanged by the organization and by the constituency.

In other words, an exchange relationship involves the offering of something of value, such as a product or service, to someone who is willing to exchange it for something else of value, such as money or time.[2] Marketing offers a structure to analyze, predict, and manage exchanges to the benefit of all concerned. In this usage, marketing is defined simply as the conscious, systematic approach to the planning, implementation, and evaluation of the exchange relationships of an organization.[3]

Marketing is based on the fundamental assumption that if each constituency can be identified and analyzed, and if each exchange can be examined and controlled, the organization will attain its objectives (profit or other) more effectively. An important corollary of the model is that exchanges are maximized if and only if supply is matched with demand—if the product (or service) of the organization coincides with the needs, wants, and desires of the consumers.

The negative connotation often attached to this subject—that marketing creates needs—results from a misconception of its modern orientation. Although it is possible to find organizations with a product orientation, that is, entities in which production precedes marketing, they are likely to fail because they are trying to impose on a market a product (or service or idea) that is not matched to the consumer's needs or wants.

To the contrary, modern theory holds that marketing's only effective form involves consumer orientation through a strategic or integrated approach in which the marketing function precedes and embodies production and in which the product is matched to needs.

Another inherent feature of modern or strategic marketing is the identification and selection of specific subgroups of the constituency, or target markets. Any attempt to serve every possible market undoubtedly will be in vain. The correct marketing process is one that includes the decision as to which possible market segments can best be served, and then focuses on them.

Marketing thus is not selling or publicity. It is not an after-the-fact way to promote a product. Rather, it is a planned activity aimed at achieving organizational objectives through the satisfaction of needs and wants of consumers (patients, in the health care field). Marketing takes place long before sales, and it precedes and directs production.

A marketing program can be developed for each of these constituencies. The hospital can engage in patient marketing, physician marketing, community marketing, donor marketing, public health marketing, and more. A hospital short of nurses can engage in nurse marketing, and so on. Although the focus here is on patient marketing, precisely the same process can be used to develop effective exchange relationships with any markets.

Marketing's Contributions to Health Services Management

The epidemiologic approach to health services management requires that it be population-based and that health be conceptualized as resulting from four broad determinants—human biology, lifestyle, environment, and health care organization. Chapter 3 discussed how these two general epidemiologic principles can be incorporated into the management process to guide what has been referred to as a global planning process. Marketing is essentially a complementary process to this global (or strategic) planning process—in effect, a set of principles and techniques that can be used to enhance planning.

Furthermore, because strategic or integrated marketing is by definition consumer oriented and geared to the needs, wants, and desires of users, it can be adopted advantageously by managers in conjunction with epidemiology to achieve sound and effective population-based operation of health services.

Figure 13-1 illustrates how the marketing process can be integrated with the global planning process described in Chapter 3 and consequently with epidemiologic-oriented management. The marketing analyses of the environment, the market, the competition, and the resources and the resulting identification of target markets all contribute to the identification of health needs and problems. The planning process then moves on to the determination of priorities and the setting of objectives, after which portfolio analysis can be conducted. Activities and programs then are planned and the marketing mix devised.

Analysis of the Market

Analysis of the market consists of three distinct parts: the market structure analysis, the market opportunity analysis (or consumer analysis), and the target market selection.

Market Structure Analysis   This refers to the identification and analysis of the organization's markets. In the initial step, the populations who are actual markets and those who realistically might become potential markets involved in an exchange relationship with the institution must be defined and identified.

For a hospital, the actual markets can be determined with a patient-origin study, whereas the potential markets can be ascertained on a geographical/political basis or on a service-capacity basis (see Chapter 11).

Actual and potential markets should then be broken down into distinct and homogeneous subgroups. This is called market segmentation. Its aim

Planning

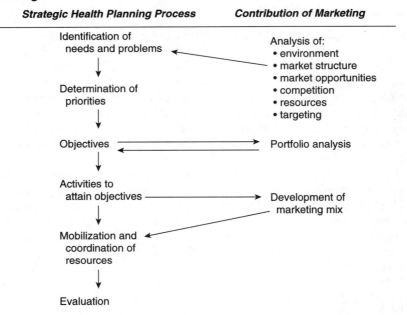

Strategic Health Planning Process   *Contribution of Marketing*

Identification of needs and problems

Determination of priorities

Objectives

Activities to attain objectives

Mobilization and coordination of resources

Evaluation

Analysis of:
• environment
• market structure
• market opportunities
• competition
• resources
• targeting

Portfolio analysis

Development of marketing mix

FIGURE 13-1 Marketing's Contribution to Strategic Health Planning. *Source:* Reprinted from "Le marketing et la planification des services de santé" by Francois Champagne with permission of *Administration Hospitalière et Sociale* 27, no. 5 (September–October 1981).

is to facilitate the analysis of actual and potential exchanges in an effort to improve their effectiveness. Because each market is composed of a wide variety of individuals (or groups or organizations), and because it is not realistic to consider each individual as a separate market, it is advisable to subdivide each market into separate groupings or segments of individuals with common characteristics.

The criteria of segmentation should be the homogeneity within each segment and the heterogeneity among the different segments. A market segment is a grouping of individuals who might be expected to behave differently than another market segment in the exchange relationship.

Three classes of variables can be used for market segmentation:

1. Geographic segmentation refers to the grouping of people according to their locations of residence or work. This can be done either on a simple geographic basis or by population density, climate, and so on.[4]

2. Demographic segmentation is the grouping of individuals on the basis of such variables as age, sex, income, occupation, education, religion, and race.

3. Psychographic segmentation uses such criteria as personal values, attitudes, opinions, personality, media usage, consumer behavior, and lifestyle.[5,6,7,8]

It has long been known that psychographic segmentation is often the most useful. Traditionally, because psychographic data was not readily available and because its collection required special market surveys, health services managers prefer to use geographic and demographic segmentation. (Information in Chapters 6, 7, and 8 on the relationships among demographic and geographic variables, health status, and service utilization can be used as the basis of patient market segmentation.) Currently, however, demographic and psychographic market segmentation is available from commercial vendors at a reasonable value.[37]

Market Opportunity Analysis   Once market structure analysis is completed, the needs, preferences, perceptions, and motivations of the individuals that compose the various market segments must be determined.

Needs assessment techniques for the determination of a population's health needs already were explained in Chapter 3. The same methods can be used for the determination of the needs of any market. Needs can be defined by the organization and/or by the markets. The institution can pinpoint the needs of its markets using any number of indicators, including trend analysis and forecasting of demand.

Epidemiologic techniques and data should be used for the organizational (or professional) definition of health needs. All epidemiologic principles and methods described earlier can thus contribute to the marketing effort by providing a scientific framework to determine the population's health needs. Needs also can be defined by consumers themselves, either through the use of surveys or through participation in consensus-reaching approaches.

In marketing, three types of surveys are used:[9]

1. **Direct surveys.** Individuals are asked to describe their needs in answering either open-ended questions (e.g., "What services would you like to see added?") or closed-ended questions (e.g., "Rate the following services in terms of your level of interest," or "Rate the following services on a scale from one to ten").

2. **Projective surveys.** Whereas the direct method assumes that consumers are aware of their needs and capable of expressing them, the projective method aims to identify needs that consumers are not really aware of or might be unable to verbalize. Psychometric techniques such as word associations, sentence completions, picture completions, and role playing are used.

3. **Prototype surveys.** The consumers are exposed to and asked to respond to a prototype of a real product or service. For example, instead of asking a group of elderly persons what they want in the way of housing, they can be shown alternative blueprints and asked to comment on what they like and dislike about each, why, what is missing, and so on.

Although all of these factors are fairly well known to health planners, market opportunity analysis also calls for the identification of preferences, perceptions, and motivation, which rarely is done in health services management. Marketers use three methods for the identification of preferences: (1) simple route ordering, (2) paired comparison, and (3) monadic, or scale, rating.[10]

The simplest method is to ask the individuals to rank services in order of preference. Such simple ordinal ranking, however, does not provide any indication of magnitude of preference or distance between services.

The second method is to present a set of services, two at a time, and ask which is preferred in each pair. From the analysis of each paired comparison, the marketer then can rank all of the services. Although this has the same disadvantages as the simple rank ordering, it is often considered a better method because people find it easier to state their preference between only two objects or services at a time and because they can concentrate better on differences and similarities.

The third method (monadic rating) consists of asking individuals to rate their liking of each service on a scale (usually of five or seven points). This method is considered easier to use (especially when there are numerous services to evaluate) and provides more information than the other methods.

The perceptions of the individuals comprising the different market segments regarding the institution and its products (services) also significantly influence their "buying behavior." Therefore it is important for the facility to identify these perceptions so that it can either concentrate in the areas where it is deemed appropriate and favorable or do something to modify and improve its image.

Many methods can be used to measure perceptions. Multidimensional scaling[11] and semantic differentials[12,13] are among the most sophisticated of such tools. For marketing purposes, Kotler proposes a simple "familiarity-favorability analysis."[14] Respondents are asked first how familiar they are with the organization (or, specifically, with one of its services) on a five-point scale from "never heard of" to "know very well." Those who have some familiarity are then asked how favorable they feel toward the institution, also on a five-point scale from "very unfavorable" to "very favorable." The results can be used to determine what further actions the organization should take.

For example, a hospital might find that some members of its constituency (or some segments of it) are not very familiar with its obstetric service, but those who are familiar have a very favorable attitude toward it. The hospital's task then should be to bring itself to the attention of more people.

Of course, it also might find that many people are familiar with it but have an unfavorable attitude toward it. The hospital then should keep a low profile (avoid news and publicity), find out why people dislike it, mend its ways, and then seek public attention again. Similarly, situations of high familiarity-favorable attitude and low familiarity-unfavorable attitude also are possible and call for still different strategies.

The final component of market opportunity analysis is the evaluation of the motivation of the various segments. The exchange relationship (for example, the utilization of a health service) depends not only on needs, preferences, and perceptions but also on some catalyst or trigger that will convert a potential user into an actual client.[15] Individuals can perceive a need for the service and have appropriate attitudes toward the organization, yet still not use it unless some specific stimulus or cue attracts them to do so.

For example, a reminder card (or phone call) informing a patient of a forthcoming appointment might be necessary to stimulate the individual to keep the appointment. Different market segments are likely to respond differently to various stimuli. The organization that can identify and predict these stimuli is likely to improve plans for and influence desired exchange.

Target Market Selection   The last component of market analysis is the selection of target segments with which the institution could or should try to establish an exchange relationship. A target market is a well-defined set of customers whose needs the organization plans to satisfy.[16] It must decide which market segments it will fit into its services. All of the analyses discussed earlier should serve as inputs in the decision as to which market segments will be targeted. This decision should be based on macroenvironmental analysis, resource analysis, market structure, market opportunity analysis, and competition analysis.

Still another element is market positioning, a method of examining a product as compared to the competition's product in relation to any number of characteristics.[17,18]

The results and conclusions of the various analyses can be fed into the planning process (Figure 13-1), where priorities can be determined (Chapter 3). It should now be clear how the use of these marketing principles and techniques can contribute, along with epidemiology, to population-based management of health services.

Marketing and Health Services Management: A Quality of Life Model for Improving Perinatal Health Status

Quality of life (QOL) assessment has been a popular theme of study among researchers in the United States and abroad.[19,20] Various instruments of QOL and health-related QOL (HR-QOL) have been developed and tested for a broad range of implications. There are usually two different approaches to QOL studies: those that seek to define a generic QOL summary and those specific to a disease or group.[21] Several well-known generic HR-QOL instruments include the SF-36,[22,23] the Sickness Impact Profile,[24,25] the Nottingham Health Profile,[26,27] and the EuroQol.[28,29] Disease-specific HR-QOL measures, such as the Health Assessment Questionnaire,[30,31] have been designed for a number of diseases, including obesity, arthritis, diabetes, asthma, pulmonary disease, cancer, epilepsy, and HIV.[32]

Until now, research has not explored the assessment of perinatal HR-QOL. Many HR-QOL instruments are recognized as valid when looking at specific health indicators such as morbidity and mortality, but they fail to portray the overall picture of public health needs and prevention outcomes.[33] A perinatal HR-QOL model that incorporates medical, lifestyle, social, and access indicators that impact perinatal health status would substantially enhance the planning and focus of prevention efforts. Although HR-QOL measures can be used to make comparisons among geographical units such as the national, state, and local levels, mechanisms for this level are currently lacking.[34] The Perinatal Health QOL Model, a unique nontraditional marketing/business model that also uses traditional QOL measures, was developed to assess perinatal health status on a microgeographic level.

The Georgia Department of Community Health's Division of Health Planning and the Health Strategies Council (HSC) devised a plan (DCH) that designated Perinatal Health Regions that were developed to better implement obstetric and neonatal health care services in Georgia (MAP). The result was six regions. The focus of this marketing approach is on Perinatal Region 6—the south-central area of Georgia. Perinatal Region 6 contains three of the nineteen Georgia Department of Public Health districts (Macon-District 5-1, Dublin-District 5-2, and Valdosta-District 8-1).

The geographical scope of this marketing strategy includes region, district, county, census tract, and block group analysis. One of the significant aspects of this approach is that the Perinatal Health QOL Model can be applied at various levels of geography in the United States—from a small area such as block group or to a macro analysis such as a state or a region. Perinatal Region 6 in Georgia is composed of thirty-six counties and 207 census tracts. Only five of the thirty-six counties are defined as urban counties by Metropolitan Statistical Area (MSA) designation. In 2000, the total population for this perinatal region was 888,679.[35] The perinatal health status QOL model for Georgia's south-central region utilized data for 1994 to 1999. During this period, the region experienced 74,662 births, 941 infant deaths, 6,655 low birth weight births (< 2500 grams), and 8,972 preterm births (< 37 weeks gestation). The region's perinatal health services for impacting these events include eighteen hospitals, thirty-nine health departments/clinics, and ninety-seven physicians.

The development of a new Perinatal Health QOL Marketing Model will enhance policy and program efforts by identifying the high-risk areas in the region on a microgeographic level. This will link these areas with marketing strategies, most notably, as provided by the Claritas PRIZM Cluster system. The Claritas system is a widely used social, economic, demographic, and psychographic marketing program in the United States for targeting populations in order to understand the business and marketing aspects of population groups. The purpose of using this system is to focus on prevention and health promotion strategies that are based more on business and marketing perspectives. It is clear the traditional medical model utilized to improve the outcomes related to perinatal health status has had limited success. Therefore, a new marketing model is appropriate for creating an opportunity to reduce the burden of illness on the perinatal population. Thus, we define a Perinatal Health QOL Marketing/Business Model.

The Perinatal Health Quality of Life (QOL) Marketing/Business Model (Figure 13-2) illustrates an algorithm design for impacting and improving perinatal health status in the south-central region of Georgia.

Quality of Life Indexes

Spatial Analysis   The marketing model as presented is capable of analyzing various levels of geography, such as might be related to small-area analysis (i.e., block groups and census tracts) (see Chapter 10). The model is also designed to analyze macro markets, such as a county, state, or region. In this application we focus on a perinatal region that represents three of the nineteen Georgia health districts: Macon, Dublin, and Valdosta. Therefore, the spatial analysis for the model represents a region that is composed of three districts, thirty-six counties, and 207 census tracts (a smaller geographic division of a county). The perinatal region in reference to the United States and Georgia is shown in Figure 13-3. Given the broad application of this approach, health services managers will have opportunities to apply this methodology on various geographic market areas.

Medical, Lifestyle, and Access Indexes   Three factors were defined reflecting twenty-six variables that are risk criteria associated with perinatal health status. These factors reflect outcomes and represent the marketing strategy to be developed for implementation on the status of perinatal health. The three factors are Medical, Lifestyle, and Access Indexes. The criteria for selecting the risk factors for the medical, lifestyle, and access variables were based on demonstrated relationships that influence perinatal health as supported in the literature, as noted in Table 13-1.[36,37,38,39,40,41,42,43,44,45,46,47,48,49] Eight variables make up the Medical Index. Examples include the infant

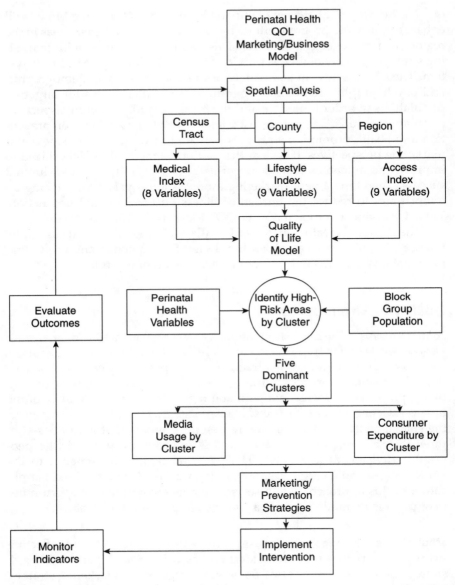

FIGURE 13-2 Marketing and QOL model for improving perinatal health status.

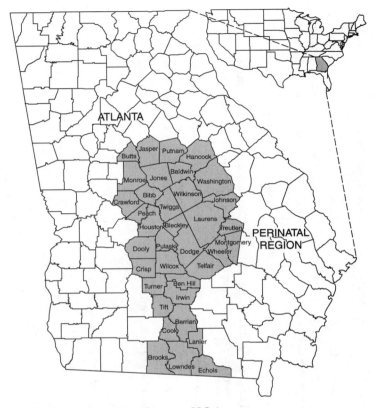

FIGURE 13-3 Perinatal region, Georgia, U.S.A.

mortality rate and the percentage of low birth weight births. Nine social indicators such as education level and drug use define the Lifestyle Index. The Access Index comprises nine variables. Examples of the Access Index include access to perinatal physicians and insurance status. Table 13-1 displays a complete listing of the risk variables for the Medical, Lifestyle, and Access Indexes that were included in calculating the overall Perinatal Health QOL Index.

Marketing—Methodology All variables for each of the factors were standardized into z-scores to produce a simple z-score additive model. The classic method for "standardizing" a set of values (finding a common metric or scale) is the calculation of z-scores. Z-scores are anchored by the mean and standard deviation of the original values and are rescaled such that the

TABLE 13-1 Medical, Lifestyle, and Access Variables Used to Create the Perinatal Health QOL Index

Medical[a]	Lifestyle[a,b]	Access[b,c,d]
Infant mortality (rate)	Mother's education level—Did not finish high school (%)	Drive-time to nearest perinatal physician (avg-min)
Birth weight <2500 grams (%)	Mother's marital status: Single (%)	Drive-time to nearest hospital (avg-min)
Gestation <37 weeks (%)	Alcoholic drinks per week: None (%)	Drive-time to nearest clinic (avg-min)
Apgar score at 1 minute (avg)	Smoked cigarettes during pregnancy (%)	Distance to nearest perinatal physician (avg-mi)
Apgar score at 5 minutes (avg)	Father's education level: Did not finish high school (%)	Distance to nearest hospital (avg-min)
Mothers having <12 prenatal visits (%)	Attended health education classes (%)	Distance to nearest clinic (avg-mi)
No prenatal care (%)	Unemployment rate (per 1,000 population)	Lack personal transportation (%)
Maternal weight gain (avg-lbs)	Health status score	Perinatal physician rate (per 10,000 population)
	Socioeconomic status score	No household insurance (%)

[a]Data from Georgia Department of Human Resources, Division of Public Health. Vital Records. 1994–1999.

[b]Data from Inforum, a Division of Claritas, Inc. ©2000.

[c]Data from Georgia Board for Physician Workforce Database. 2000.

[d]Data from Georgia Department of Community Health. Annual Hospital Questionnaire. 2000.

new mean is 0 and the new standard deviation is 1. The resulting z-scores correspond to points on the standard normal curve, with a theoretical range of approximately −3 to +3. The actual range for each indicator, however, will be different. Z-scores can be calculated for individual-level or aggregate-level data. In either case, each value is treated as an "individual" member of a sample. The z-score standardization process does not alter the distribution of the data. If the data set is abnormally or normally distributed, the z-score does not impact the distribution.

A separate z-score, Infant Health Risk Score, for each Medical, Lifestyle, and Access Index was calculated and summed for the thirty-six counties and 207 census tracts in the perinatal region. Table 13-2 displays the results of calculating the z-scores of one medical variable, the infant mortality rate. Table 13-2 also shows how the Medical Index was calculated by adding the z-scores of all eight medical variables. A numeric rank from 1 to 36 was given to every county, and a rank of 1 to 207 was given to every census tract, reflecting lowest to highest risk, respectively. The census tract analysis is not shown. After the counties and census tracts were ranked, a grading scale of A-B-C-D-F was given to every county and census tract. As shown in Table 13-2, each county was given a grade for the Medical Index by calculating the mean and standard deviation for the *z-score of the Medical z-scores* column. The grades were assigned based on the plus and minus deviations from zero so that an almost normal distribution resulted. For example, a value greater than −1.0 standard deviation received a grade of A, whereas a value of greater than 1.0 standard deviation received a grade of F (the former reflecting five counties and the latter representing seven counties). Thus, there were five A counties, eight B counties, twelve C counties, four D counties, and seven F counties. The formulas used to calculate the z-score, rank, and grades of the Medical Index were likewise used to calculate and determine the Lifestyle and Access Indexes. An example of the z-score methodology applied to the Lifestyle Index is shown in the appendix of this chapter.

Quality of Life Index

The Perinatal Health QOL Index was calculated by summing the z-scores of the Medical, Lifestyle, and Access Indexes, which is shown in Table 13-3. A numeric rank from lowest to highest risk (1 to 207 for census tracts, and 1 to 36 for counties) was provided for the respective geographies. The mean and standard deviation was calculated for the z-score of Medical, Lifestyle, and Access z-scores column to determine the grading scale, A-B-C-D-F. The resulting grades represent the Infant Health Risk Score for each census tract and county in the perinatal region as determined by the Perinatal Health QOL Index. In this instance, the results show three counties with a grade of A, five with B, eighteen with C, eight with D, and two with a grade of F.

TABLE 13-2 Z-Score Calculation of Medical Index by County

| County | Z-Score and Rank of One Medical Variable | | | Z-Score and Rank of All Medical Variables | | | |
	Infant Mortality Rate[a]	Z-Score	Rank	Medical Z-Scores (Sum)[b]	Z-Score of Medical Z-Scores[c]	Rank	Grade
Wheeler	7.5	-1.1	4	1.32	-1.67	1	A
Treutlen	11.3	-0.2	19	1.90	-1.55	2	A
Montgomery	6.5	-1.3	2	1.98	-1.53	3	A
Berrien	8.0	-1.0	6	4.15	-1.08	4	A
Laurens	16.2	0.9	33	4.21	-1.06	5	A
Dodge	7.3	-1.1	3	4.86	-0.93	6	B
Irwin	5.9	-1.4	1	4.86	-0.93	7	B
Johnson	10.3	-0.4	11	5.07	-0.88	8	B
Houston	9.9	-0.5	8	5.14	-0.87	9	B
Jones	10.3	-0.4	12	5.39	-0.81	10	B
Crawford	15.7	0.8	32	6.15	-0.65	11	B
Cook	10.1	-0.5	9	6.43	-0.59	12	B
Butts	11.2	-0.2	17	6.52	-0.58	13	B
Jasper	14.2	0.5	27	7.68	-0.33	14	C
Lanier	10.2	-0.4	10	7.69	-0.33	15	C
Twiggs	10.8	-0.3	16	8.12	-0.24	16	C
Lowndes	12.3	0.0	21	8.18	-0.23	17	C
Bleckley	10.5	-0.4	14	8.24	-0.21	18	C
Telfair	8.6	-0.8	7	8.44	-0.17	19	C
Pulaski	10.6	-0.4	15	8.64	-0.13	20	C
Ben Hill	12.3	0.0	22	8.78	-0.10	21	C
Brooks	7.8	-1.0	5	9.39	0.03	22	C

TABLE 13-2 (continued)

| County | Z-Score and Rank of One Medical Variable | | | Z-Score and Rank of All Medical Variables | | | |
	Infant Mortality Rate[a]	Z-Score	Rank	Medical Z-Scores (Sum)[b]	Z-Score of Medical Z-Scores[c]	Rank	Grade
Wilkinson	14.4	0.5	28	9.44	0.04	23	C
Monroe	10.4	-0.4	13	11.03	0.38	24	C
Putnam	13.8	0.4	26	11.51	0.48	25	C
Washington	12.9	0.2	25	12.24	0.63	26	D
Wilcox	16.9	1.1	34	13.23	0.84	27	D
Peach	15.3	0.7	30	13.58	0.91	28	D
Bibb	14.7	0.6	29	13.61	0.92	29	D
Turner	12.4	0.0	23	14.97	1.21	30	F
Tift	12.9	0.2	24	15.46	1.31	31	F
Dooly	11.7	-0.1	20	15.75	1.37	32	F
Hancock	11.3	-0.2	18	16.79	1.59	33	F
Baldwin	17.5	1.2	35	17.25	1.69	34	F
Crisp	15.4	0.7	31	17.25	1.69	35	F
Echols	31.0	4.3	36	17.82	1.81	36	F

[a]Infant Mortality Rate is one of the eight medical variables that create the Medical Index.

[b]All eight medical variable z-scores were added together.

[c]Represents the Infant Health Risk Score for medical variables ranked from lowest- to highest-risk county.

TABLE 13-3 Z-Score and Integer Ranking of the Perinatal Health QOL Index by County

County	Medical Z-Score (Sum)	Lifestyle Z-Score (Sum)	Access Z-Score (Sum)	Medical, Lifestyle, and Access Z-Scores (Sum)	Z-Score of Medical, Lifestyle, and Access Z-Scores[a]	Rank	Grade
Houston	5.1	-12.4	-7.3	-14.5	-2.5	1	A
Jones	5.4	-7.8	-4.5	-6.9	-1.7	2	A
Lowndes	8.2	-7.2	-7.4	-6.5	-1.7	3	A
Cook	6.4	1.0	-7.1	0.3	-0.9	4	B
Irwin	4.9	0.7	-5.2	0.4	-0.9	5	B
Bleckley	8.2	-0.9	-5.0	2.3	-0.7	6	B
Laurens	4.2	-3.3	1.6	2.5	-0.7	7	B
Crawford	6.2	-1.6	-2.0	2.6	-0.7	8	B
Wheeler	1.3	0.8	3.1	5.2	-0.4	9	C
Dodge	4.9	0.6	-0.1	5.4	-0.4	10	C
Peach	13.6	-1.3	-6.7	5.7	-0.4	11	C
Treutlen	1.9	3.1	1.6	6.6	-0.3	12	C
Berrien	4.1	2.9	-0.1	6.9	-0.2	13	C
Montgomery	2.0	-1.7	7.0	7.2	-0.2	14	C
Wilkinson	9.4	-3.8	1.7	7.3	-0.2	15	C
Monroe	11.0	-5.0	1.3	7.4	-0.2	16	C
Ben Hill	8.8	6.2	-6.8	8.2	-0.1	17	C
Pulaski	8.6	-1.6	1.3	8.4	-0.1	18	C
Lanier	7.7	4.8	-3.7	8.8	0.0	19	C
Bibb	13.6	-5.4	1.1	9.3	0.0	20	C
Baldwin	17.2	-4.3	-3.1	9.8	0.1	21	C
Brooks	9.4	0.3	0.5	10.3	0.1	22	C
Washington	12.2	-0.8	-0.7	10.8	0.2	23	C

TABLE 13-3 (continued)

County	Medical Z-Score (Sum)	Lifestyle Z-Score (Sum)	Access Z-Score (Sum)	Medical, Lifestyle, and Access Z-Scores (Sum)	Z-Score of Medical, Lifestyle, and Access Z-Scores[a]	Rank	Grade
Tift	15.5	0.9	-5.5	10.9	0.2	24	C
Putnam	11.5	-3.8	3.2	10.9	0.2	25	C
Johnson	5.1	3.7	4.2	13.0	0.4	26	C
Crisp	17.3	2.9	-6.1	14.1	0.5	27	D
Butts	6.5	1.0	7.0	14.6	0.6	28	D
Turner	15.0	3.5	-3.9	14.6	0.6	29	D
Jasper	7.7	3.0	4.3	15.0	0.6	30	D
Twiggs	8.1	4.7	3.6	16.4	0.8	31	D
Wilcox	13.2	2.6	0.8	16.7	0.8	32	D
Telfair	8.4	4.7	7.9	21.0	1.2	33	F
Echols	17.8	-0.7	5.8	22.9	1.4	34	F
Dooly	15.7	7.6	4.4	27.7	1.9	35	F
Hancock	16.8	6.8	13.8	37.4	3.0	36	F

[a]Represents the Infant Health Risk Score for the Perinatal Health QOL Index ranked from lowest- to highest-risk county.

Dominant Clusters

Identify High-Risk Areas by Cluster   As noted in the previous section and reflected in Table 13-3, the high- and low-risk counties were identified. Utilizing the PRIZM cluster system, we tagged these high- and low-risk counties with the cluster that dominates the specific geographic area. PRIZM clusters are a lifestyle segmentation system developed by Claritas, Inc., in order to group neighborhoods together that exhibit similar social, demographic, and behavioral characteristics. These neighborhood clusters can be used to identify and locate targets for marketing. In the PRIZM system every U.S. neighborhood/block group is defined according to sixty-two distinct clusters. (A block group is a smaller division of a census tract, and a census tract is a smaller division of a county.) The perinatal region is represented by thirty-four of the nation's sixty-two clusters at the block-group level, and twenty-nine of the thirty-four PRIZM clusters can be linked to the region's census tracts. Because census tracts can have several block groups and each block group could represent a different cluster, it was determined that the cluster with the greatest population and/or most "like" clusters would be selected to represent the census tract cluster group.

Three components were combined to determine the five dominant PRIZM clusters for the region. However, the number of clusters chosen for further analysis is not necessarily limited to five. The number is very much dictated by the degree of problem that is encountered as the data is summed across all clusters. In this instance, the marketing approach shows that the majority of the problems in the region are reflected in five dominant clusters that are examined further for marketing and prevention strategies. The three components used for determining the five dominant clusters in this analysis were the following:

1. The cluster block group population
2. The cluster rank of the perinatal health variables (births, infant mortality, low birth weight births, and preterm births)
3. The cluster rank of the QOL Indexes (Medical, Lifestyle, Access) denoted as the Quality of Life Marketing Index

Block Group Population. The PRIZM clusters are defined by block groups, smaller divisions of a census tract. To qualify as a top-five high-risk PRIZM cluster, each cluster in the region must comprise at least 5 percent of the region's total block group population. The clusters with the highest percentage population in the region are Scrub Pine Flats, Norma Rae-ville, Southside City, Shotguns and Pickups, and Grain Belt.

Perinatal Health Variables. Four medical variables—births, infant mortality, low birth weight births, and preterm births—were selected to determine their impact on perinatal health status in the region by PRIZM cluster. Although these four variables are included in the Medical Index, they are analyzed separately to examine their impact at the cluster level, which then can be used to target the marketing efforts.

The birth rate, infant mortality rate, percentage of low birth weight births, and the percentage of preterm births were determined by cluster group. For example, the PRIZM cluster Southside City has the highest birth rate (20.1), and the PRIZM cluster Family Scramble has the highest infant mortality rate (24.0). After the rates and percentages were determined for each medical variable by PRIZM cluster, the clusters were linked to the census tracts for each medical variable by summing the z-scores of each variable and ranking the sum by highest- to lowest-risk PRIZM cluster. Cluster rank and percentage of total block group population were taken into consideration when choosing the top-five high-risk clusters. The top-five high-risk clusters for selected medical variables listed from highest to lowest risk are Norma Rae-ville, Scrub Pine Flats, Southside City, New Homesteaders, and Grain Belt (Table 13-4).

Quality of Life Index. To review, the Perinatal Health QOL Index was developed by combining the twenty-six variables from the Medical, Lifestyle, and Access Indexes. The PRIZM clusters were linked to the census tracts of the QOL Index by summing the z-scores of the census tracts in the QOL Index and ranking the sum based on risk from highest to lowest by PRIZM cluster. In Table 13-5 the z-score of the twenty-one census tracts of Southside City is 22.7, which is the highest z-score of all the clusters for the QOL Index. Therefore, Southside City ranks the highest for perinatal health risks related to medical, lifestyle, and access variables. Again, cluster rank and percentage of total block group population were taken into consideration when choosing the top-five high-risk clusters. The top-five high-risk clusters for QOL Indexes listed from highest to lowest risk are Southside City, Scrub Pine Flats, Grain Belt, Norma Rae-ville, and Family Scramble (Table 13-4).

Five Dominant Clusters   The top-five high-risk clusters are finalized by adding the rank of each cluster for the percentage block group population, selected medical variables, and the QOL Marketing Index. Table 13-5 shows how the cluster ranks were added to get the final top-five PRIZM clusters for the region. The five dominant clusters that ranked from highest to lowest risk are shown in Table 13-6. This table highlights the social, economic, and demographics of the five dominant clusters that represent high risk in terms of perinatal health status. Therefore, these clusters were identified as marketing and health promotion targets for the region for impacting health status of the perinatal population.

Results—Quality of Life Indexes

An Infant Health Risk Score was created for each county (36) and census tract (207) by calculating the z-scores of selected medical, lifestyle, and access variables in order to construct a Perinatal Health QOL Index. Table 13-7 gives a

TABLE 13-4 PRIZM Cluster Rank for Combined Block Group Population, Medical Variables, and Quality of Life Indexes; Perinatal Region 6, Georgia 1994-1999

PRIZM Cluster*	%Prizm Cluster Population by Block Group	Cluster Rank from High to Low Risk				Combined PRIZM Cluster Rank
		Population	Medical Variables	Quality of Life Index	Sum of Ranks	
Scrub Pine Flats	18.1	1	2	2	5	1
Norma Rae-ville	12.6	2	1	4	7	2
Southside City	5.9	3	3	1	7	3
Grain Belt	5.1	5	5	3	13	4
Shotguns & Pickups	5.5	4	7	6	17	5
Back Country Folks	4.7	6	8	11	25	6
Starter Families	2.3	15	6	16	37	7
New Homesteaders	3.6	8	4	29	41	8
Middle America	2.3	14	13	14	41	9
River City, USA	3.6	9	9	24	42	10
God's Country	3.7	7	11	28	46	11
Blue Highways	2.7	11	25	10	46	12
Sunset City Blues	2.2	16	12	19	47	13
Red, White & Blues	2.5	13	14	21	48	14
Rustic Elders	1.4	23	18	7	48	15
Big Fish, Small Pond	2.8	10	17	22	49	16
Middleburg Managers	2.5	12	10	27	49	17
Big Sky Families	1.7	18	27	9	54	18
Upward Bound	1.8	17	23	17	57	19
Family Scramble	0.6	31	22	5	58	20
Military Quarters	1.6	19	15	25	59	21

TABLE 13-4 (continued)

| | %Prizm Cluster Population by Block Group | Cluster Rank from High to Low Risk | | | | Combined PRIZM Cluster Rank |
| | | Population | Medical Variables | Quality of Life Index | Sum of Ranks | |
PRIZM Cluster						
New Eco-topia	1.6	20	21	18	59	22
Mines & Mills	0.8	30	24	8	62	23
Agri-Business	1.5	21	29	13	63	24
Country Squires	1.1	25	16	23	64	25
Hard Scrabble	1.1	26	26	12	64	26
Greenbelt Families	1.5	22	28	15	65	27
Towns & Gowns	0.9	29	19	20	68	28
Second City Elite	1.3	24	20	26	70	29
Rural Industria	1.1	27				30
Boomtown Singles	0.9	28				31
Hometown Retired	0.5	32				32
Smalltown Downtown	0.3	33				33
Golden Ponds	0.2	34				34

Note: High-risk cluster groups are bold.

TABLE 13-5 PRIZM Cluster Rank for QOL Index; Perinatal Region, 1994–1999

PRIZM Cluster*	# Census Tracts Where Cluster Is Dominant	QOL Index Z-Scores by Census Tract (Sum)	Cluster Rank from High to Low Risk	% PRIZM Cluster Population by Block Group
Southside City	21	22.7	1	5.9
Scrub Pine Flats	45	18.2	2	18.1
Grain Belt	16	8.1	3	5.1
Norma Rae-ville	26	7.7	4	12.6
Family Scramble	1	2.2	5	0.6
Shotguns & Pickups	11	2.0	6	5.5
Rustic Elders	3	1.9	7	1.4
Mines & Mills	1	0.7	8	0.8
Big Sky Families	1	0.3	9	1.7
Blue Highways	2	0.0	10	2.7
Back Country Folks	16	-0.7	11	4.7
Hard Scrabble	2	-0.8	12	1.1
Agri-Business	3	-0.9	13	1.5
Middle America	2	-1.1	14	2.3
Greenbelt Families	1	-1.2	15	1.5
Starter Families	5	-1.3	16	2.3
Upward Bound	1	-1.3	17	1.8
New Eco-topia	2	-1.4	18	1.6
Sunset City Blues	4	1.7	19	2.2
Towns & Gowns	3	-1.9	20	0.9
Red, White & Blues	4	-3.7	21	2.5
Big Fish, Small Pond	3	-4.1	22	2.8
Country Squires	2	-4.4	23	1.1
River City, USA	7	-4.5	24	3.6
Military Quarters	3	-5.2	25	1.6
Second City Elite	3	-6.7	26	1.3
Middleburg Managers	6	-7.3	27	2.5
God's Country	6	-7.8	28	3.7
New Homesteaders	7	-7.9	29	3.6
Rural Industria	0			1.1
Boomtown Singles	0			0.9
Hometown Retired	0			0.5
Smalltown Downtown	0			0.3
Golden Ponds	0			0.2
Perinatal Region	**207**			**100.0**

*Note: High-risk cluster groups are bold.

TABLE 13-6 PRIZM Cluster Demographics

Cluster Name	Type	Description	Age Group	Race
Scrub Pine Flats	Rustic Living	Older African-American Farm Families	Under 18, 18–24, 65+	Predominantly Black
Norma Rae-ville	Working Towns	Young Families, Bi-racial Mill Towns	Under 18, 18–24, 25–34	Predominantly Black
Southside City	2nd City Blues	African-American Service Workers	Under 18, 18–24, 25–34	Predominantly Black
Shotguns & Pickups	Country Families	Rural Blue-Collar Workers and Families	Mixed	Predominantly White
Grain Belt	Heartlanders	Farm Owners and Tenants	Under 18, 55–64, 65+	Predominantly White, High Hispanic, Some Native American

Source: Data from Inforum, a Division of Claritas, Inc. ©2000.

TABLE 13-7 Distribution of Index Grades and Percentage of Population by Medical, Lifestyle, Access, and Quality of Life Scores by County and Census Tract; Perinatal Region 6, Georgia, 1994–1999

Grades	Medical				Lifestyle				Access				Quality of Life			
	Number of Counties	% of County Population	Number of Census Tracts	% of CT Population	Number of Counties	% of County Population	Number of Census Tracts	% of CT Population	Number of Counties	% of County Population	Number of Census Tracts	% of CT Population	Number of Counties	% of County Population	Number of Census Tracts	% of CT Population
A	5	9.3	30	14.4	3	25.5	23	17.7	5	29.2	17	8.1	3	25.5	17	12.6
B	8	24.7	47	27.0	6	33.1	30	18.2	8	18.8	61	36.3	5	10.7	49	27.4
C	12	26.9	69	32.9	14	24.3	90	41.9	12	38.4	72	34.3	18	50.5	82	36.3
D	4	23.3	28	12.9	10	12.7	50	18.4	7	8.0	32	11.9	6	9.2	48	21.3
F	7	15.8	33	12.8	3	4.4	14	3.8	4	5.6	25	9.4	4	4.1	11	2.4

summary of the grade distribution for the indexes of the Perinatal Health QOL Index.

Results—Medical, Lifestyle, and Access Indexes

Nearly one-third of the counties in the perinatal region received a grade of D or lower for the Medical Index variables. Sixty-one census tracts, representing 26 percent of the perinatal region's population, received grades of D or lower for the Medical Index variables. Geographically, the medical grade results are quite randomly distributed throughout the region (Figure 13-4). However, pockets of poor medical status, grades of D and F, are clustered and more evident in the northwest urban tracts of Baldwin, Bibb, and Peach counties and the west-central rural counties of the region.

Lifestyle variables, those that pertain to education, alcohol use, cigarette smoking, socioeconomic status, and health status, reflect the overall behavioral characteristics of the perinatal population. Thus, the Lifestyle Index shows that thirteen counties and sixty-four census tracts, 22 percent of the region's population, received grades of D or lower. The Lifestyle Index of High Risk by census tract (Figure 13-5) illustrates that high-risk tracts are scattered randomly throughout the region with a concentration of the high-risk tracts in the region's south to central regional counties.

Twenty-one percent of the region's population has problems with access to perinatal health care services. About one-third of the counties and fifty-seven census tracts received grades of D or lower for Access variables of high risk. Problems with access or tracts that received grades of D or lower are evident around the region's periphery as well as the suburbs of the metropolitan counties such as Bibb, Baldwin, Laurens, and Lowndes (Figure 13-6). A primary reason for this peripheral pattern of lack of access is because the counties contiguous to the region were not evaluated for access to services within the region. It has been suggested to the policymakers that a statistical assessment of access should be conducted so as to overcome this deficiency noted at the regional level.

Quality of Life Index

The Quality of Life Index was calculated by using the z-score additive model, thereby combining the three indexes (Medical, Lifestyle, and Access). As a result of this analysis, ten counties and fifty-nine census tracts, 23 percent of the region's population, are identified and are targeted as high-risk perinatal health "hot spots." The overall QOL grades are shown in Figure 13-7.

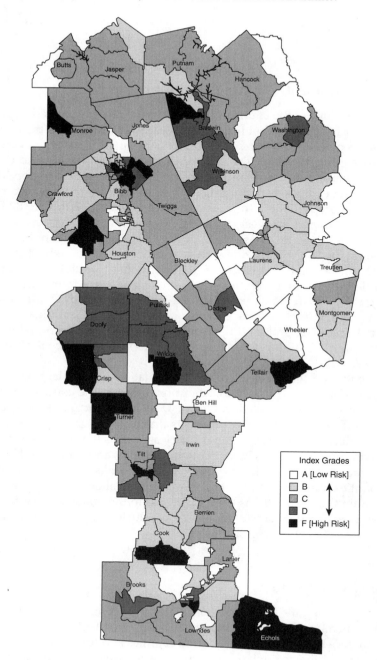

FIGURE 13-4 Medical Index of High Risk by Census Tract; Perinatal Region 6, Georgia, 1994–1999.

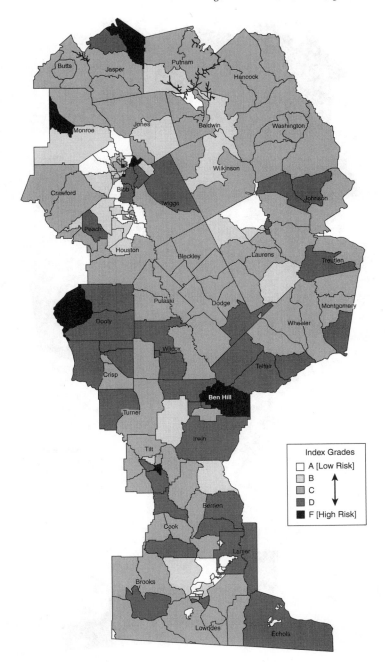

FIGURE 13-5 Lifestyle Index of High Risk by Census Tract; Perinatal Region 6, Georgia, 1994–1999.

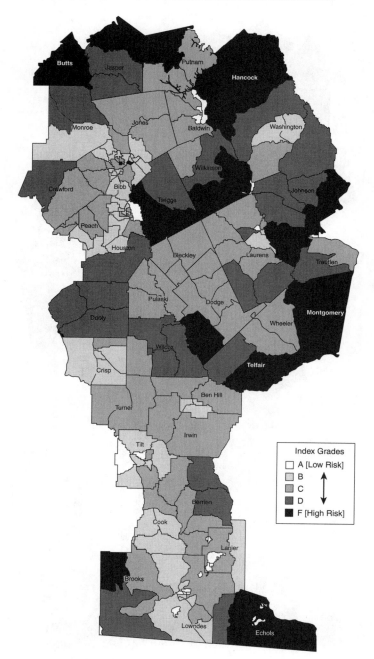

FIGURE 13-6 Access Index of High Risk by Census Tract; Perinatal Region 6, Georgia, 1994–1999.

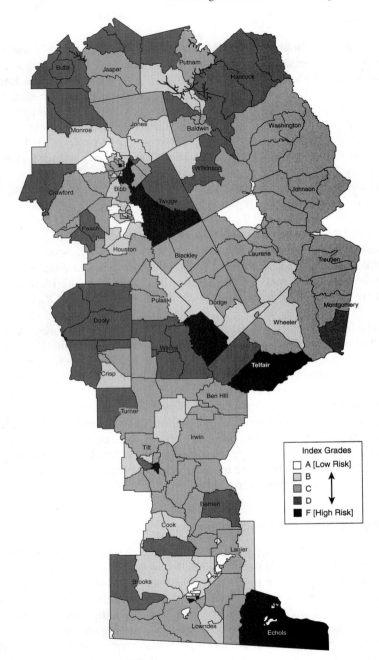

FIGURE 13-7   QOL Index of High Risk by Census Tract; Perinatal Region 6, Georgia, 1994–1999.

Five Dominant Clusters

Selected Medical Variables/Births, IM, LBW, Preterm   As previously mentioned, the top-five high-risk clusters for selected medical variables were identified for the region. Listed from highest to lowest risk they are Norma Rae-ville, Scrub Pine Flats, Southside City, New Homesteaders, and Grain Belt. Norma Rae-ville comprises 13 percent of the region's population. As seen previously, the total of Norma Rae-ville's z-scores for birth rate, infant mortality rate, percentage of low birth weight births, and percentage of preterm births was the highest in the region. For instance, Norma Rae-ville experienced 18.4 infant deaths per 1,000 population for the years 1994 to 1999. The cluster with the lowest overall score for selected medical variables was Agri-Business, which comprises 2 percent of the region's population.

Quality of Life Indexes   The top-five PRIZM clusters for the Quality of Life Indexes were previously identified as Southside City, Scrub Pine Flats, Grain Belt, Norma Rae-ville, and Shotguns and Pickups. Sixty-six percent of Southside City's tracts exhibit grades of D and F for the region, and six of the twenty-one Southside City tracts received an F for QOL.

Five Dominant Clusters   The top-five high-risk clusters, or five dominant clusters based on the calculated scores and rankings of the Block Group Population, Medical Variables, and Quality of Life Indexes were Scrub Pine Flats, Norma Rae-ville, Southside City, Shotguns and Pickups, and Grain Belt. Aggregated, these five dominant clusters of the perinatal region make up 47 percent of the region's population and represent 119 census tracts throughout the region. Figure 13-8 displays the distribution of the clusters in the region. The birth rate, infant mortality rate, percentage of low birth weight births, and percentage of preterm births for the top-five high-risk clusters are all higher than the region rates and percentages, and these rates and percentages are shown in Table 13-8.

Marketing/Prevention Strategies

As a result of identifying the five dominant clusters that experience the worst or most significant perinatal health problems, the focus now turns to a method for intervening in the natural history of disease pathway. Clearly, the natural history of the perinatal disease process is not well understood and the medical model has been weak in advancing any new causal or behavioral changes to improve outcomes. Marketing strategies focused on media usage and consumer behavior patterns among the previously identified top-five high-risk clusters were thus implemented. PRIZM clusters were geographically linked with the high-risk QOL geography and population counts for the estimated utilization of media usage and consumer behavior

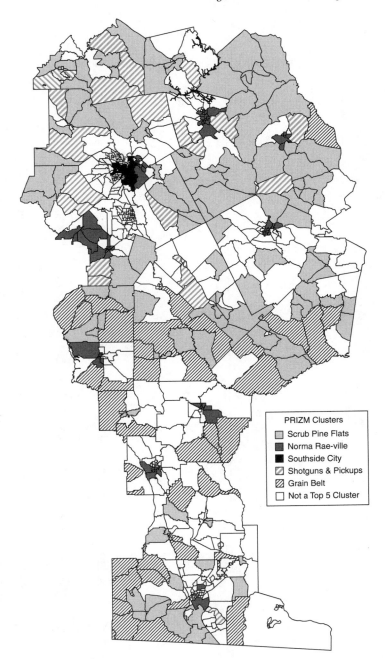

FIGURE 13-8   Top-Five High-Risk PRIZM Clusters; Perinatal Region 6, Georgia, 1994–1999.

TABLE 13-8 Top-Five High-Risk Clusters, Rate and Percentage in Perinatal Region 6, Georgia 1994–1999

PRIZM Cluster	2000 Population		1994–1999 Births				1994–1999 Deaths			1994–1999 Low Births Weight Infants			Preterm		
	#	%	#	%	# per Year	Rate	#	% per Cluster	Infant Mortality Rate	#	% per Cluster	LBW %	#	% per Cluster	Preterm Birth %
Scrub Pine Flats	184,556	20.8	14,680	19.7	2,447	13.3	160	17.0	10.9	1,482	19.9	10.1	2,004	20.0	13.7
Norma Rae-ville	121,593	13.7	11,144	14.9	1,857	15.3	205	21.8	18.4	1,421	19.1	12.8	1,867	18.7	16.8
Southside City	55,019	6.2	6,624	8.9	1,104	20.1	116	12.3	17.5	948	12.8	14.3	1,158	11.6	17.5
Grain Belt	48,952	5.5	3,644	4.9	607	12.4	36	3.8	9.9	355	4.8	9.7	523	5.2	14.4
Shotguns & Pickups	45,965	5.2	3,298	4.4	550	12.0	41	4.4	12.4	297	4.0	9.0	413	4.1	12.5
Top-5 High-Risk	456,085	51.3	39,390	52.8	6,565	14.4	558	59.3	14.2	4,503	60.6	11.4	5,965	59.7	15.1
Perinatal Region 6	888,679	100.0	74,662	100.0	12,444	14.0	941	100.0	12.6	7,430	100.0	10.0	9,997	100.0	13.4

patterns were identified (Inforum/Claritas). The media and consumer categories are estimated based on a percent usage by the United States. Therefore, every cluster media and consumer expenditure pattern of percent usage can be compared with the corresponding percentages for the nation.

The categories for media usage are television, radio, and magazines; and the categories for consumer behavior are restaurants, food items, shopping locations, and other. The overall media usage and consumer behavior patterns for each high-risk cluster were summarized several different ways to ensure the focus of unique intervention marketing efforts.

Media Usage and Consumer Behavior Patterns—Combined All available media usage and consumer behavior topics that were practiced by the top-five high-risk clusters were combined and ranked. In order to be included, all five clusters and at least 25 percent of the cluster population must participate in the media or consumer topic. Seventy-five percent of the top-five high-risk clusters watch Turner Broadcasting System (TBS), which is 55 percent higher than the national average that watch TBS. Likewise, 94 percent eat at fast-food restaurants—6 percent more than the nation.

Media Usage and Consumer Behavior Patterns—Unique (>25 Percent Population) Unique media usage and consumer behavior patterns detected among the top-five high-risk clusters were calculated. The purpose of this analysis was to determine which topics were unique to each cluster. The media usage and consumer behavior categories must have been observed in only one or two clusters and used by at least 25 percent of the cluster population to be included in the marketing and prevention strategy. For example, 35 percent of Norma Rae-ville readers prefer to read news magazines. The other four clusters do not read news magazines, or they read this magazine less than 25 percent of the time. Table 13-9 illustrates the unique media and consumer topics viewed and/or practiced by the Norma Rae-ville cluster.

Media Usage and Consumer Behavior Patterns—Unique (>125 Propensity) Propensity is the percentage above the national usage rate for each of the topics considered where the national usage rate is set to equal 100 percent or 100 propensity. For instance, a 125 propensity score is a topic usage that is 25 percent greater than the national usage or the topic is 1.25 times more likely to be used than the national usage. The purpose of this type of analysis was to identify media and consumer topics used by the clusters that were 25 percent higher than the national use rate. Unique media usage and consumer behavior patterns detected among the top-five high-risk clusters in which there is greater than a 125 percent propensity for the cluster were identified. The media usage or consumer behavior pattern must have only been observed in one cluster to be included in this analysis. An example of propensity usage patterns in the Norma Rae-ville cluster is provided in

TABLE 13-9 Example of Unique Media Usage and Consumer Behavior for PRIZM Cluster: Norma Rae-Ville

Media Usage			Consumer Behavior		
Pattern (U.S. Average %)	% Usage (>25%)	Propensity (>125)	Pattern (U.S. Average %)	% Usage (>25%)	Propensity (>125)
News Magazines Net Aud (24.3%)	35		Attend Theater/Concerts	29	
Special Appeal Mags Net Aud (26.3%)	31		Own 35mm Camera (26.6%)	28	
Computer Mags Net Aud (4.2%)		156	Purch Athltc Shoes-Nike (23.1%)	33	
Elle (1.3%)		159	Shop at CVS (19.1%)	33	
Entertainment Weekly (3.5%)		138	Eat Cap'n Crunch (17.0%)	33	
Newsweek (7.0%)		153	Drink Diet Coke (6.8%)		134
Time (9.5%)		133	Drink Diet Pepsi		135
			Drink Other Diet Soft Drinks (21.1%)		125
			Eat at Del Taco (2.5%)		189
			Exercise at YMCA/YWCA (2.7%)		262

Figure 13-9. For example, Norma Rae-villes are .89 times more likely to eat at Del Taco's than the rest of the nation. Two and a half percent of the nation, compared to 189 percent of Norma Rae-villes, eat at Del Taco's. Or most simply noted, nationally, 2.5% of the population eat at Del Taco's whereas 4.7% of the Norma Rae-ville cluster eat at Del Taco's.

A Community Marketing Application—Targeting the High Risk

County Analysis   The Perinatal Health QOL Model components must be applied to a geographic area to determine the appropriate interventions and implementation strategies. A detailed health status summary for every county in the region was provided by block group and census tract. Figure 13-9 provides an example that illustrates the following:

- Shades the location of the top-five high-risk clusters
- Plots the location of the infant deaths by block group
- Displays a table for the QOL Index grades by census tract, giving a grade for all categories Medical, Lifestyle, Access, and QOL
- Provides reference data such as city boundaries, interstates, and highways to assist with further assessment of the area

It is important to note that on the map, the reference data boundaries are layered above the census tracts and block groups. For example, some census tract boundaries might be "hidden" due to the U.S. highway boundaries.

The idea is that the community application can be approached in several different ways, depending on the clusters involved, infant deaths by block group, and QOL Index grades by census tract.

Number of Infant Deaths   The infant deaths from 1994 to 1999 were geocoded to each block group in the perinatal region. *Geocoding* is the assignment of spatial coordinates based on a given street address, county, census tract, block group, or ZIP code so that the location can be referenced in the map software and displayed on a map. The symbols on the map represent 1 infant death, 2 to 3 infant deaths, and greater than 3 infant deaths. The numbers on the map represent the census tract and block group numbers. For example, 1–1 refers to census tract 1, block group 1, and 1–2 refers to census tract 1, block group 2. To estimate the number of infant deaths by census tract, simply add the number of deaths for each block group within the census tract. Remember to consider the population of the census tract when reviewing infant deaths because a high number of deaths might only reflect a high number of births and not a high-risk area.

There are two ways of examining the impact of the infant deaths. First, note the infant deaths by block group and census tract on the map, and compare these tracts in the table to identify if the same tracts are high risk

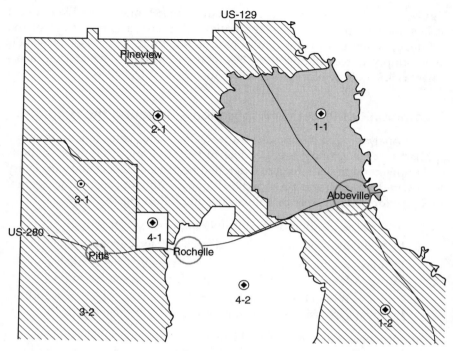

Composite Index Grades	Risk Category for Tracts		
	Low	Medium	High
	A, B	C	D,F
Medical	3	0	1-2-4
Lifestyle	0	1-3	2-4
Access	0	3	1-2-4
Quality of Life	0	3	1-2-4

Legend:
- Scrub Pine Flats
- Norma Rae-ville
- Southside City
- Shotguns & Pickups
- Grain Belt
- Not a Top 5 Cluster
- ⊙ 1 Infant Death
- ◉ 2–3 Infant Deaths
- Ⓞ >3 Infant Deaths
- —— City Boundary
- —— US Highway
- – – Block Group Boundary
- ······ Census Tract Boundary

FIGURE 13-9   Perinatal Health Status Assessment; Wilcox County, Public Health District 5-1, Perinatal Region 6, Georgia, 1994–1999

(grades D and F). Second, note the infant deaths by block group and census tract on the map in relationship to the PRIZM clusters by block group or census tract. This last option is explained in greater detail in the following section, "Identify the Clusters."

For instance, Wilcox County has 4 census tracts and 7 block groups. The county has experienced infant deaths in 7 of the 8 block groups and in all 4 census tracts. Of these census tracts, tracts 1, 2, and 4 are high risk for Medical, Lifestyle, and QOL indicators in the Perinatal Health QOL Index, which can be viewed in the table on the map.

High-Risk Census Tracts—Grades D and F   A summary for the perinatal heath status index grades (Medical, Lifestyle, Access, and QOL) is provided for each county in a table on the map. Every census tract in the region was given a grade for Medical, Lifestyle, Access, and QOL indicators. The grades range from A to F or from low to high risk, respectively. Grades A and B are low risk (good), grade C is medium risk (fair), and grades D and F are high risk (poor). The numbers in the table represent the census tracts in the county. Census tracts that score in the high-risk category should be targeted for health promotion and disease prevention strategies.

There are two ways of assessing the information in the QOL Index table. First, look at the high-risk tracts in the table (grades D and F) and compare these tracts to the tracts on the map to see if the same tracts display high numbers of infant deaths. Second, look at the high-risk tracts in the table (grades D and F) in relationship to the PRIZM clusters by block group or census tract.

Wilcox County has 4 census tracts and 7 block groups. Tracts 1, 2, and 4 have been rated as high-risk tracts because they scored grades of D and F for Medical, Lifestyle, Access, and QOL indicators in the Perinatal Health QOL Index. All of these tracts should be examined because they all experienced infant deaths during the six-year period, 1994 to 1999.

Identify the Clusters   Utilizing the high-risk areas as defined, the cluster groups are tagged to these areas. The PRIZM clusters are identified so as to decide on the appropriate marketing strategies for an area such as the region, district, census tract, or block group. After the steps have been taken to decide which tracts and/or block groups should be targeted, by looking at the number of infant deaths and high-risk tracts, the tracts and block groups must be linked to the clusters. If the block groups are shaded, that means they can be linked to a high-risk cluster, Scrub Pine Flats, Norma Rae-ville, Southside City, Shotguns and Pickups, or Grain Belt. If a block group is white, it is not a top-five high-risk cluster for the region and should be investigated if necessary; however, the yield will be low because the remaining clusters represent a very small percentage of the problem, given the magnitude of the issue in the entire region. This analysis has been designed to create a marketing method that is targeted and positioned to yield a high return on intervention and further conserve resources for maximum impact.

Six of the seven block groups in Wilcox County are defined by two high-risk clusters, Scrub Pine Flats, shaded in dark gray and Grain Belt, shaded in light gray. Only one block group, 4–2, is defined by a different PRIZM cluster. Because the majority of the county is composed of the two clusters, the marketing and prevention model should be based on the media usage and consumer behavior topics exhibited by the two cluster groups Scrub Pine Flats and Grain Belt. The media usage and consumer behavior for these two cluster groups is shown in Tables 13-10 and 13-11.

Future Considerations

The Perinatal Health QOL Model enabled the assessment of the perinatal health status in the region. This analysis encompassed a broad range of indicators that determined infant health status directly and indirectly related to the medical health of the infant and mother, socioeconomic and lifestyle indicators, as well as issues associated with access to care. These variables were combined to create a holistic approach to defining perinatal health.

The Perinatal Health QOL Model can be utilized with other geographic units such as at the national, state, and local levels. The local areas such as the counties, census tracts, and block groups were identified as high-, medium-, or low-risk areas for overall QOL, as well as medical, lifestyle, and access indicators. The result of this approach creates an Infant Health Risk Score that was assigned to every county and census tract in the region.

Using the data from the Perinatal Health QOL Model, the local areas that were identified as high risk were linked to a marketing tool, PRIZM clusters. Five of the sixty-two PRIZM cluster groups were selected to represent the target groups of the perinatal region. The top-five high-risk PRIZM cluster selections were based on percentage population, perinatal health variables, and the QOL Index.

The PRIZM cluster marketing system is able to identify various demographic and lifestyle variables that separate one group of consumers from another. The clusters within a target group show similarities in behavior and in fundamental lifestyle characteristics such as media habits and product usage. In other words, the high-risk census tracts can be linked to consumer-specific data such as what individuals watch, listen to, read, and buy as well as where they eat and shop. This specific marketing approach is needed to determine the focus of health promotion and disease prevention strategies for the region.

TABLE 13-10 Example of Unique Media Usage and Consumer Behavior for PRIZM Cluster: Scrub Pine Flats

Media Usage			Consumer Behavior		
Pattern (U.S. Average %)	% Usage (>25%)	Propensity (>125)	Pattern (U.S. Average %)	% Usage (>25%)	Propensity (>125)
TV 7 am–9 am M-F (19.7%)	27		Own CD-ROM Drive (32.6%)	30	
TV 11 pm–11:30 pm M-F (23.4%)	26		Own Word Process Software (37.6%)	29	
Watch TV Food Network (15.1%)	26		Ban Polluting Products (19.3%)	28	
CNN Your Money (3.9%)		167	Full-Size SUV Bought New (1.2%)		271
7th Heaven 2–4 M (4.8%)		166	Use Pills for Diet (3.3%)		263
TV Soccer (1.8%)		153	Use Low-Fat Cold Cuts (11.7%)		183
CMT Country Music Videos (8.3%)		150	Use Baby Foods (8.8%)		167
Better Homes & Gardens (11.3%)		142	Drink Sport/Activity Drinks (34.3%)		128
Home Services Mags Net Aud (25.9%)		127	Drink Bourbon (12.0%)		127

TABLE 13-11 Example of Unique Media Usage and Consumer Behavior for PRIZM Cluster: Grain Belt

Media Usage			Consumer Behavior		
Pattern (U.S. Average %)	% Usage (>25%)	Propensity (>125)	Pattern (U.S. Average %)	% Usage (>25%)	Propensity (>125)
Watch FX Network (18.2%)	40		Go Hunting (10.9%)	26	
Watch E! Entertainment TV (21.1%)	33		Medicare/Medicaid (18.2%)	26	
Watch Encore (11.1%)	29		Bght Western Boots LY (2.3%)		218
Watch CNN (40.9%)		186	Veh Shock Absorber/Strut LY (9.3%)		181
Oprah Winfrey 3–5 S (6.8%)		161	Remodel Bathroom (10.0%)		157
General Hospital 3–5 W (4.0%)		158	Order Items from Magazine (12.6%)		144
JAG 2–4 M (8.6%)		135	Own a Cat (27.0%)		144
King of Queens 2–4 M (7.2%)		135	Use Canned Chili (18.2%)		139
20/20 Friday 2–4 M (10.1%)		129	<$50 Grocery Shopping Wkly (15.1%)		138

Combining the high-risk groups with specific marketing information creates an ideal situation for identifying consumer targets and developing interventions using a marketing-message model. The goal of formative research in public health is to understand the target audience for behavior change.[50] The Perinatal Health QOL Model uses the PRIZM cluster marketing data to understand the behaviors and characteristics of the people living in the high-risk areas so that creative public health messages and interventions based on prevention and behavior change can be framed to address social changes that will improve perinatal health status.

A perinatal planning committee for the region can develop strategies to implement the media usage and consumer behavior marketing information to focus their prevention efforts to the high-risk areas in the region. The results of the Perinatal Health QOL Model can be followed by additional research to determine the success of this proposed small-area marketing/prevention analysis.

Summary

This chapter examined the contributions of marketing to health services management. Marketing was described as a process complementary to planning that could enrich the managerial task of adapting an organization's services to the needs, wants, and desires of the population.

The marketing approach is essentially similar to the epidemiologic approach to health services management in that both promote and call for population-based management. Both of these approaches also can contribute to a more comprehensive understanding of health and its determinants and consequently to more effective management of health services.

Health services managers can use marketing to plan and manage their organization's relationships with other groups such as physicians, employees, suppliers, and community supporters, as well as for health education and promotion. The Perinatal Health QOL Model is an approach to improve perinatal health that is much different than the traditional medical model of treatment. By encompassing a number of complex characteristics, such as biologic, social, and psychologic factors, the Perinatal Health QOL Model is relative to the biopsychosocial model of health.[51] The perinatal model is broad in its holistic approach to improve perinatal health status but narrow in its focus on creating health promotion themes to target groups in the region.[52,53] The Perinatal Health QOL Model is an approach of significant value in the planning and focus of prevention efforts to link marketing business intervention methods with a perinatal epidemiologic health needs assessment.

References

1. R. E. MacStravic, *Marketing Health Care* (Rockville, Md.: Aspen Systems Corporation, 1977), 7.
2. J. G. Keith, "Marketing Health Care: What the Recent Literature Is Telling Us," Special 2, *Hospital and Health Services Administration* (1981):66–94.
3. MacStravic, *Marketing Health Care*, 16.
4. D. Finlay, "Geographic Targeting," *American Demographics* (October 1980):39–41.
5. A. S. Boote, "Mind over Matter," *American Demographics* (April 1980):26–29.
6. E. J. Forrest et al., "Psychographic Flesh, Demographic Bones," *American Demographics* (September 1981):25–27.
7. H. Assael, "Segmenting Markets by Group Purchasing Behavior: An Application of the Aid Technique," *Journal of Marketing Research* 7 (May 1970):153–158.
8. Mercer University School of Medicine, Department of Community Medicine, *Regional Perinatal Assessment: Health Status, Prevention, and Marketing Study— District, County, and Census Tract Overview Perinatal Region 6, Georgia*, Monograph (2003).
9. P. Kotler, *Marketing for Nonprofit Organizations*, 2d ed. (Englewood Cliffs, N.J.: Prentice Hall, Inc., 1982), 240–241.
10. Kotler, *Marketing for Nonprofit Organizations*, 245.
11. P. E. Green and V. R. Rao, *Applied Multidimensional Scaling* (New York: Holt, Rinehart and Winston, Inc., 1972), 292.
12. C. Osgood, G. Suci, and P. Tannenbaum, *The Measurement of Meaning* (Urbana: University of Illinois Press, 1967), 346.
13. J. Snider and C. Osgood, eds., *Semantic Differential Technique: A Sourcebook* (Chicago: Aldine Publishing Co., Inc., 1969), 681.
14. Kotler, *Marketing for Nonprofit Organizations*, 57–58.
15. MacStravic, *Marketing Health Care*, 95–97.
16. P. Kotler, *Principles of Marketing*, 2d ed. (Englewood Cliffs, N.J.: Prentice Hall, Inc., 1983), 64.
17. P. Kotler, *Marketing Management* (Englewood Cliffs, N.J.: Prentice Hall, Inc., 1980), Chapter 3.
18. R. E. MacStravic, *Marketing by Objectives for Hospitals* (Rockville, Md.: Aspen Systems Corporation, 1980), Chapter 9.
19. A. E. Bomoni et al., "Quality of Life Measurement. Will We Ever Be Satisfied?" *Journal of Clinical Epidemiology* 53 (2000):19–23.
20. K. O. Morgan and S. E. Morgan, "Quality of Life," *State Statistical Trends* VI, no. 1 (2003).
21. Bomoni et al., "Quality of Life Measurement."
22. R. D. Crosby, R. L. Kolotkin, and G. R. Williams, "Defining Clinical Meaningful Change in Health-Related Quality of Life," *Journal of Clinical Epidemiology* 56 (2003):395–407.
23. A. Garratt et al., "Quality of Life Measurement: Bibliographic Study of Patient Assessed Health Outcome Measures," *BMJ*, 324 (2002):1417. Available at *http://bmj.com/cgi/content/full/314/7351/1417.*

24. Crosby, Kolotkin, and Williams, "Defining Clinical Meaningful Change in Health-Related Quality of Life."
25. Garratt et al., "Quality of Life Measurement."
26. Crosby, Kolotkin, and Williams, "Defining Clinical Meaningful Change in Health-Related Quality of Life."
27. Garratt et al., "Quality of Life Measurement."
28. Crosby, Kolotkin, and Williams, "Defining Clinical Meaningful Change in Health-Related Quality of Life."
29. Garratt et al., "Quality of Life Measurement."
30. B. Bruce and J. F. Fries, "The Stanford Health Assessment Questionnaire: Dimensions and Practical Applications," *Health and Quality of Life Outcomes* 1, no. 1 (2003):20. Available at *http://www.pubmedcentral.nih.gov/articlerender.fcgi?tool=pubmed&pubmedid=12831398.*
31. Garratt et al., "Quality of Life Measurement."
32. Crosby, Kolotkin, and Williams, "Defining Clinical Meaningful Change in Health-Related Quality of Life."
33. C. H. Hennessy et al., "Measuring Health-Related Quality of Life for Public Health Surveillance," *Public Health Reports* 109, no. 5 (1994):665–672.
34. G. E. A. Dever et al., "Health Status and Socioeconomic Status in Georgia: A Quality of Life Perspective," *Journal of the Medical Association of Georgia* 89, no. 1 (2000):30–35.
35. U.S. Census Bureau, *http://www.census.gov* (for data, accessed July 2003).
36. Georgia Department of Human Resources, Division of Public Health, Vital Records, data from 1994–1999.
37. Inforum, a Division of Claritas, Inc., ©2000.
38. Georgia Board for Physician Workforce Database, data from 2000.
39. H. L. Brown, K. Watkins, and A. K. Hiett, "The Impact of the Women, Infants and Children Food Supplement Program on Birth Outcomes [See Comments]," *American Journal of Obstetrics and Gynecology* 174, no. 4 (1996):1279–1283.
40. P. A. Buescher et al., "Prenatal WIC Participation Can Reduce Low Birth Weight and Newborn Medical Costs: A Cost-Benefit Analysis of WIC Participation in North Carolina," *Journal of the American Dietetic Association* 93, no. 2 (1993):163–166.
41. T. R. Collins et al., "Supplemental Food Program: Effects on Health and Pregnancy Outcome," *Southern Medical Journal.* 78, no. 5 (1985):551–555.
42. A. V. Graham et al., "A Clinical Trial to Reduce the Rate of Low Birth Weight in an Inner-City Black Population," *Family Medicine* 24, no. 6 (1992):439–446.
43. A. A. Herman et al., "Evaluation of the Effectiveness of a Community-Based Enriched Model Prenatal Intervention Project in the District of Columbia," *Health Services Research* 31, no. 5 (1996):609–620.
44. S. E. Jacobs, "'Our Babies Shall Not Die:' A Community's Response to Medical Neglect," *Human Organ* 38, no. 2 (1979):120–133.
45. G. Julnes et al., "Community-Based Perinatal Care for Disadvantaged Adolescents: Evaluation of the Resource Mothers Program," *Journal of Community Health* 19, no. 1 (1994):41–53.

46. M. L. Poland et al., "Effects of a Home Visiting Program on Prenatal Care and Birthweight: A Case Comparison Study," *Journal of Community Health* 17, no. 4 (1992):221–229.

47. W. Reguero and M. Crane, "Project MotherCare: One Hospital's Response to the High Perinatal Death Rate in New Haven, Conn.," *Public Health Reports.* 109, no. 5 (1994):647–652.

48. D. Rush, Z. Stein, and M. Susser, "A Randomized Controlled Trial of Prenatal Nutritional Supplementation in New York City," *Pediatrics* 65, no. 4 (1980):683–697.

49. A. M. Spitz et al., "The Impact of Publicly Funded Perinatal Care Programs on Neonatal Outcomes, Georgia, 1976–1978," *American Journal of Obstetrics and Gynecology.* 147, no. 3 (1983):295–300.

50. M. Siegel and L. Doner, *Marketing Public Health: Strategies to Promote Social Change* (Gaithersburg, Md.: Aspen Publishers, Inc., 1998).

51. L. G. Pol and R. K. Thomas, *The Demography of Health and Health Care* (New York: Plenum Press, 1992).

52. G. E. A. Dever, *Social Indicators Research* 2 (1976):455.

53. G. E. A. Dever, *Community Health Analysis: Global Awareness at the Local Level,* 2d ed. (Gaithersburg, Md.: Aspen Publishers, Inc., 1991).

Appendix

APPENDIX Z-Score Calculation Example—Lifestyle Index

	[1]		[1]		[1]		[1]		[1]		[1]		[1]		[1]		[1]		[2]	[3][4]	[5]	[6]
	Mothers that did not finish high school (%)		Single mothers (%)		Mothers that did not drink alcohol during pregnancy (%)		Mothers that did not smoke cigarettes during pregnancy (%)		Fathers that did not finish high school (%)		Mothers that attended health education classes (%)		Unemployment rate by county (per 1,000 population)		Health status index by county		Socio-economic status score by county		Lifestyle Index			
County	%	z-score	%	z-score	%	z-score	%	z-score	%	z-score	%	z-score	%	z-score	%	z-score	%	z-score	Sum of Lifestyle z-scores	Z-score of Sum of Lifestyle z-scores	Rank	Grade
Houston	23.4	−1.7	32.7	−1.5	98.7	0.8	12.6	−0.1	9.9	−1.6	14.2	−3.0	18.2	−0.7	39.7	−2.2	50.0	−2.4	−12.4	−2.8	1	A
Jones	25.8	−1.3	33.6	−1.4	99.5	−0.8	13.2	0.1	15.2	−0.5	11.8	−1.1	22.1	0.0	32.2	−0.7	49.0	−2.1	−7.8	−1.8	2	A
Lowndes	28.4	−0.9	39.0	−0.7	98.9	0.4	10.1	−1.0	12.8	−1.0	13.1	−2.1	22.8	0.2	33.9	−1.1	46.0	−1.0	−7.2	−1.7	3	A
Bibb	31.4	−0.3	51.9	0.8	98.7	0.8	9.8	−1.1	10.9	−1.4	12.9	−1.9	23.7	0.3	32.8	−0.9	48.0	−1.7	−5.4	−1.2	4	B
Monroe	29.8	−0.6	38.1	−0.9	99.1	0.0	14.4	0.6	13.5	−0.9	11.2	−0.6	17.6	−0.8	30.3	−0.4	47.0	−1.4	−5.0	−1.1	5	B
Baldwin	31.0	−0.4	51.5	0.7	98.9	0.4	11.1	−0.6	11.8	−1.2	12.3	−1.5	21.3	−0.1	31.2	−0.6	46.0	−1.0	−4.3	−1.0	6	B
Wilkinson	26.0	−1.3	47.4	0.2	99.2	−0.2	8.0	−1.8	11.3	−1.3	10.1	0.2	19.5	−0.5	23.1	1.1	44.0	−0.3	−3.8	−0.9	7	B
Putnam	31.3	−0.4	48.1	0.3	99.0	0.2	11.9	−0.4	14.4	−0.7	10.5	−0.1	17.9	−0.8	31.8	−0.7	47.0	−1.4	−3.8	−0.9	8	B
Laurens	32.1	−0.2	43.9	−0.2	99.4	−0.6	10.1	−1.0	14.2	−0.7	10.8	−0.4	21.5	−0.1	27.7	0.1	44.0	−0.3	−3.3	−0.8	9	B
Montgomery	36.1	0.5	37.7	−0.9	99.7	−1.3	10.0	−1.0	21.2	0.7	9.4	0.7	16.4	−1.0	27.2	0.2	42.0	0.4	−1.7	−0.4	10	C
Pulaski	24.2	−1.6	51.0	0.7	99.5	−0.8	11.5	−0.5	12.9	−1.0	9.8	0.4	33.8	2.2	30.2	−0.4	45.0	−0.6	−1.6	−0.4	11	C
Crawford	24.0	−1.6	36.7	−1.0	99.4	−0.6	16.5	1.3	17.7	0.0	10.3	0.0	25.9	0.8	29.1	−0.1	44.0	−0.3	−1.6	−0.4	12	C
Peach	31.4	−0.3	46.6	0.1	99.0	0.2	12.2	−0.2	16.9	−0.2	11.9	−1.2	28.8	1.3	28.1	0.1	46.0	−1.0	−1.3	−0.3	13	C
Bleckley	29.9	−0.6	43.6	−0.2	98.4	1.5	11.9	−0.4	15.9	−0.4	9.5	0.7	17.0	−0.9	30.0	−0.3	44.0	−0.3	−0.9	−0.2	14	C
Washington	30.0	−0.6	52.2	0.8	99.2	−0.2	8.6	−1.6	11.8	−1.2	10.2	0.1	25.8	0.7	23.3	1.0	43.0	0.1	−0.8	−0.2	15	C

APPENDIX (continued)

| | [1] | | [1] | | [1] | | [1] | | [1] | | [1] | | [1] | | [1] | | [1] | | Lifestyle Index | | | |
| | Mothers that did not finish high school (%) | | Single mothers (%) | | Mothers that did not drink alcohol during pregnancy (%) | | Mothers that did not smoke cigarettes during pregnancy (%) | | Fathers that did not finish high school (%) | | Mothers that attended health education classes (%) | | Unemployment rate by county (per 1,000 population) | | Health status index by county | | Socio-economic status score by county | | [2] | [3][4] | [5] | [6] |
County	%	z-score	%	z-score	%	z-score	%	z-score	%	z-score	%	z-score	%	z-score	%	z-score	%	z-score	Sum of Lifestyle z-scores	Z-score of Sum of Lifestyle z-scores	Rank	Grade
Echols	42.6	1.6	38.0	-0.9	100.0	-1.9	14.7	0.7	22.5	0.9	8.9	1.1	13.5	-1.6	34.0	-1.1	42.0	0.4	-0.7	-0.2	16	C
Brooks	36.0	0.5	51.0	0.7	99.3	-0.4	10.7	-0.8	19.6	0.3	9.6	0.6	20.4	-0.3	33.5	-1.0	41.0	0.8	0.3	0.1	17	C
Dodge	31.2	-0.4	39.0	-0.7	99.1	0.0	13.9	0.4	17.6	-0.1	9.6	0.6	18.2	-0.7	24.7	0.7	41.0	0.8	0.6	0.1	18	C
Irwin	34.5	0.2	41.2	-0.5	99.0	0.2	12.9	0.0	23.6	1.2	10.0	0.3	28.4	1.2	40.2	-2.3	42.0	0.4	0.7	0.2	19	C
Wheeler	35.8	0.4	36.5	-1.0	99.8	-1.5	13.5	0.2	18.8	0.2	8.7	1.3	19.3	-0.5	25.4	0.6	40.0	1.2	0.8	0.2	20	C
Tift	44.1	1.8	46.6	0.1	99.4	-0.6	11.7	-0.4	25.7	1.6	11.5	-0.9	22.7	0.2	31.5	-0.6	44.0	-0.3	0.9	0.2	21	C
Butts	31.4	-0.3	45.4	0.0	98.7	0.8	14.8	0.7	14.6	-0.7	9.8	0.4	19.6	-0.4	22.9	1.1	45.0	-0.6	1.0	0.2	22	C
Cook	39.5	1.1	39.8	-0.7	99.4	-0.6	13.5	0.2	28.0	2.0	10.0	0.3	15.2	-1.3	30.7	-0.5	42.0	0.4	1.0	0.2	23	C
Wilcox	33.1	0.0	46.6	0.1	98.2	1.9	14.7	0.7	21.8	0.8	8.8	1.2	14.3	-1.4	35.2	-1.3	41.0	0.8	2.6	0.6	24	D
Crisp	42.8	1.6	57.9	1.5	99.3	-0.4	11.3	-0.6	22.7	1.0	11.4	-0.8	19.4	-0.5	26.9	0.3	41.0	0.8	2.9	0.7	25	D
Berrien	34.0	0.1	30.6	-1.7	99.1	0.0	18.6	2.1	21.7	0.8	9.3	0.8	22.2	0.1	26.3	0.4	42.0	0.4	2.9	0.7	26	D
Jasper	29.9	-0.6	44.9	-0.1	98.2	1.9	16.7	1.4	17.3	-0.1	10.2	0.2	25.5	0.7	26.9	0.3	45.0	-0.6	3.0	0.7	27	D
Treutlen	37.5	0.7	43.0	-0.3	99.8	-1.5	13.6	0.3	23.6	1.2	9.9	0.4	21.6	-0.1	22.3	1.2	40.0	1.2	3.1	0.7	28	D
Turner	40.4	1.2	49.1	0.4	99.9	-1.7	10.9	-0.7	20.4	0.5	9.8	0.4	35.1	2.5	29.8	-0.3	40.0	1.2	3.5	0.8	29	D
Johnson	39.8	1.1	53.6	1.0	99.0	0.2	10.7	-0.8	18.1	0.0	9.5	0.7	15.6	-1.2	20.8	1.5	40.0	1.2	3.7	0.8	30	D

APPENDIX (continued)

		[1]		[1]		[1]		[1]		[1]		[1]		[1]		[1]		[1]	[2]	[3] [4]	[5]	[6]
		Mothers that did not finish high school (%)		Single mothers (%)		Mothers that did not drink alcohol during pregnancy (%)		Mothers that did not smoke cigarettes during pregnancy (%)		Fathers that did not finish high school (%)		Mothers that attended health education classes (%)		Unemployment rate by county (per 1,000 population)		Health status index by county		Socio-economic status score by county			Lifestyle Index		
County		%	z-score	%	z-score	%	z-score	%	z-score	%	z-score	%	z-score	%	z-score	%	z-score	%	z-score	Sum of Lifestyle z-scores	Z-score of Sum of Lifestyle z-scores	Rank	Grade
Twiggs		32.2	−0.2	47.7	0.3	99.2	−0.2	14.7	0.7	18.2	0.1	10.0	0.3	30.0	1.5	21.0	1.5	41.0	0.8	4.7	1.1	31	D
Telfair		36.9	0.6	47.4	0.2	98.4	1.5	13.0	0.0	20.1	0.4	9.0	1.1	18.0	−0.7	26.5	0.4	40.0	1.2	4.7	1.1	32	D
Lanier		38.1	0.8	38.7	−0.8	99.4	−0.6	19.5	2.4	24.4	1.3	9.2	0.9	20.3	−0.3	27.1	0.3	41.0	0.8	4.8	1.1	33	D
Ben Hill		42.2	1.5	50.3	0.6	98.9	0.4	17.4	1.6	23.2	1.1	10.9	−0.4	20.8	−0.2	22.5	1.2	42.0	0.4	6.2	1.4	34	F*
Hancock		24.0	−1.6	75.6	3.5	98.4	1.5	15.6	1.0	8.0	−2.0	9.7	0.5	25.8	0.7	18.5	2.0	40.0	1.2	6.8	1.5	35	F
Dooly		40.4	1.2	57.7	1.4	98.4	1.5	9.3	−1.3	22.7	1.0	9.2	0.9	30.1	1.6	25.5	0.6	41.0	0.8	7.6	1.7	36	F

Instructions for calculating the z-score:

1. Z-score formula: *(value − mean)/standard deviation*
2. Sum the total z-scores for each lifestyle indicator
3. Calculate the mean and standard deviation for the sum of the z-scores
4. The total z-score was ranked from lowest to highest risk (−2.8 to 1.7)
5. A numeric rank from 1 to 36 was given for each county
6. The mean and standard deviation were calculated for the "z-score of the sum of the z-scores" column to determine the grading scale. For example:

   a. Mean = −0.0008

   b. 1 standard deviation from the mean = 1.0

   c. ½ standard deviation from the mean = + or − 0.5

   d. Between ½ and 1½ standard deviations from the mean = + or − 0.5 to 1.5 (B or D)

   e. 1 and ½ standard deviations from the mean = + or − 1.5 (A or F*)

*Because of the natural break between Lanier (1.1) and Ben Hill (1.4), Ben Hill is given an "F" for lifestyle.

Index